ACKNOWLEDGEMENTS

I wish to thank my family for allowing me to take the many extra hours of time for all of my "physical therapy projects." Their understanding and help has been invaluable to me. I also want to thank those physical therapists and physicians with whom I have worked, who have challenged, criticized, encouraged and supported me in my endeavors.

I am indebted to my daughter, Robin, for her help with editing and typesetting, to Mary Albury-Noyse for the illustrations and, especially, to Allyn Woerman for his advice and help in writing and organizing the entire content of the book.

Evaluation, Treatment and Prevention of Musculoskeletal Disorders

H. Duane Saunders, M.S., P.T.

In collaboration with

Allyn L. Woerman, M.M.S., P.T.
Lieutenant Colonel, Army Medical Specialist Corps
Chief, Physical Therapy Section
Reynolds Army Community Hospital
Fort Sill, Oklahoma 73502

Contributing author

Steven L. Kraus, P.T.
Williamsburg Professional Center
1989 North Williamsburg Drive — Suite H
Decatur, Georgia 30033

Illustrations by
Mary Albury Noyes

Edited by
Robin L. Saunders

Educational Opportunities
by H. Duane Saunders, M.S., P.T.
7750 West 78th Street
Bloomington, Minnesota 55435
Phone: (612) 944-1656

Library of Congress Number 84-091301

ISBN Number 0-9616461-0-1

PRINTED IN THE UNITED STATES OF AMERICA

BY VIKING PRESS INC./MINNEAPOLIS, MN

4th PRINTING SEPTEMBER, 1989

page layout: Mary Jestrab Schultz

CONTENTS

PREFACE

This book is the result of 20 years of experience I have had in clinical practice, association with physicians and fellow physical therapists, self-study and attendance of numerous educational seminars and courses.

I do not have a great deal of capacity for academic achievement. I believe that my accomplishments have been because of hard work, a dissatisfaction and frustration in the way we have cared for our patients and a willingness to try new ideas before passing judgement.

Two years ago, I published the first edition of this book and, although it was an amateurish publication in many ways, I am extremely pleased with the reception my collegues have given it. With very little promotion, that edition sold over 7,000 copies in less than two years and many schools of physical therapy have adopted it as a textbook for their programs. Some allopathic and osteopathic physicians have shown interest in the book, but more especially, some chiropractors. All of this pleases me very much and has encouraged me to undertake this second edition in an effort to improve and expand the original work. This book truly says what I want to say and how I want to say it, at least for the present.

I have always been impressed with the desire we physical therapists have demonstrated to improve our skills and with the sincerity we demonstrate in our approach to patient management, but I have been disappointed with our lack of professional self-esteem and frustrated that we have not achieved a level of practice and recognition that our skills and knowledge justly deserve. If this book contributes in some way to the improvement of patient care and the raising of standards of practice in physical therapy, my goals will have been accomplished.

CHAPTER 1
INTRODUCTION

The role of the physical therapist in evaluation and treatment of musculoskeletal disorders is broadening to assume a position of greater responsibility in the medical field. No longer can a physical therapist responsibly practice without a proper data base from which to plan the treatment of a musculoskeletal problem. The physician, due to the logarithmic proliferation of knowledge, can no longer encompass the totality of medical knowledge. Physicians are not, except in a few cases, skilled in musculoskeletal evaluation, assessment and treatment planning. The high level of activity of their practices has forced some to turn to nurse clinicians, physician assistants and other ancillary personnel to screen and treat their patients. Since the physical therapist already possesses many of the skills necessary to carry out musculoskeletal evaluation, assessment and treatment, it seems obvious that he should seek this role since it is the physical therapist who continues to see the patient as the treatment plan is carried out. Therefore, it is paramount that the training of physical therapists be expanded in order that they become experts in the area of problem assessment and conservative management of disorders which affect the musculoskeletal system.

A void presently exists in this area described by James Cyriax, M.D., as the "vacuum in orthopaedic medicine[1]." His reference is to the gap between prescription of a drug for a particular problem on the one extreme and surgical intervention on the other. It is from this "vacuum" that the orthopaedic physical therapy specialization has emerged. When the physician and the physical therapist who specializes in orthopaedics develop a complementary working relationship, the patient truly receives effective and efficient management of his problem. In order for this management to be effective, the treatment planning must involve the physical therapist, for it is the physical therapist who has the most thorough knowledge of the indications for, the contraindications to and the effects of physical therapy techniques and modalities at his disposal.

Today, most patients treated by a physical therapist soon realize that physical therapy is not just the application of modalities and exercises, but the application of a comprehensive, systematic approach to the patient's problem. This approach involves the areas of: 1) Patient evaluation, both subjective and objective; 2) Problem assessment, i.e. correlation of compatible signs and symptoms; 3) Treatment planning; 4) Application of treatment techniques based on the evaluation and assessment; 5) Reassessment to determine the treatment's effect; 6) Modification of the treatment program according to changes in the patient's signs and symptoms; 7) Long-term rehabilitation and education of the patient after the acute episode has been resolved; and 8) Prevention.

In weighing the relative importance of each of the above components in this systematic approach, we must recognize that the evaluation is a vital part. Evaluation, through a series of pointed questions and objective tests, provides a data base from which assessment of the problem can occur.

Perhaps of greatest importance is the assessment of the patient's problem based upon correlation of comparable signs and symptoms arising from the objective and subjective aspects of the evaluation. The assessment is a continual process during the evaluation and leads the physical therapist to a working diagnosis. A well-organized and meaningful evaluation and assessment builds the confidence of the patient in the physical therapist and is time well spent. The patient will thus have confidence in the subsequent treatment regimen planned for him, recognizing that it is based on a thorough understanding of his particular problem. It should be noted that all pieces of the puzzle may not fall into place or be apparent during the initial evaluation and assessment process. A written record of the patient's signs and symptoms is imperative to the successful management of the problem.

Following the initial evaluation and assessment, treatment is instituted based on the assessment. After all, selection of modalities and techniques, no matter how skillfully applied, will be ineffective if applied inappropriately to a particular problem. Thus, treatment, in relation to evaluation and assessment, is of lesser importance, lying in the psychomotor domain more than in the cognitive.

Reassessment begins during and following the initial treatment according to patient response. Reassessment takes place prior to any subsequent treatment, for as the patient's condition changes, his signs and symptoms may be altered dramatically,

1

sometimes implicating a totally different area or structure than first assessed. Thus, treatment may have to be modified according to these noted changes in the data base. The therapist's experience, skill, judgement and knowledge all come into play during these phases, with reassessment and modification ongoing as the patient's condition resolves. Also, as the condition is resolving, the therapist is educating the patient in management and preventative measures, helping the patient assume responsibility for the ultimate management of his own condition to the greatest extent possible.

Most musculoskeletal disorders, especially those of the spine, are recognized to be the result of an accumulative effect of poor posture, faulty body mechanics, stressful living and working conditions, loss of flexibility and a decline in the general level of physical fitness. These disorders are rarely the result of a single traumatic event[2,3,4,5,6] (Fig. 1-1). Months or years may pass before these factors result in an actual pathological disorder. An analogy may be used to compare musculoskeletal disorders and heart disease in that they both occur in much the same way. In both cases, the problem develops over time due to one's lifestyle long before an acute episode actually occurs. If one accepts the contention that most musculoskeletal disorders are the results of these cumulative factors, the overall management concepts for the patient will change dramatically, shifting the emphasis from the acute phase to the long-term rehabilitation/education/

**Musculoskeletal Disorders are
Seldom Caused by a Single Traumatic Injury**

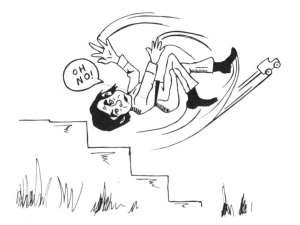

Fig. 1-1. Musculoskeletal disorders are seldom caused by a single traumatic injury. Many are the result of the accumulated effects of poor posture, faulty body mechanics, stressful living and working habits, loss of flexibility and a general decline of physical fitness.

prevention phase. While attention must be given to the disorder when it is in an acute or subacute stage, the primary focus should be directed toward teaching the patient what *he* can do to effect a lasting "cure".

The physical therapist must always guard against the patient becoming dependent upon passive treatment and/or modalities, and should try to shift the responsibility for management of the disorder to the patient as soon as is appropriate. Thus, patient education with the restoration of normal posture, strength, flexibility and fitness become the ultimate goals of treatment. It is ironic that many of the experts of today blindly accept the notion that once a musculoskeletal disorder develops, particularly one of the spine, it will always exist. A frequently seen statement in many orthopaedic texts and journals is that "once a lower back problem is experienced, the patient is eight times more likely to experience a second episode than someone who has never had a problem." Such statements imply that a real cure cannot be effected once a problem has developed. While in the past this may have been true, it does not necessarily have to remain the case today with an emphasis in long-term rehabilitation and educational programs.

Increased emphasis must also be placed on prevention. One must recognize that there are limitations as to what can be done in the presence of certain degenerative processes, especially if in advanced stages. Only three cents of every medical dollar spent in America is for preventative measures[7]. While there seems to be unlimited resources to treat many apparently hopeless disorders, there is often no financial support for preventative diagnostic procedures and educational programs. This trend seems to be slowly reversing, but much more needs to be accomplished in order to put into effect the many advances which have been made in preventative physical therapy during the past few years. Prevention is basically an educational process, thus physical therapists must become expert teachers as well as treaters. Robin McKenzie has said, "Let's make physical therapy known as the profession that teaches patients to help themselves[8]." This trend is beginning and physical therapy is truly the profession that can lead the way.

References:

1. Cyriax J:Textbook of Orthopaedic Medicine; Treatment by Manipulation, Massage and Injection, Vol 2, 10th ed, Bailliere-Tindall, London, 1980.

References: (Continued)

2. Cady, L, et al: Strength and Fitness and Subsequent Back Injuries in Firefighters, Joul of Occ Med, 21:269-272, 1979.

3. Nachemson, A: Toward a Better Understanding of Low Back Pain: A Review of the Mechanics of the Lumbar Disc, Rheumatology and Rehabilitation, 14:129-143, 1975.

4. Nordby, E: Epidemiology and Diagnosis in Low Back Injury, Occupational Health and Safety, 50:38-42, Jan, 1981.

5. Nachemson, A: Low Back Pain, It's Etiology and Treatment, Clinical Medicine, 18-24, 1971.

6. Chaffin, D:Manual Materials Handling, Joul of Environmental Pathology and Toxicology, 2:31-66.

7. Cooper, K: The Aerobics Way, Bantam Books, New York, 1977.

8. McKenzie, R: The Lumbar Spine, Spinal Publications, Waikanae, New Zealand, 1981.

CHAPTER 2

PRINCIPLES OF ORTHOPAEDIC PHYSICAL THERAPY

Basically, two approaches may be used when determining the basis for evaluation, assessment and treatment of musculoskeletal disorders. The **first approach** uses the idea that the problem assessment and treatment plan are based upon the **specific pathology** identified in the evaluation. Each pathological entity presents a unique clinical picture (signs and symptoms.) When this clinical picture is clear and a specific pathological entity or process can be identified, the most effective treatment for that disorder can be selected based upon previous successful clinical experiences. Although this first approach is ideal and may be utilized successfully in many cases, it is somewhat limited because often a clear clinical picture of some pathological processes may not always immediately emerge. In this case, treatment of signs and symptoms becomes the viable alternative approach.

This **second approach** requires that the therapist identify the **signs and symptoms** which can be treated. Treatment for such manifestations of pathology as pain, decreased joint mobility or abnormal posture, can be administered even if the underlying pathological entity is not understood or fully recognized. For example, a patient's low back pain may be so acute initially that much of the objective evaluation cannot be performed. In such a case, the pain can be treated with medication, rest and various modalities. After the pain is controlled, the patient can be examined more throughly, enabling the pathological process to be better identified so that more specific treatment can be instituted. Another example might be the case of a patient who has vague pain in the neck and upper back but presents no clear clinical picture of a specific pathological process. However, his most obvious finding is a definite forward head posture. In this case, the physical therapist may proceed to use corrective exercises, posture training and patient education to correct the faulty posture without a clear understanding of what the underlying pathological process may be. The patient's pain and/or other signs and symptoms may subside when this abnormal posture is corrected. Thus, the physical therapist will have successfully treated the patient and may have not gained a clear understanding if whether the disc, ligaments or muscles were in a "pathological" state. Since there often exists considerable disagreement even among experts concerning which structures may be at fault when certain signs and symptoms are present, this approach has considerable merit.

When using this second treatment approach, the physical therapist must be knowledgeable as to what can be accomplished with the various treatment regimens possible and must administer them appropriately. The following principles apply:

A. **Treatment to relieve pain** falls under one of the following schemes:
   1. Immobilization and rest — Many acute strains, sprains and inflammations involving soft tissues need rest and immobilization to initiate the healing process. Any movement that causes lingering pain is thought to aggravate the already injured tissue. Immobilization may take the form of bed rest, positions of comfort or supportive slings, braces and splints. For lumbar strain, this may mean restriction of certain activities and the use of a lumbar roll or a lumbosacral corset. For ankle or knee injuries, this may mean crutch walking and/or an elastic/tape support. A severe sprain or strain of the cervical spine may require a soft collar for support.
   2. Modality therapy — Modality therapy has long been effectively used for relief of pain. The various forms of heat, cold and hydrotherapy are usually effective as are electrotherapy and massage. Many of these modalities have the added benefit of increasing circulation which speeds the healing of injured tissue and promotes relaxation of muscle spasm and guarding, factors which almost always have to be reduced before treatment of the primary disorder can be instituted.
   3. Mobilization — Mobilization is often effective in relieving pain. The techniques employed usually consist of gentle tractions and/or other graded movements in the pain-free range.

B. **Treatment to increase mobility** is of primary importance. As soft tissue and joint injuries begin to heal, stiffness is inherent. The joints may become hypomobile as a result of the healing process if not treated. Hypomobility of joints may further lead to early degenerative changes. To avoid this possible chain of events, mobilization techniques should be used. The earlier mobilization is instituted, the more beneficial it can be, provided that it is done without aggravating any concomitant soft tissue injury.
   1. Exercises — Soft tissue and connective tissue massage, contract-relax techniques, passive stretch and active and passive range of motion exercises all increase mobility of soft tissue.
   2. Correction of postural or biomechanical stresses — Joints, even those not a site of a pathological process, can become hypomobile through abnormal postural and biomechanical stresses. For example, cervical mobility in patients with a chronic forward head posture is often reduced. Correction of the faulty posture allows for increased mobility and the efficacy of other, more specific treatments.
   3. Mobilization — Specific and general joint mobilization techniques are used to restore mobility of joints.

C. **Treatment to reduce mobility** is indicated if the joints are hypermobile or unstable.
   1. Exercises — If the muscles around a hypermobile or unstable joint are strengthened, the support of the joint will be improved for most physical activities. In some cases, it is also possible to reduce joint mobility by muscle strengthening. Isometric and/or short arc isotonic exercises can be used for this purpose. Strong (heavy resistive) contractions with few repetitions are quite effective for building such strength.
   2. Correction of postural or biomechanical stresses — Joint hypermobility can also sometimes be related to postural or biomechanical stresses. When this is the case, attempts should be made to make corrections through patient education, exercises and/or orthotic devices. For example, chronic foot strain may be corrected with a simple foot orthosis. Genu valgus may be corrected in much the same way. Excessive lumbar lordosis, which can be a contributing factor in development of lumbar hypermobility into extension, may be corrected using a combination of strengthening exercises, posture training and/or a lumbosacral corset. It must be recognized, however, that in the spine especially, a joint can be hypermobile in one direction (in this case extension) and hypomobile in the opposite direction (flexion.) Such a situation will require a balance in treatment.
   3. Supports — Braces, slings and splints are sometimes used to reduce joint mobility. Usually, one would attempt management with muscle strengthening exercises and/or postural training, but if these methods fail, supports are often necessary. For example, a patient with a hypermobile spondylolisthesis will often need a "chair-back" brace or a lumbosacral corset if he is to avoid strain and aggravation during physical activity. Or, a patient with an unstable ankle joint may always need to wear a supportive device or use tape before engaging in vigorous activity. Sacroiliac hypermobility may be effectively managed with a belt or corset specially made to reduce strain across the joint.

D. **Treatment to restore anatomical relationships** may be limited to a few specific conditions — in particular, disc lesions and joint dislocations, subluxations and impingements.
   1. Traction — Mechanical and/or manual traction techniques are effective in reducing a disc protrusion. Traction techniques can also stretch adaptively shortened soft tissues such as capsules, ligaments and muscles.
   2. Exercises — Certain corrective exercises can also be used to reduce a disc protrusion and restore normal physiological length to soft tissues.
   3. Posture — Certain specific posturing techniques can be used to maintain correction of reduced disc protrusions and maintain normal length of soft tissues.
   4. Mobilization — Mobilization techniques can be used to restore the normal anatomical relationship of joints, both intra- and extra-articularly. The ultimate purpose of any mobilization technique is, however, to restore full, free, painless active range of motion, i.e. normal physiological function.

There is much confusion over the use of the word "subluxation". To the chiropractor, it simply means any anatomical or physiological alteration within the joint. **Dorland's Medical Dictionary** defines subluxation as "a **partial** dislocation of the joint[1]." Used in this context, one can reason that such conditions do indeed occur. Such a condition is particularly well suited to treatment with mobilization. The sacroiliac joint is a common joint which can become subluxed and can be successfully treated in this manner. The subtalar joint is frequently subluxed during ankle sprains and is easily treated with mobilization. Some authorities believe that soft tissue (synovial lining), particularly of the spinal facet joints, can become entrapped or "nipped" between the joint surfaces causing the joint to "block" or become "stuck". Although such conditions are not true subluxations, mobilization techniques are thought to release the entrapped tissue, thus restoring the normal anatomical relationship within the joint.

E. **Treatment to restore active function** is what the practice of orthopaedic physical therapy is all about. It is not within the scope of this text to teach or review all possible techniques which may have application in this context. Any or all of these treatment approaches can be combined in the treatment of the whole patient. One approach does not necessarily replace another. The best aspects of one approach should complement the best aspects of another. Treatment to restore active function may thus involve various types of muscle strengthening and re-education techniques such as proprioceptive neuromuscular facilitation (PNF), muscle energy techniques, mobilization and modalities.

F. **Treatment to promote healing** — Since mechanical injuries and/or inflammatory processes are often involved in musculoskeletal disorders, it may be necessary to treat to promote healing.

1. Immobilization and rest — Activities that are vigorous enough to further injure healing tissue or which inhibit the healing process must be avoided. Orthotic devices and/or supports may be required to accomplish this.

2. Modalities — Ice, heat, electrical stimulation (high voltage and low intensity direct current), intermittent positive pressure sleeves, whirlpool, contrast bath, massage and other modalities are all useful in some way to promote healing. Such healing is accomplished by reducing edema, promoting circulation and stimulating cellular activity.

G. **Treatment to correct poor posture** may be all that is required in order to treat some musculoskeletal disorders. It has been previously mentioned that posture correction can aid in reducing a bulging disc or lessening a biomechanical stress that may be contributing to joint hyper/hypomobility. Pain, secondary to injury, will cause one to modify his posture. As the injury heals and as the pain subsides, the subtle posture change that has occurred may have become habitual and may not be noticed. This adaptive posture may later become the source of a new mechanical stress causing an entirely different musculoskeletal problem. An example of this phenomenon is the forward head posture which develops secondary to cervical strain. Patients can continue to suffer one or two years after the initial injury. But do they still have the muscular strain and inflammatory response that resulted from the injury? The answer is no! Healing will have taken place within a few weeks. What the patient may now have is an abnormal posturing that, when corrected, will alleviate the chronic stress which has developed secondary to the original injury.

H. **Treatment to improve general physical and mental fitness** may have a direct effect upon musculoskeletal problems. Since many physical activities influence or are influenced by general strength, coordination, endurance, flexibility and cardiovascular fitness, one must not overlook treatment in these areas. Obesity, drug dependence, nutritional health and emotional health are also factors which can affect the chronicity and severity of musculoskeletal disorders. In fact, individuals in a poor state of general physical fitness cannot undertake certain strenuous physical activities without an undue risk of injury. For example, there is evidence that general physical fitness testing is perhaps the single most accurate way to determine a person's vulnerability to low back injury[2,3].

I. **Treatment to train and instuct** must not be overlooked. The cost of medical care today makes it necessary that home self-treatment be part of the patient's care. The therapist must be skilled at designing an individualized home program and motivating the patient to carry out the program. This treatment may take the form of specific exercises. Of equal or more importance, however, is instruction in good body mechanics and activities of daily living. The patient must be taught which activities are potentially harmful and which ones are helpful to his situation. If the therapist fully understands the patient's problem(s) and has an appreciation of the biomechanics involved, he is indeed in the best position to provide this instruction. Since most musculoskeletal disorders are the result of the accumulative effects of months or even years of poor posture, faulty body mechanics, stressful living and working habits, loss of joint flexibility, muscular weakness and a general decline in the level of physical fitness, this aspect is usually the single most important part of the total treatment regimen. What has been accomplished if the patient's pain has been relieved, the joint sprain healed or the disc bulge reduced and he returns to the same activity or posture that caused the problem in the first place?

Because lower back disorders are epidemic, special mention is made here of the dilemma that exists today and of some thoughts concerning what can be done to improve the management and prevention of this problem. Regardless of the area of medical practice (family practice, orthopaedic surgery, neurosurgery, internal medicine, occupational medicine, chiropractic, osteopathy or physical therapy), there is concrete evidence of failure of the traditional approach to the management of lower back problems. Every year, more and more money is spent on treatment of lower back disorders, yet the number and severity of cases continues to increase (Fig. 2-1). This fact alone should cause one to take a critical look at the treatment approaches currently used. Recognizing that the reasons for failure are often complex, the following criticisms seem valid:

1. Most medical practitioners have a basic lack of understanding and little interest in conservative (non-surgical) management techniques for lower back disorders. Many new concepts of conservative management have been introduced in the past few years. Many physical therapists believe that they possess the knowledge to prevent and/or manage most lower back disorders. Yet, most patients are

---

FACT: Back injuries are the most CHRONIC and EXPENSIVE disability in industry.

FACT: Once a person has had an attack of lumbago or sciatica, he is EIGHT TIMES as likely to have another attack.

FACT: BILLIONS OF DOLLARS are spent in the U.S. each year on occupational back injuries.

FACT: IN INDUSTRY, roughly 34% to 44% of all payments made to individuals as settlement for injury are the result of back injuries.

FACT: BILLIONS OF DOLLARS are paid in disability claims and lawsuits. Individual suits now range from $750,000 to $1,500,000.

FACT: 8 of every 10 people will be seen by a physician for back pain during their lifetimes.

FACT: 70% to 90% of these people will have a significant problem.

FACT: 7.5 MILLION new victims are added to this each year.

FACT: 5 MILLION of this group are partially disabled.

FACT: 2 MILLION are completely disabled.

FACT: 93 MILLION workdays are lost each year in the U.S. because of back problems.

FACT: Low back pain is SECOND only to the common cold and respiratory problems as the cause of work absenteeism.

FACT: 17 BILLION DOLLARS were spent in 1983 on industrial back injuries.

Fig. 2-1. Back injury fact sheet[4,5].

being treated by practitioners who do not have the time or interest to learn about or apply these techniques.

2. Many medical practitioners tend to stereotype persons with lower back pain into two or three general categories rather than recognizing that there are many different causes of lower back pain and each patient must be evaluated as an individual. For example, lower back pain without neurological signs is usually thought of as being a muscle strain by these practitioners. Lower back pain with neurological signs is automatically considered a herniated disc, unless an x-ray happens to show a minor defect or anomaly which, all too often, becomes the diagnosis. "Arthritis" is often blamed for lack of any real finding because the practitioner is at a loss to give an explanation and the patient is looking for an answer.

3. Treatment regimens have varied, largely because of the training and philosophy of the practitioner rather than being based on the specific signs and symptoms displayed by the patient (Fig. 2-2).

My Treatment is:	Therefore 90% of My Patients Have
Manipulation	Fixations and Subluxations
Disc Surgery	Disc Disease
Exercise	Weakness, Stiffness
Muscle Relaxants	Muscle Spasm
Anti-depressants	Depression
Rhizotomy	Facet Disease
Pain Medication	Pain
Anti-Inflammation Medication	Inflammation
Nothing	Hysteria or Malingering

Fig. 2-2. Medical practitioners tend to stereotype persons with lower back pain into one or two groups that fit their methods of treatment rather than recognize that there are many different disorders and that each should have its own unique treatment approach.

4. There is a general tendency to perform complex and expensive diagnostic tests and exams in the early stages of the problem. Having multiple tests and exams may make the patient believe that his condition is more serious than it actually is. As previously noted, some tests may identify a degenerative or arthritic process, or perhaps a congenital defect such as a spine bifida occulta, which probably has little or nothing to do with the patient's real complaint. Such findings tend to absolve the physician of any further real involvement with the patient's problem and tend to make the patient believe that he is helpless and unable to manage his own problem. After all, "How can exercise, posture or good body mechanics help if I have a defect or arthritis in my back?" In most cases, the patient and the physician are better off if they do not know that these conditions exist. There is always time for these tests and exams if the patient does not respond to common sense, conservative management of the problem (eliminating abnormal stresses, patient education and exercises to restore normal posture, strength, flexibility and fitness.)

5. There has been a lack of emphasis on preventative and patient self-help programs.

6. Treatment is often limited to the acute phase only, treating the pain and muscle guarding, with little or no effort being made to improve strength, flexibility and posture. This is often true even following surgery.

7. Although some workers do take advantage of worker's compensation benefits, unjustly seeking time off from work and sometimes seeking disability and medical compensations that are out of pro-

portion to their injuries, many workers who have legitimate problems are treated unfairly with suspicion and harassment by supervisors and medical practitioners alike. This leads to resentment by the worker and he soon develops the attitude that he will have to "prove" that he has a real problem.

Recognizing the need for a new, positive approach to the management of lower back disorders, the following suggestions are offered (Fig. 2-3):

1. Prevent lower back problems rather than treat them after they occur. Back injury prevention programs offered by industry have shown that reduction in the number and severity of lower back injuries occurs following the initiation of such programs[6-9].

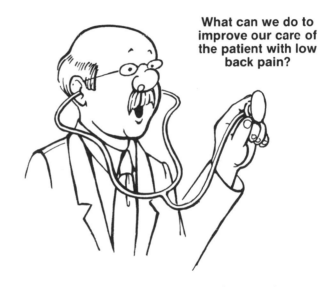

What can we do to improve our care of the patient with low back pain?

Fig. 2-3. A new approach is needed.

2. Keep back injuries "low profile" by avoiding extensive diagnostic tests and examinations unless the need for such services is truly indicated (Fig. 2-4). When the patient is sent to several specialists and/or given many tests, he begins to think of his injury as being much more serious than it may actually be (Fig. 2-5). This also tends to make the patient dependent upon the doctor to find a "cure" for the problem and often detracts from what the patient can do to help himself.

3. Show a sincere interest in the patient and treat him as if he has a real problem until proven otherwise.

4. Do something early in the way of positive treatment for the patient. Avoid sending the patient

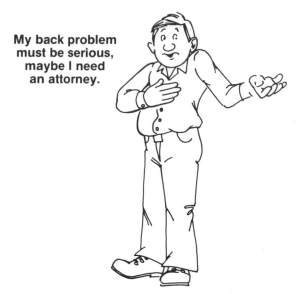

My back problem must be serious, maybe I need an attorney.

Fig. 2-4. Keep back injuries "low profile".

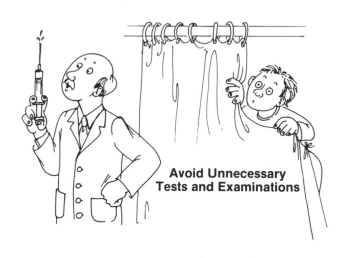

Avoid Unnecessary Tests and Examinations

Fig. 2-5. Too many specialists and too many tests may cause the patient to think he has a serious problem.

home for "rest" with no other treatment or instructions. This does not mean that everyone should receive physical therapy modalities right away. In fact, indiscriminant use of hot packs, massage, ultrasound and other modalities can also make the patient think that the therapist will "cure" the problem. Early treatment should emphasize posture correction, proper resting positions, mild corrective exercises, patient education, home treatment and rest (Fig. 2-6).

5. Keep the patient at work if possible. Company management should be made to recognize the economic advantages of providing light duty policies without harassment for employees with minor problems.

6. Recognize that there are many types of lower back disorders and that treatment programs must be individualized to meet unique situations.

7. Recognize that lower back problems are usually caused by a combination of poor posture, faulty body mechanics, stressful living and working habits, loss of flexibility and a general decline in physical fitness rather than by a single traumatic event.

8. Recognize that tension, nutrition, rest and self-image also play a part in management of lower back problems.

9. Treatment should involve correcting the cause (posture, body mechanics, flexibility and fitness) as well as including measures to manage acute episodes.

10. Treatment should focus on the patient's responsibility for management of the problem and what can be done to prevent recurrence.

11. Look for and treat the obvious first (Fig. 2-7). In many cases, such things as postural cor-

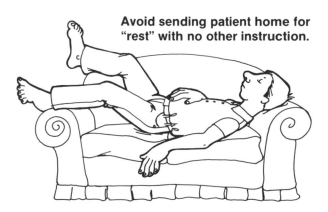

Avoid sending patient home for "rest" with no other instruction.

Fig. 2-6. Do something positive early.

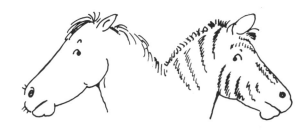

"When you hear hoofbeats, think horses, not zebras."

Fig. 2-7. Look for and treat the obvious, simple things such as poor posture, stiffness and weakness first.

rection, home exercises, rest and patient education are all that is necessary to treat a back disorder, yet these simple things are often overlooked when a patient initially complains of back pain.

12. Stop looking for magic answers (Fig. 2-8). The patient is often under the mistaken impression that sooner or later something is going to "pop" in his back and he will be well, or that some doctor or therapist is going to come along with a pill, injection, manipulation or surgery that will cure him. Patients have this attitude because medical practitioners have, to a certain degree, conditioned them to think this way. The first point that often needs to be made with many patients is that there are no magic answers for lower back problems and that only they themselves can effect a lasting "cure".

Stop Looking for Magic Answers.

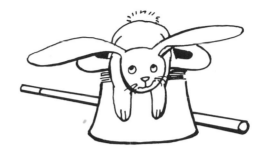

Fig. 2-8. Both medical practitioners and patients alike spend too much time looking for a magic answer to back disorders. This attitude often distracts the patient from the simple, common sense things that he should be doing to help himself.

References:

1. Dorland's Medical Dictionary: 23rd ed. Saunders, Philadelphia, 1957.
2. Cady, L. et al: Strength and Fitness and Subsequent Back Injuries in Firefighters, Joul of Occ Med, 21:260-272, 1979.
3. Biering-Sorenson, F: Physical Measurements as Risk Indicators for Low Back Trouble Over a One-Year Period, Spine 9:106-119, 1984.
4. Nachemsom, A: Low Back Pain, It's Etiology and Treatment, Clinical Medicine, 18-24, 1971.
5. Nordby, E: Epidemiology and Diagnosis of Low Back Injury, Occupational Health and Safety, 50:38-42, Jan 1981.
6. Lepore, B, Olson, C, and Tomer, G: The Dollars and Sense of Occupational Back Injury Prevention Training, Clinical Management, 4:38-41, 1984.
7. Fisk, J, DiMonte, P, Courington, S: Back Schools, Clinical Orthopaedics, 179:18-23, Oct 1983.
8. Fitzler, S, Berger, R: Attitudinal Change: The Chelsea Back Program, 51:24-26, 1982.
9. Fitzler, S, Berger, T: Chelsea Back Program: One Year Later, 52:52-54, 1983.

CHAPTER 3

EVALUATION OF A MUSCULOSKELETAL DISORDER

The role of the physical therapist in the examination and treatment of musculoskeletal disorders is developing greater responsibility in the medical field. Therefore, to competently practice, the therapist must prepare a proper data base from which to make a proper assessment and plan an effective treatment regimen for a particular musculoskeletal problem. This chapter discusses the important steps in evaluating a musculoskeletal disorder.

THE EVALUATION PROCESS

In physical therapy, evaluation is an ongoing process. Thus, even though it may be possible to complete a full and thorough evaluation during the patient's first examination, signs and symptoms must be rechecked during the course of treatment to determine the patient's progress or lack of progress. This ongoing evaluation and assessment forms the basis for treatment modification.

The need to continue the evaluative process is also a key factor in total patient management. The initial examination, no matter how thorough, cannot be expected to provide all the answers. A trial treatment should be administered and its effects assessed to determine whether a more definitive treatment program is necessary.

EXAMINATION

The examination is the foundation upon which effective treatment rests. The examination findings should guide the therapist in selecting appropriate treatment techniques. Because many different tests, measurements and sequences for collecting the required data are available, the format chosen largely depends upon individual preference. However, the internalizing of a methodical and complete examination process is essential to the therapist's success.

When performing a musculoskeletal examination, the therapist should adhere to one method. This will allow full development of the therapist's intuitive skills. Several recognized methods of evaluation are taught in orthopaedic physical therapy settings. While there are some differences in the order of questioning and emphasis, the essentials of the examination differ little. The emphasis, of course, should always be on thoroughness and accuracy.

The only exception to the rule of performing a complete examination and assessment of the patient's status on the initial visit is in the case of acute, severe pain. In this case the practitioner must determine if the problem is of a musculoskeletal nature, ruling out such things as fractures or dislocations if trauma is involved. A complete history should be taken and, if the history does not contraindicate the objective information available, the therapist can proceed with treatment of the symptoms both to relieve pain and to expose its underlying cause. However, when the symptoms of acute pain have subsided sufficiently, the therapist must carry out a complete evaluation.

COLLECTING DATA

In performing an evaluation, the physical therapist must collect data which are relevant, accurate and measurable. It is most desirable to measure and record data as objectively as possible. For example, it is essential to measure and record a positive straight leg raise test in degrees and to take actual circumference measurements and state restrictions of movement in degrees or inches. These data need to be accurately determined since they will be used later to assess changes brought about by treatment.

Any subjective information must be collected and recorded in an objective manner also. This seemingly contradictory task can be accomplished by recording some objectively measurable factors which correlate with the subjectively described symptoms such as the length of time the symptoms persist after a certain activity or the distance the patient can walk before the onset of symptoms.

Subjective questioning protocol and objective tests must be individualized by the therapist to maximize the information obtained. The therapist should ask the patient only purposeful questions that are directed at determining the patient's problem. In addition, objective tests should be used that are geared to the therapist's individual size, dexterity, physique and experience. Similarly, certain questions and tests will have more or less meaning with individual patients. For example, the result of an individual test or the answer to a question can lead to further questioning and testing to determine the relevance of the item to the present signs and symptoms. Correlation of compatible signs and symptoms is the key.

The tendency to jump to conclusions during the data collection phase of the evaluation process must be resisted. Only careful, accurate, thorough collection coupled with proper interpretation will ensure correct assessment and treatment.

RECORDING DATA

In performing an examination, it is important to record data in a format that can be easily interpreted by physicians and other health professionals. The recommended format is that of the S-O-A-P note. S-O-A-P stands for the elements of Subjective, Objective, Assessment and Plan. This format can be used for all patient's seen in a physical therapy clinic. The subjective portion contains the patient's pertinent past medical history and present complaint. The objective portion is a summary of all the clinical tests which the therapist performs to evaluate the problem. The assessment portion lists the problems determined in the subjective and objective sections and gives a working diagnosis. The planning section consists of an outline of the treatment plan, goals and prognosis.

Progress notes and the discharge summary should also follow the S-O-A-P format and, in combination with the initial examination, assessment and treatment plan, they become the complete physical therapy record for most patients. Special tests that require an additional form, such as a complete muscle test or a nerve conduction study, can be attached to the initial evaluation. There also may be occasions when a separate data base and/or problem list will be needed.

The use of dictation equipment and a typewriter aids efficiency and clarity in record keeping.

The examination report can be an effective communication instrument, but to achieve this, it must be concise and clear. A handwritten examination report is seldom as neat, easy to read, concise and complete as one that is typewritten. In addition, physicians and other health care personnel are less likely to read an evaluation if it is over one page in length, particularly if it is handwritten. However, thoroughness should not be sacrificed in order to keep the written evaluation brief. Material should always be arranged in the same order so others will know where to find certain information, and reference must be made to negative as well as to positive findings. For example, if the therapist should note that, "The neurological exam was within normal limits," he has said very little that is meaningful to a physician, for what constitutes a normal neurological exam to the therapist may not constitute a normal exam to the physician. If, however, the therapist records all tests done as positive or negative, this will assure the physician that the patient was being well evaluated and managed.

To assure that all important parts of the evaluation are performed and recorded, a worksheet should be used (Fig. 3-1). Even the most experienced practitioner may not recall all of the pertinent questions and tests that are necessary for a complete and thorough examination. Therefore, a worksheet is used to record all findings during the examination and as a reference when the formal written examination is dictated.

SEQUENCE OF EXAMINATION

When conducting an examination, the therapist should follow a sequential list of tests and questions to avoid unnecessary movement of the patient (Fig. 3-2). This sequence is simply performing all tests at one time which can be done in the standing, sitting, supine, side lying and prone positions. This sequence assures that nothing is overlooked or forgotten and it keeps the physical therapist moving along in an organized and efficient manner. This sequencing should be applied to examination of all major musculoskeletal areas, and data gathering sheets should be developed for use as a reference to assure thoroughness in testing. The sequence begins with the subjective examination.

PHYSICAL THERAPY WORKSHEET

PATIENT DATA

Subjective:
   Patient complaint:
   Nature:
   Location:
   Onset:
   Behavior:
   Course and Duration:
   Other Medical Problems:

OBJECTIVE:
   Structural:
   Mobility:
   Neurological:
   Palpation:
   Special Tests:
   Doctor's Report, Lab, & X-ray:

ASSESSMENT:
   Problem List:
   Goals:

PLAN:

Fig. 3-1. Worksheet used to record findings during the evaluation. The physical therapist dictates the initial evaluation (subjective and objective findings, assessment and plan) from this worksheet and then it is discarded.

SUBJECTIVE EXAMINATION (SYMPTOMS)

In conducting the initial subjective examination, the therapist should at all times be in control of the situation. Some questions, particularly those directed to the chronic pain patient, lend themselves to long discourses by the patient. The therapist must develop the fine art of not appearing to be rushed, yet he must be able to direct the interview so as to not waste time in superfluous information volunteered by some patients.

Each musculoskeletal disorder presents a unique history. The physical therapist must possess a thorough understanding of musculoskeletal pathology and the clinical picture that each disorder presents. Even with this in mind, it is a mistake to consider treating a pathological disorder such as degenerative disc disease with a routine or "cookbook" approach. The signs and symptoms of a specific disorder in one patient may differ significantly from those in another, or signs and symptoms may alter from treatment to treatment in the same patient.

It is essential to good practice to sit down with the patient in the examination room and obtain a detailed history of the condition and events that led to the onset of symptoms. It is a mistake to blindly

---

A   SEQUENCE OF SPINAL EVALUATION LUMBAR, MID & LOWER THORACIC SPINE

Standing
Gait
Posture
Structural base
Correct lateral shift
Aids and assistive devices
Active FB & BB
Repeated FB and BB
Active SB
Heel-toe raises
Weight shift test
Active ROM SI joints

Sitting
Posture
Active rotation (overpressure)
Knee, ankle reflex
SLR's
Resisted knee extension
Clear knee
Resisted ankle-dorsiflexion
Great toe extension
Clear ankle
Distraction test

Supine
Passive FB (knees to chest)
Repeated passive FB
Long-sitting vs. supine leg length test
SLR's
Check for hip flexor & hamstring
   tightness
SI spring test
SI mobility test
Sensation
Resisted hip flexion
Clear hip (ROM & compression)
Babinski's test

Side-Lying
Passive FB & Rotation
Palpate ligament and bone

Prone
A-P mobility test
Passive BB
Repeated passive BB
Palpate skin, subcutaneous, muscle,
   ligament & bone
Femoral nerve stretch

B   SEQUENCE OF SPINAL EVALUATION CERVICAL & UPPER THORACIC SPINE

Standing
Posture
Aids & assistive devices
Structural base

Sitting
Active ROM neck with over pressure
Resisted cervical muscle tests
Resisted shoulder elevation
Resisted shoulder abduction
Clear shoulder
Resisted elbow flexion
Resisted elbow extension
Clear elbow
Resisted wrist extension
Resisted wrist flexion
Resisted thumb extension
Resisted finger abduction
Distraction/compression test
Palpation
   skin, subcutaneous, muscle,
   ligament, & bone
Thoracic outlet tests (3)

Supine
Vertebral artery test
Passive cervical ROM
   side bend — rotation —
      backward bend
   forward bend — side glide
Babinski's test
Distraction test

Prone
Active upper thoracic rotation

Fig. 3-2. Sequence of spinal evaluation. A) Lumbar, mid and lower thoracic spine; B) Cervical and upper thoracic spine.

accept sketchy or inadequate information, even if it came from a physician. Very often, the therapist asks an entirely different set of questions based on his knowledge of mechanics, posture and activities of daily living than does the physician. With the history completed, the therapist may sometimes wish to leave the room to finish recording the history, review the notes from the subjective examination and plan the objective examination. Although one cannot always assign more importance to the subjective examination than the objective examination, in many cases much of the information needed to make a correct assessment can be elicited from the patient during the subjective examination.

The following is a step-by-step description of some common areas of questioning that should be part of the subjective examination done by the therapist to obtain an adequate patient history:

Patient complaint — When taking the history, the first question to ask is simply, "What is your complaint?" This gives the patient a chance to tell in his own words anything which he believes is important. This first question facilitates the rest of the interview by placing both the therapist and the patient at ease.

Nature of symptoms — If the patient has not mentioned the nature of his symptoms in answering the therapist's first question, it is important to find these out now. Pain, weakness, numbness, stiffness and hypersensitivity are common symptoms. The therapist should ask for a specific description of the symptoms such as a "constant deep ache", "intermittent pain" or "sharp stab of pain", but should not lead the patient by suggesting descriptions.

It is important to carefully differentiate between "pins and needles" and/or "tingling" or "numbness" descriptions. The patient should be asked if there is an area of skin that can be pinched or pricked with a pin and not be felt. If this is the case, nerve root impingement or peripheral nerve entrapment is a probability. "Pins and needles" and/or "tingling" are often non-specific descriptions that many patients use regardless of the disorder involved.

Weakness that is present without pain suggests a neurological deficit unless it is generalized and associated with prolonged disuse. Painless weakness associated with a peripheral nerve entrapment or spinal nerve root compression often follows a specific dermatome or myotome distribution. If weakness is present with pain, it is sometimes difficult to determine if the pain alone is causing the weakness or if there is also an underlying neurological deficit.

Often the patient will describe a slipping, popping or clicking sensation that is associated with certain movements. It is important to determine if this sensation occurs repeatedly every time the particular movement is repeated. If it cannot be repeated it is probably the vacuum popping effect that one experiences if the joint surfaces are separated suddenly. This phenomenon is similar to the "pop" that is heard when a rubber suction cup is pulled suddenly from a flat surface. It is simply the sudden filling of the vacuum that is momentarily created as the two surfaces are separated. Once this type of pop occurs, it cannot be repeated for a certain period of time. This is a normal phenomenon. If a joint cannot be popped it is an indication that it is hypomobile and if a joint seems to pop quite easily it is an indication that the joint is hypermobile.

If the patient describes a joint noise that can be repeated over and over again it is an indication of: 1) an unstable joint that may be subluxing or partially subluxing with certain movements, 2) a mechanical roughness or abnormality of the joint surfaces such as a meniscus tear or osteophytosis or 3) thickening and scarring of the soft tissue (ligament and capsule) that surrounds the joint.

Location of symptoms — The patient should be asked to indicate the location of the symptoms, but it should be remembered that the location of the pain is not necessarily a reliable indicator of the actual site of pathology[1]. For example, most disc or nerve root syndromes cause bilateral pain in the spine, while most spinal facet joint problems are unilateral. Pain limited to one spinal segment is suggestive of a joint or nerve root disorder whereas pain over several spinal segments is more descriptive of a muscular inflammation or systemic disorder.

Pain and other symptoms are often referred distally and are rarely referred proximally. For example, cervical pain is often felt in the rhomboid muscle area, shoulder pain in the upper arm, and lower back pain in the buttocks and posterior thigh.

Pain that migrates from one joint to another suggests a systemic disease rather than a musculoskeletal disorder. Pain that spreads from the original site to the surrounding tissues is usually caused by inflammation and/or muscle spasm, both of which are often secondary reactions to the primary disorder.

Onset of symptoms — The original onset of symptoms as well as the most recent episode should be considered. Knowing the exact mechanism of injury can be helpful. For example, joint locking is often caused by a sudden, unguarded movement, whereas sprains and strains involve aggravation or trauma. Inflammatory and systemic disorders present a more subtle onset. Disc disorders usually have an insidious onset caused by repeated activities related to slumped sitting, forward bending and lifting; however, the patient may perceive the onset as a sudden event related to one particular activity in which he was engaged when the pain was first noticed.

It is important to realize that the patient will always try to remember some incident that caused the problem. This may not be reliable and it is often misleading to place too great an emphasis on the onset as described by the patient. The patient may also attempt to relate present complaints to old injuries. This can be very misleading.

Since many musculoskeletal disorders are caused by the accumulative effects of poor posture, faulty body mechanics, stressful working and living habits, loss of flexibility and a general state of poor physical condition, one should be certain that these areas are discussed in detail with the patient. Many times the answers to both the cause and the cure of the problem are found in this area of questioning.

Behavior of symptoms — Closely related to the nature of the symptoms is the behavior of the symptoms. Do the symptoms occur with certain activities or positions? Does the patient wake up with the pain in the morning? Is the pain worse while sitting, standing or walking? Does the weakness appear only after walking? Is there a pattern to the symptoms over a 24-hour period? The patient should be asked to explain how the symptoms are aggravated and how they are eased. Musculoskeletal symptoms are usually aggravated by certain movements and positions and are generally relieved with rest. If the symptoms are unrelated to movement or position and are not relieved with rest, one should suspect a systemic disease or visceral disorder and should seek consultation with a physician.

The effect of position can be an important clue to the cause of pain. For example, spinal pain arising from the disc is aggravated by sitting and forward bending, whereas walking tends to give relief. Pain arising from the facet joints will often be relieved by sitting and forward bending and walking is likely to be painful. Pain associated with acute injury and/or inflammation will often be present if a joint is moved in any direction, whereas simple joint dysfunction

and disc pain are often aggravated by movements in only one or two directions. Pain while resting suggests the presence of an inflammatory process. Night pain is suggestive of a possible tumor. Peripheral nerve entrapments, such as carpal tunnel and thoracic outlet syndromes, often worsen at night[1].

Course and duration of symptoms — It is important that the therapist consider the length of time since the onset of the symptoms in order to determine whether the condition is in an acute, subacute or chronic state. Determination of the degree of acuteness or chronicity will influence treatment.

The natural progression of the condition should also be considered. Was the pain greatest when the injury first occurred, or did it worsen on subsequent days? Has there been improvement? Has the patient continued to work since the onset of the symptoms? Is there a workman's compensation claim or litigation pending?

Effect of previous treatment — It is important to know the effect of any previous treatment. If the patient has been to a chiropractor or other medical practitioner, did the treatment affect the condition? If the patient has had a previous episode of this condition and a certain treatment helped, such treatment should again be considered as a possible means of treatment. Medication and home treatment are also important to note at this time.

Other related medical problems — Special questions involving other medical problems such as general health, bowel and bladder problems, any recent, unexplained weight loss or any recent illnesses must also be considered. Previous surgery should be noted and a special note should be made if the patient has had a history of malignancy.

OBJECTIVE EXAMINATION (SIGNS)

Screening examination — Sometimes the exact location of the disorder is unclear. The patient complaining of arm symptoms may have a cervical disorder. Leg symptoms may be referred from the lumbar spine or the hip joint. The screening examination should be a quick overview of several areas to provide the physical therapist with enough information to decide what specific areas must be examined in detail. If the screening examination proves negative, it must be repeated since there is the possibility that something was missed. If no abnormalities are found and symptoms persist, the therapist should consult with a physician and further medical diagnosis should be pursued[1].

Screening exams are especially helpful when the patient initially complains of symptoms in the extremities. One must always consider that extremity symptoms may be related to spinal pathology. The neck should always be examined if the patient is complaining of an upper extremity symptom. Similarly, the lower back should always be examined if the patient is complaining of a lower extremity symptom. The screening exams are ideally suited for these cases. If, on the other hand, the patient's original complaint centers in the spine, one should go directly to the complete evaluation of that area. Since the complete evaluation of a spinal area also includes the extremities, the screening exam would simply be a duplication of effort.

The screening exam begins with the therapist's initial observations of how the patient carries himself, his posture, gait and balance even prior to entering the examination room. The patient is unaware that he is being evaluated and may show inconsistent patterns, particularly if there is secondary gain.

1) Upper quarter screening examination — The upper quarter screening examination consists of a series of mobility and neurological tests to identify problem areas in the cervical spine, shoulder, elbow, wrist and hand (Fig. 3-3). The testing is done with the patient sitting in a straight backed chair or on the edge of a treatment table.

First, a postural assessment should be made, then the cervical spine is taken through the active ranges of motion as the therapist watches for signs of pain, muscle spasm and/or limited range of motion. If no signs or symptoms are observed with active range of motion and passive overpressures, the joints of the cervical spine are considered "clear" and are not the causal structures involved.

Next, resisted pressures are exerted in all planes of motion with the cervical spine held in a neutral mid-range position. If these isometric resisted muscle tests produce no pain and no weakness is observed, the musculature of the cervical spine is considered "clear". Resisted rotation of the cervical spine is also a neurological test of spinal level C1. Resisted shoulder elevation is a test for a disorder in the upper trapezius, levator scapulae and rhomboid muscles and neurological involvement of the spinal levels C2 through C4.

1. Postural assessment
2. Active range of motion of cervical spine
3. Passive over pressures if symptom-free
4. Resisted muscle tests cervical spine (rotation C-1)
5. Resisted shoulder elevation (C-2,3,4)
6. Resisted shoulder abduction (C-5)
7. Active shoulder flexion and rotations
8. Resisted elbow flexion (C-6)
9. Resisted elbow extension (C-7)
10. Active range of motion of elbow
11. Resisted wrist flexion (C-7)
12. Resisted wrist extension (C-6)
13. Resisted thumb extension (C-8)
14. Resisted finger abduction (T-1)
15. Babinski's reflex test (UMN)

Fig. 3-3. Upper quarter screening exam (adopted from Cyriax[1].)

The patient is then asked to hold the arms abducted to 90° with the elbows flexed while downward resistance is applied, testing the deltoid and supraspinatus musculature and spinal level C5. This is followed by active shoulder flexion and external and internal rotation with overpressure to clear the shoulder joint. Resisted elbow flexion and extension tests the musculature of the upper arm and spinal levels C6 and C7. Active range of motion completes clearing of the elbow. The wrist and hand are cleared by resisted testing of wrist flexion and extension, thumb extension and finger abduction, testing simultaneously spinal nerves C7 to T1. The upper quarter screening is completed by doing a Babinski reflex test for upper motor neuron involvement.

2) Lower quarter screening examination — The lower quarter screening examination consists of a series of mobility and neurological tests to identify problem areas in the lumbar spine, sacroiliac area, hip, knee, ankle and foot (Fig. 3-4). The examination begins with the patient standing so that posture can be observed. The lumbar spine is taken through active forward, backward and lateral bending as the therapist watches for signs of pain, muscle spasm and/or limited movement. Heel and toe walking is then completed, which is a neurological test for L4 and L5 (heel) and S1 (toe). It also clears the ankle and foot when no pain or limitation of movement is observed. A quick technique to clear all joints of the lower extremity is to ask the patient to squat and then stand.

1. Postural assessment
2. Active forward, backward and lateral bending of lumbar spine.
3. Toe raises (S-1)
4. Heel walking (L-4,5)
5. Active rotation of lumbar spine
6. Over pressure if symptom-free
7. Straight leg raise (L-4, 5, S-1)
8. Sacroiliac spring test
9. Resisted hip flexion (L-1,2)
10. Passive range of motion to hip
11. Resisted knee extension (L-3,4)
12. Knee flexion, extension, medial and lateral tilt
13. Femoral nerve stretch
14. Babinski's reflex test (UMN)

Fig. 3-4. Lower quarter screening exam (adopted from Cyriax[1].)

Active lumbar rotation is checked with the patient sitting. The patient is asked to extend the arms directly in front with the hands held together and then to twist to the right and left as far as possible. If no signs or symptoms are observed with active range of motion, passive overpressures are applied. If rotation along with forward, backward and lateral bending produces no signs or symptoms when done both actively and with passive over-pressure in rotation, the joints and muscles of the lumbar spine are considered clear for those movements.

Next, the patient is positioned supine for straight leg raising, which is a neurological test of spinal levels L4 through S1. Differentiation between tightness of hamstrings and sciatic pain is critical. Spring tests for sacroiliac involvement are also done at this time.

The hip is clear if passive flexion, medial and lateral rotation and resisted hip flexion do not produce any signs or symptoms. Resisted hip flexion is also a neurological test of spinal levels L1 and L2.

Resisted knee extension is a neurological test of spinal levels L3 and L4. Clearing of the knee is completed by passively testing flexion and extension and applying varus and valgus stresses.

A femoral nerve stretch in the prone position may be indicated if the patient has described symptoms in the anterior hip, thigh and/or groin area. The lower quarter screening is completed by doing a Babinski reflex test for upper motor neuron involvement.

SPECIFIC OBJECTIVE EXAMINATION

Areas of specific complaint or areas that have shown some questionable signs during the screening examination should be examined in detail. The detailed objective examination of a specific area begins with general observation of the patient. The way the patient responds to the therapist's questions should be noted. What kind of attitude does the patient seem to have toward his condition-apprehensive, resentful or depressed? Since the behavioral attitude of the patient often has a bearing on the success of the treatment, the therapist should take time to think about this important aspect of the patient's condition.

How does the patient walk and sit? Does he seem to be in excruciating pain? Are there any obvious abnormalities in the way he moves and carries himself? Such observations are important for the therapist to note, as they may later tell more about the patient's progress than direct questioning does.

SPINE AND SACROILIAC JOINTS

Structural Examination

The structural exam involves a closer, more specific inspection of the area of complaint. Inspection involves the observation of bony, joint and muscular structures in the areas involved. It is essential that the parts to be examined be adequately free of clothing. Gym shorts and haltertops (females) are helpful because they allow adequate observation, yet avoid embarrassment.

Posture — Postural assessment should be made considering the entire spine even if the patient's complaint concerns only one area of the spine. There should be a gentle continuation of anterior-posterior curves the entire length of the spine. An excessive curve in one area will usually cause an increased curve in an adjacent area. For example, excessive lumbar or cervical lordosis may be accompanied by increased thoracic kyphosis. Suboccipital muscle and/or joint tightness will cause backward bending of the head and upper cervical spine, which causes the patient to forward bend the lower cervical and upper thoracic spine in order to achieve a level head position. The characteristic feature seen with this syndrome is the forward head position and rounded upper thoracic spine. The forward head posture is often seen following cervical strains and can become the major cause of symptoms in the chronic stages of these injuries. Forward head posture is also often seen as a result of certain working positions and habits.

The lumbar and cervical spine should show a mild lordotic curve and the thoracic spine should have a mild kyphotic curve. Absence of any of the curves may indicate restriction of mobility, whereas excessive lordotic curves may indicated the presence of any of a variety of structural and postural problems. Many pathological processes present certain predictable changes in lordosis and kyphosis and can be important clues to aid in diagnosis[1,2]. Increased lumbar lordosis may be associated with joint hypermobility, weak abdominal muscles and/or tight hip flexor muscles. The pelvis is anteriorly rotated. If this is the case, the patient may have a chronic postural strain and should be treated with a corrective exercise program. Absence or decrease of lumbar lordosis should be noted as it may be an indication of a disc disorder or may be the result of

living and working in the sitting or forward bending posture over a long period of time. The patient with flat back posture often has very little lumbar extension mobility and often has tight hamstring muscles. The pelvis is posteriorly rotated.

The sway-back posture is often mistaken for the hyperlordotic posture, however it is quite different. The sway-back posture is characterized by forward displacement of the hip joint, posterior rotation of the pelvis, a flat lower lumbar spine, a slight lordotic curve in the upper lumbar spine and a long slightly increased thoracic kyphosis[3]. The forward head posture is seen with all three of the posture abnormalities described above (Fig. 3-5) [1,2,4].

It is also very important to observe the patient's sitting posture. Often the slumped lumbar flexion posture contributes to loss of lumbar extension and to the development of a posterolateral disc protrusion. This posture may be the first clue as to what the problem may be (Fig. 3-5)[5].

Scoliotic curves in the spine are abnormal and are classified as either functional or structural or as caused by a specific pathological process. A

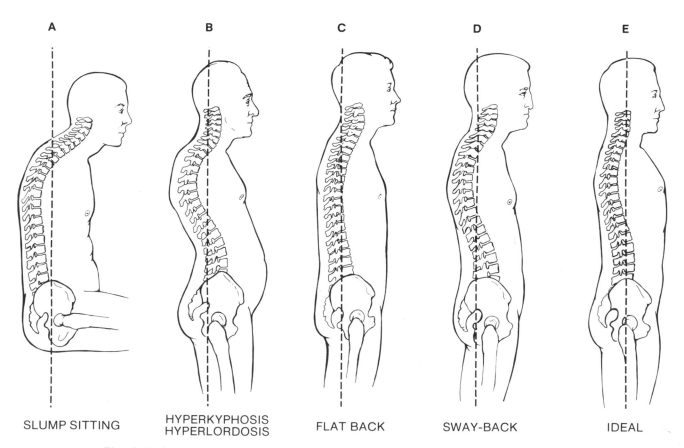

A	B	C	D	E
SLUMP SITTING	HYPERKYPHOSIS HYPERLORDOSIS	FLAT BACK	SWAY-BACK	IDEAL

Fig. 3-5. Common postural disorders. A) Forward head, rounded shoulders; B) Hyperlordosis — Hyperkyphosis; C) Hypolordosis (flat back); D) Sway-back; E) Ideal posture.

structural scoliosis is caused by a defect in the bony structure of the spine such as wedging of the vertebral bodies. A structural scoliosis is characterized by the fact that it does not straighten during forward bending or side bending into the convexity of the spine. Because lateral bending is always accompanied by rotation, the patient will have a "lumbar bulge" and/or "rib hump" when he forward bends if a structural scoliosis is present (Fig. 3-6). A functional scoliosis can be caused by a non-spinal defect such as unequal leg length, muscle imbalance or poor postural habits. Generally, a functional scoliosis of this type will straighten during forward bending and sidebending into the convexity; however, this may not be true if moderate to severe muscle spasm and guarding is present. The patient should always be asked to hold his hands together when forward bending. This eliminates some chance of error in determining if a rib hump is a true structural scoliosis or just active rotation of the spine.

Although consideration should be given to structural scoliosis, the therapist should remember that when seen in an adult, it will be a long-standing condition and may be only indirectly related to the patient's present complaint. Long-standing structural scoliosis may cause early degenerative joint/disc disease as well as indirectly contributing to a variety of disorders. When seen in children and early adolescents, structural scoliosis has much more significance. It must be managed by someone knowledgeable and competent to give the special treatment required.

Facet joint impingement may cause an acute scoliosis in any area of the spine. This disorder involves the entrapment of soft tissue within the facet joint. If this happens, the patient may shift to the opposite side of impingement to take the weight off of the painful structure.

A more common type of lateral curve seen with acute disorders in the lumbar spine is the "lateral shift" or "protective scoliosis" (Fig. 3-7). According to McKenzie, a lateral shift will often occur as the nucleus pulposus moves posterolaterally. For example, if the nucleus moves posterolaterally to the right, the patient is likely to shift his body weight anteriorly and to the left. Thus, the patient would appear to have a flattened lumbar lordosis and a left lateral shift[5]. Finneson advances another explanation for an acute lateral curve in the lumbar spine, which he calls the "protective scoliosis". If a protective scoliosis is present, he theorizes that it is

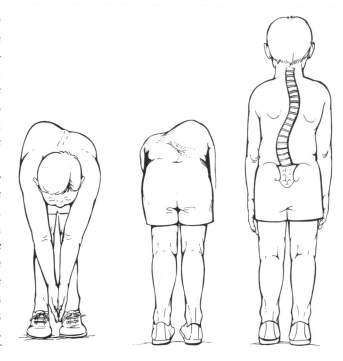

Fig. 3-6. Structural scoliosis. This example shows side bending to the right and rotation to the left in the lumbar spine and side bending to the left and rotation to the right in the thoracic spine.

caused by the patient moving the spinal nerve root away from the bulge of a disc herniation with protrusion. If the bulge is lateral to the nerve root it is encroaching upon, the patient will shift to the opposite side (most common.) If the bulge is medial to the nerve root it is encroaching upon, the patient will shift to the same side (uncommon) (Fig. 3-8)[4,6].

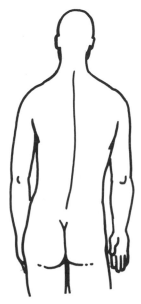

Fig. 3-7. Lumbar scoliosis.

Sacral base and leg length — Close attention is paid to the sacral base during the structural examination. With the patient standing straight with the feet slightly spread apart and weight equally distributed, the height of the iliac crests, posterior-superior iliac spines (PSIS), anterior-superior iliac spines (ASIS), trochanters, gluteal folds and fibular heads are checked to determine if the sacral base is uneven and, if so, where the discrepancy lies (Fig. 3-9). For example, if the PSIS's are uneven and the trochanters are even, the discrepancy lies between the two structures. In this case, the sacroiliac joint, the angulation of the femoral neck or the hip joint itself are possible areas of dysfunction.

Leg length differences that cannot be corrected by treatment should be corrected with a shoe lift. If left uncorrected, an uneven sacral base will cause a lumbar scoliosis which will contribute to uneven weight distribution on the facet joints and the intervertebral disc. This may lead to early degenerative changes in the lumbar spine and hip.

The height of the iliac crests should also be checked in the sitting position because it is possible for one side of the pelvis to be larger than the other. This will cause an uneven sacral base and a lumbar scoliosis while sitting. It can be corrected by using a seat cushion that is thicker on one side.

The sacral base should be checked closely even in patients with complaints in the cervical spine because compensatory scoliotic curves are often present in the cervical spine that may need to be treated by correcting the sacral base. The shoulders

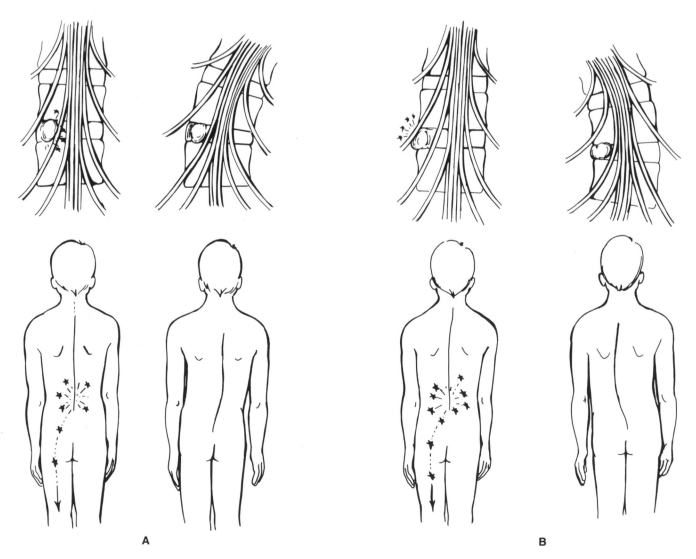

A   B

Fig. 3-8. Protective scoliosis sometimes seen in patients with herniated disc with protrusion (adopted from Finneson[6].)

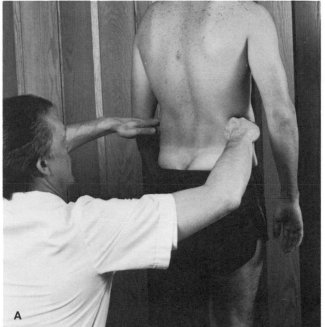

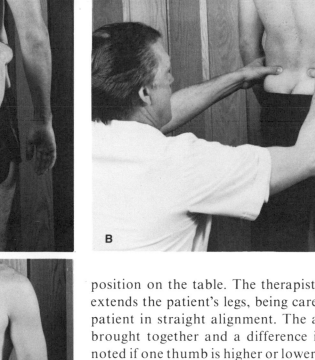

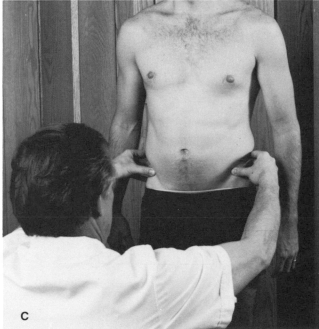

Fig. 3-9. Sacral base test to check: A) Height of iliac crests; B) Height of posterior superior iliac spines; C) Height of anterior superior iliac spines.

position on the table. The therapist then passively extends the patient's legs, being careful to keep the patient in straight alignment. The ankles are then brought together and a difference in leg length is noted if one thumb is higher or lower than the other. This finding should agree with the standing sacral base test. If findings of the standing and the supine leg length test do not agree it is because of error in testing or because there is a discrepancy that only shows up during weight bearing. Now, the patient is asked to come to the long sitting position and the malleoli are again observed. If this time the leg length becomes more equal or reverses, the test for possible sacroiliac (iliosacral) involvement is positive. This is an indication of a rotational defect in one of the innominates on the sacrum (Fig. 3-10). Some authors refer to these rotational defects as iliosacral rather than sacroiliac since the description of the dysfunction involves movement of the innominate on the sacrum (see discussion in Chapter 5.)

Assistive devices and supports — Any special assistive devices or supports, such as a knee brace, lumbar corset, cervical collar or cane that the patient uses, should be noted at this time. Care should be taken to assess if the device has been properly fitted and if it is being utilized correctly.

Mobility Examination

The mobility exam consists of posture correction and active, passive, resistive and special mobility tests. It is done to determine if the disc,

and the base of the cervical spine (C7) should also be examined to determine if they are level.

The long sitting versus supine leg length test is done to determine sacroiliac (iliosacral) involvement. The patient lies supine and flexes his knees and hips as the therapist grasps the ankles with his thumbs under the medial malleoli. The patient then lifts his buttocks from the table and returns to the resting position. This is done to equalize the patient's

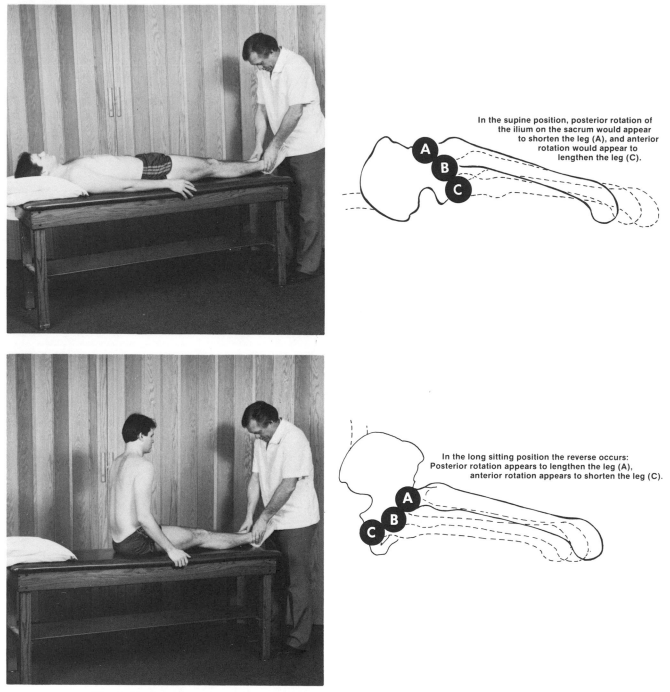

In the supine position, posterior rotation of the ilium on the sacrum would appear to shorten the leg (A), and anterior rotation would appear to lengthen the leg (C).

In the long sitting position the reverse occurs: Posterior rotation appears to lengthen the leg (A), anterior rotation appears to shorten the leg (C).

Fig. 3-10. Supine vs. long sitting leg length test to determine sacroiliac subluxation.

facet joints and/or muscles are involved and, if so, to what extent. During the mobility exam, the therapist is looking either for joint hyper or hypomobility, general flexibility and to see if movement causes a change in the patient's symptoms. The examination must include all tissues from which the patient's symptoms might arise. Tension must be applied on all of these tissues to note which movements provoke or change the patient's symptoms or otherwise appear abnormal.

Since posture often plays an important role in both the cause and treatment of many musculoskeletal disorders, an important part of the mobility exam involves observation of the effects of correcting postural abnormalities. **Posture correction** is done to determine if return to normal posture is possible and if the patient's symptoms are altered when posture is corrected. This may help find which structures are at fault and will also help the therapist determine to what extent the postural deformity is involved with the patient's current complaint. Clinical observation shows that many spinal musculoskeletal disorders start as local pain in the neck or lower back but as the condition worsens, the pain and other symptoms begin to spread toward the periphery (arm or leg.) Therefore, as a general rule, a neck or lower back movement or position that tends to increase arm or leg pain is harmful, whereas a neck or lower back movement or position that tends to increase local pain may not be causing harm (see further discussion in Chapter 5.)

The tissues may be divided into two groups-noncontractile (inert) and contractile. The noncontractile tissue group includes capsules, ligaments, bursae, nerves and their sheaths, cartilages, intervertebral discs and dura mater. These structures can have tension applied to them by passive stretching (passive movements.) The contractile tissue group includes muscles and tendons with their attachments. These structures may also have tension applied to them by passive stretching, but it is more effective to make them contract against resistance as a test of provocation.

Active range of motion of the spine is performed to give the therapist a general assessment of available range of motion. The specific level of hyper or hypomobility cannot be determined, but a general impression of problem areas can be gained. Pain arising from active movements may occur in certain predictable patterns that are helpful in determining the origin of such pain. For example, a painful recovery from forward bending indicates a disorder of muscular origin, whereas pain only at the end of range is more indicative of joint restriction. Active movements of the spine give the therapist a general assessment of the available range of motion and/or the patient's willingness to move. Such movements combine joint range of motion and muscle contraction and should be done only within the limits of pain.

Resisted movements are static contractions. They are usually done in a comfortable neutral position within the available range of motion. If no pain or weakness is observed at the joint, the muscle group (contractile) has been tested and the inert structures have not been disturbed. If contractile tissue is at fault, the appropriate resisted movement will be painful and/or weak. The joints are placed in a neutral midrange position and the patient is asked to hold against resistance in each direction. The therapist attempts to elicit a strong muscle contraction with very little or no joint movement. If the test causes increased pain, the muscles are primarily implicated. While this method of testing is very helpful in examining the extremity joints, it has very little application in testing the lumbar and thoracic spine because of the difficulty in isolating muscle contraction without the occurrence of joint movement in these areas. Resisted muscle tests can be helpful in determining muscular involvement in the cervical spine.

Passive movements test the specific range of motion available in a joint or spinal segment. These tests determine if the joint range is reduced (hypomobile), increased (hypermobile) or normal. If noncontractile tissue is at fault, passive movements may be painful and/or restricted and conversely, contractile tissue will be undisturbed.

Passive movement testing is an extremely valuable procedure to use when testing the spine because it provides the therapist with specific information about each individual spinal segment. It requires considerable practice and experience before competence is achieved. Passive range of motion tests are done to assess movement at the specific segmental level. An attempt is made to grade the movement using the following scale:[7]

0 — Ankylosed
1 — Considerable restriction
2 — Slight restriction
3 — Normal
4 — Slight increase
5 — Considerable increase
6 — Unstable

Special mobility tests are done to assess mobility or to determine if the structure being tested (stressed) is painful, indicating a pathological process.

Cervical and Upper Thoracic Spine — Mobility Exam

Postural correction in the cervical and upper thoracic spine often involves the slumped sitting, rounded shoulders, forward head posture which is often seen in patients complaining of a variety of musculoskeletal disorders. If correction of the poor posture can be accomplished, it should be done. However, if posture correction causes increased pain or other symptoms in the arm, attempts to

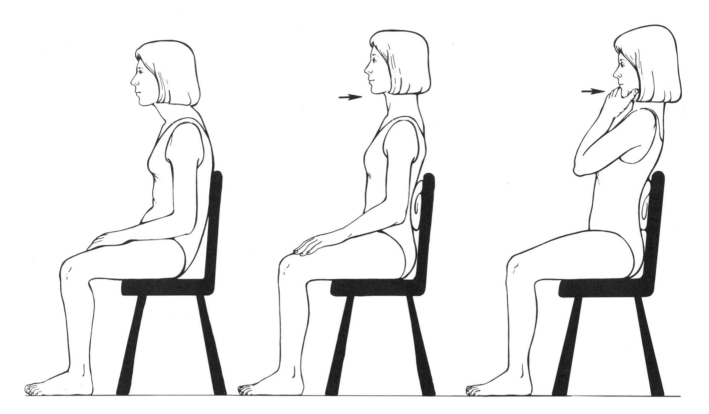

Fig. 3-11. Method of correction of forward head, rounded shoulder posture. If correcting the posture causes an increase in central neck pain, it may be acceptable to continue. If, however, an increase in peripheral signs and symptoms is noted, the attempts at correction should be discontinued.

correct the poor posture should be discontinued (Fig. 3-11).

Upper Cervical Spine

Atlanto/Occipital Joint — The vast majority of the motion which takes place at the A/O joint is in the sagittal plane in the form of nodding of the head on the cervical spine. The joint can be tested actively and passively.

For **active** motion, the joint can be tested with the patient seated or supine by simply asking the patient to nod his head. The cervical spine should be in neutral or in axial extension (head back, chin in) for this test. The therapist may then use the nose and the midline of the face for reference and observe for any lateral deviations of the head during the movement. Deviation to one side indicates a restriction in movement of the A/O joint on that side.

To palpate **passive** mobility of the A/O joint, the examiner stands at the head of the table with the patient lying supine. The head is fully supported under the occiput by both hands while contact is made with the transverse processes of the atlas by the index or middle fingertips. This contact is indirectly made through soft tissue between the mastoid and the ramus of the mandible. This hand support and palpatory technique can be used by the examiner for forward/backward bending, side bending and rotational movements.

1) Forward/Backward Bending — The examiner passively moves the head in a nodding movement. The transverse processes should move symmetrically or not at all.

2) Side Bending — The examiner passively side bends the head on the neck. The transverse process of the atlas will become more prominent on the side opposite the direction of side bending.

3) Rotation — The transverse process keeps a constant relationship between the mastoid and ramus during the first few degrees of rotation. However, at the end of rotation range, the transverse process may be felt to approximate or even disappear behind the mastoid or the ramus depending which way the head is turned. For example, if the examiner turns the head to the left, the right transverse process will approximate/disappear be-

hind the right mastoid. In right rotation, the opposite should occur. The two sides are compared for symmetry of movement.

When testing mobility of the **Atlanto-Axial joint,** one should remember that this joint is oriented in the horizontal plane. Rotation is facilitated here. There are only small components of side bending and forward/backward bending.

The examiner stands at the head of the table with the patient lying supine. He uses the same hand placement as in the A/O evaluation. Holding the head in a neutral position, he then fully side bends the cervical spine to one side or the other. The A/A joint may then be tested for a restriction in its ability to rotate by the examiner rotating the head on the newly created axis in the opposite direction of the side bending. For example, to test the right A/A joint, the cervical spine would be side bent to the left. Rotation would then be imparted to the right. The examiner tests for both quantity and quality of motion.

Mid-Lower Cervical and Upper Thoracic Spine

Active range of motion of the mid-lower cervical and upper thoracic spine is examined with the patient sitting. The therapist asks the patient to forward and backward bend, side bend and rotate in each direction. Any movements that are limited or that change the patient's symptoms are noted.

In the cervical spine, the therapist can feel movement at the individual segments by holding his thumb and index finger on the articular pillar at each level as the patient performs the active movements (Fig. 3-12A). In a slender patient, cervical movements can also be felt by placing the finger between the spinous processes (Fig. 3-12B).

In the upper thoracic spine, movement can be felt by placing the finger between the spinous processes as the patient forward and backward bends. Active rotation can be assessed by placing the thumbs on the spinous processes at two levels and watching and feeling the movement between the levels. This test can also be done with the patient lying prone, rotating the head from one side to the other (Fig. 3-13).

If all active range of motion is within normal limits and is symptom free, the movements are repeated and passive overpressures are given at the end of range of each movement. If no pain or other symptoms arise, even when overpressures are

applied, the area is clear of musculoskeletal pathology.

The **resisted** movement tests to determine muscular involvement in the cervical and upper thoracic spine are done with the patient sitting. The head is held well supported in a neutral, midrange position as the patient is asked to hold against resistance in each range of motion direction (Fig. 3-14). Shoulder elevation is tested with the patient sitting to determine if the upper trapezius and/or rhomboid muscles are involved (Fig. 3-15). The middle and lower trapezius muscles are tested with the patient prone (Fig. 3-16). A strong muscle contraction is elicited with very little or no joint movement. A weak and painless contraction indicates neurological involvement or weakness due to prolonged disuse (see neurological examination.)

The **passive** mobility tests for the cervical spine are forward bending, backward bending, rotation, side bending and side glide. They enable the therapist to feel specific areas of hyper or hypomobility in the cervical spine.

The patient is positioned supine with his head extending over the end of the treatment plinth for all of the passive mobility tests. It is important that the therapist support the patient's head in such a way that the patient will be able to relax completely, having confidence that the therapist has full control of the movements. The treatment plinth must be adjusted to the correct height for the individual therapist. The patient's head is rested against the anterior aspect of the therapist's hip (Fig. 3-17). The therapist must observe the neck musculature (sternocleidomastoids) to be certain that the patient is relaxed. The hands are cradled to hold the patient's head and neck. The index fingers support on the articular pillar superior to the segment to be tested (Fig. 3-18).

Forward bending in the cervical spine involves superior and anterior glide of the superior articulating surface on the inferior articulating surface bilaterally. The patient's head and neck are held in 30° of forward bending. This aligns the plane of the cervical facet joints perpendicular to the floor. Forward bending is done by lifting straight upward with both hands. To start, the therapist's knees should be slightly bent. The therapist extends his knees slightly to keep the patient's head in the correct position (Fig. 3-19). Most of the force is directed through the index fingers, but contact is maintained with all of the neck and head so that it is carried along with the movement.

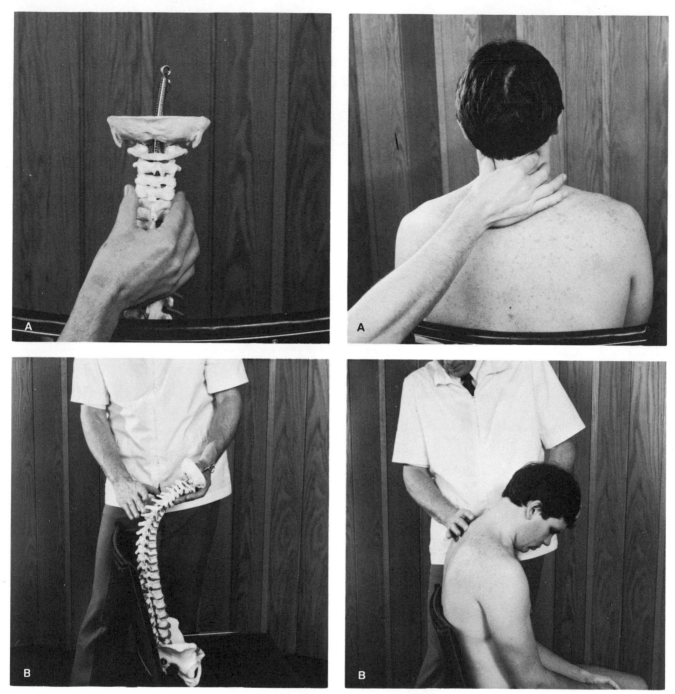

Fig. 3-12. A) Position of thumb and index finger on articular pillars of the cervical spine to palpate active movements. B) Position of finger between spinous processes to palpate active movements in cervical and upper thoracic spine.

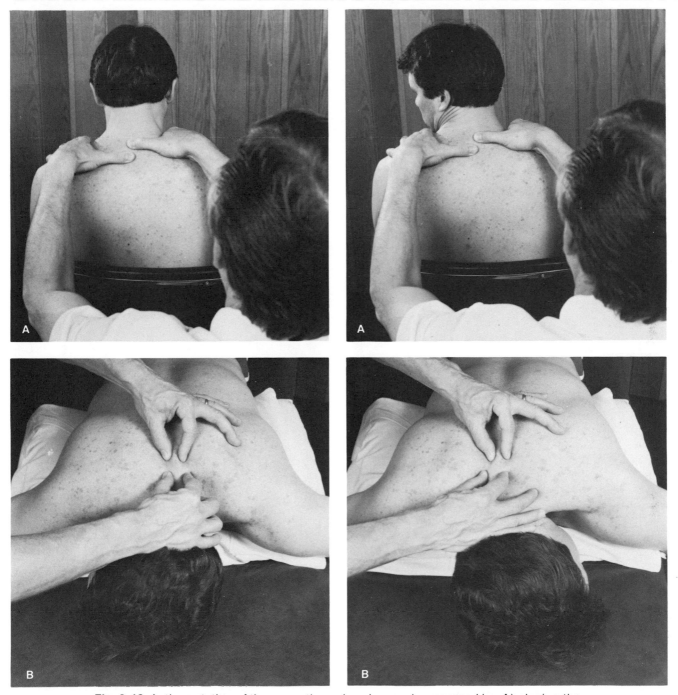

Fig. 3-13. Active rotation of the upper thoracic spine can be assessed by: A) placing the thumbs on the spinous processes as shown and feeling and observing movement or by B) pinch test of spinous processes to observe movement as patient rotates from right to left.

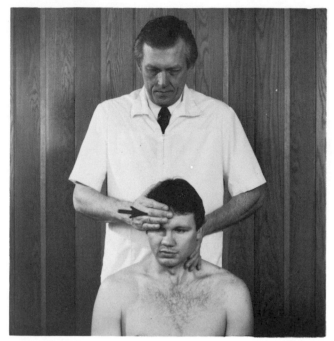

Fig. 3-14. Position to test resisted movements of the cervical spine in all planes of motion.

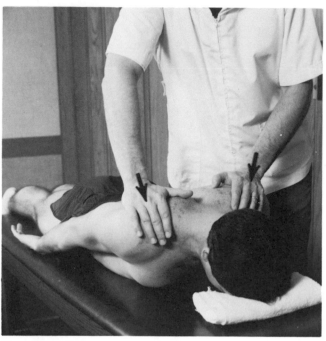

Fig. 3-16. Resisted muscle test for middle and lower trapezius muscles.

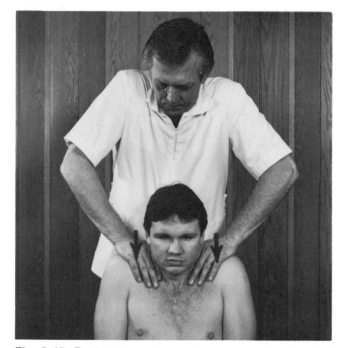

Fig. 3-15. Resisted muscle test for upper trapezius and rhomboid muscles.

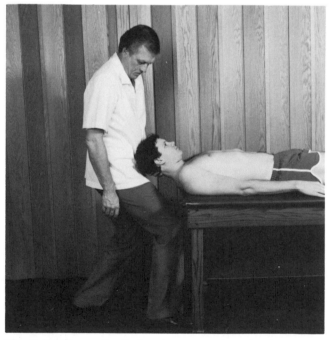

Fig. 3-17. The patient's head rests against the therapist's anterior hip for cervical passive mobility testing.

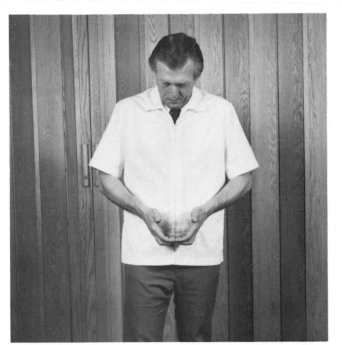

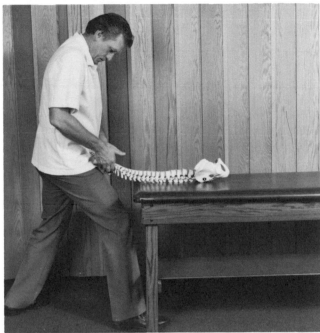

Fig. 3-18. Position of hands for cervical mobility testing.

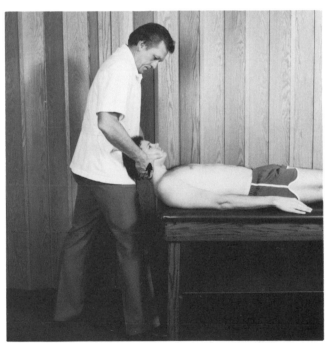

Fig. 3-19. Forward bending cervical passive mobility test.

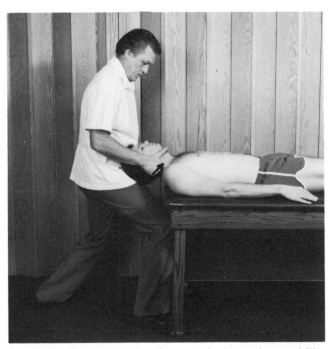

Fig. 3-20. Backward bending cervical passive mobility test.

Backward bending is performed in exactly the same manner, except that the head and neck are not carried along with the movement and the test is done with the head and neck in a neutral position. Only force through the index fingers is applied. This causes backward bending to occur at the segmental level superior to the contact (Fig. 3-20).

Cervical rotation involves superior and anterior glide of the superior articulating surface on the inferior articulating surface on one side and slight inferior and posterior glide on the opposite side. Therefore, rotation is tested in the same manner as forward bending, except to only one side at a time, and it is done from the neutral position. For example, to do left rotation, the right hand lifts upward to perform the movement, while the left hand supports (Fig. 3-21).

Passive cervical side bending utilizes the same positioning. Force is applied in a medial and slightly inferior direction through the index finger as it contacts the lateral aspect of the articular pillar. The point of contact on the index finger is lateral and slightly toward the palmar surface of the meta-carpophalangeal joint. This force causes the segment below the contact to side bend to the same side as the mobilizing force. The opposite hand supports (Fig. 3-22).

Passive cervical side gliding also utilizes the same basic position. Force is applied in a medial direction through the index finger as it contacts the lateral aspect of the articular pillar, causing movement to occur at the segment below the contact. The point of contact on the index finger is on the palmar surface of the metacarpophalangeal joint. The patient's head is carried to the side with this movement. In order to do this, the therapist must shift his hips in the direction of the mobilization (Fig. 3-23).

Lumbar and Mid-Lower Thoracic Spine — Mobility Exam

Postural correction in the lumbar spine involves either hypolordosis, hyperlordosis or a lateral

scoliosis. Hypolordosis or hyperlordosis is evaluated during active forward and backward bending testing.

When an acute lateral lumbar scoliosis is seen during the examination an attempt should be made to correct it (Fig. 3-24). If the scoliosis is caused by a mild to moderate disc protrusion (lateral shift, McKenzie), the correction procedure will often

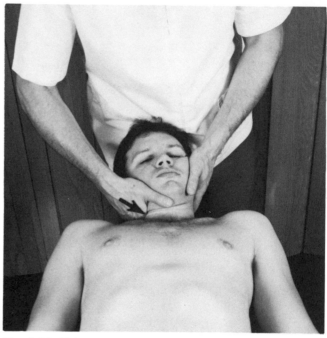

Fig. 3-22. Side bending cervical passive mobility test.

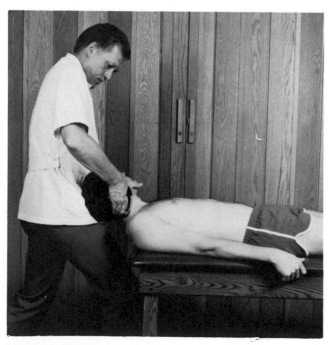

Fig. 3-21. Rotation cervical passive mobility test.

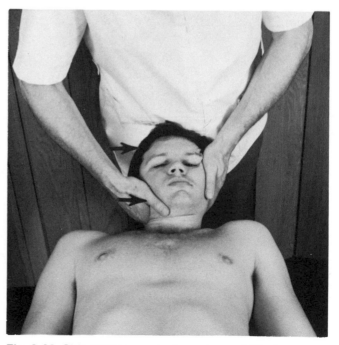

Fig. 3-23. Side gliding cervical passive mobility test.

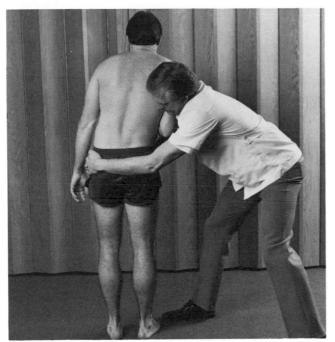 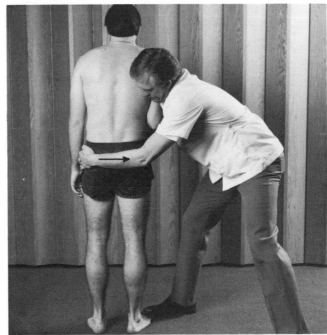

Fig. 3-24. Method of correcting a lumbar scoliosis.

cause centralized pain in the lumbar spine but no increase of peripheral symptoms. An exception to this would involve a large bulge in which some of the disc material is being trapped outside the postero-lateral edge of the vertebral bodies. In this case, attempted correction would probably cause increased pain or other symptoms in the lower extremity.

If the scoliosis is a protective scoliosis as described by Finneson, any attempt at correction will increase pain and other symptoms in the lower extremity. At this point in the examination, the following rule applies: *If the acute lateral lumbar scoliosis can be corrected without increasing pain or other symptoms in the lower extremity, it should be done. If, on the other hand, attempted correction increases the pain or other symptoms in the lower extremity, attempts to correct the shift should be discontinued (see discussion in Chapter 5.)*

All **active** range of motion is tested with the patient standing as he was for the sacral base test. If the sacral base is uneven, it should be leveled by placing the correct thickness of books or magazines under the short side. If this is not done during active range of motion testing, an accurate assessment of true range of motion in the lumbar spine cannot be made.

When examining active movements of the spine, a general assessment of movement is made first. Next, the therapist observes closely the exact area of the patient's complaint. In addition to observing movement, the patient is asked if he experiences any pain, stiffness or any other symptoms with the movement.

Active forward bending is checked by having the patient bend forward as the therapist assesses the general and specific mobility of the spine (Fig. 3-25).

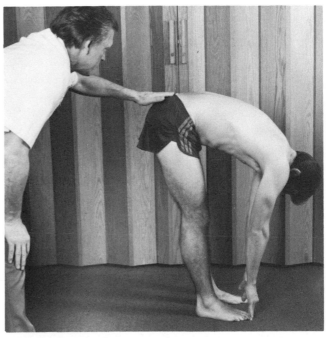

Fig. 3-25. Active forward bending of lumbar, mid and lower thoracic spine.

Does the normal lordosis in the lumbar spine straighten (normal range of motion) or become slightly kyphotic (hypermobility) during forward bending? If the lordosis does not straighten completely, hypomobility is noted. Does the thoracic spine show increased kyphosis? Is the movement smooth and does it seem to be uniform throughout the length of the spine? Does the patient experience pain, stiffness or any other symptoms? If so, is it central in the lower back or does it radiate into the lower extremity? If the patient experiences increased pain when recovering from the forward bent position, he is said to have a "tortuous recovery", which indicates an active lesion in the spinal muscles[8]. The patient with a tortuous recovery will often "crawl" his hands up his thighs to regain the standing position. Does the patient drift to the left or right instead of bending straight forward? If this is found it indicates unilateral hypomobility of the facet joint(s), unilateral muscular tightness or postero-lateral disc protrusion. It is often necessary to ask the patient to forward bend with his eyes closed before this drift can be seen because it is natural for the patient to fix his eyes on the floor and guide himself straight down, thus overriding any tendency to drift laterally. Having the patient close his eyes will eliminate this chance of error.

Active backward bending is also checked with the patient standing (Fig. 3-26). Restrictions of backward bending are usually associated with disc protrusion, facet joint hypomobility or facet joint pain.

During mobility testing it is important to note what movements (changes in lordosis) cause the patient's pain to move centrally and what movements cause the pain to move to the periphery. According to McKenzie[5], for patients with lumbar disc protrusion, movements that centralize the pain are helpful and ones that move the pain to the periphery are harmful. When testing repeated lumbar forward and backward bending in standing, if the symptoms move toward the periphery, it is an indication that the movement is making the condition worse. For example, it may be causing further disc bulging. If movements cause the pain to move centrally, it is not necessarily an indication that the condition is getting worse. When a stiff joint is moved it will be painful but it must be moved to regain mobility. The most common example is that repeated forward bending will cause the pain to move away from the midline and into the buttock and thigh while repeated backward bending will

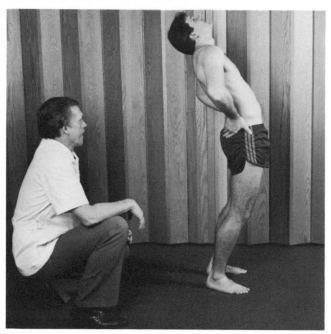

Fig. 3-26. Active backward bending of lumbar, mid and lower thoracic spine.

cause increased pain in the center of the lumbar spine. When this reaction is seen, it is an indication that the patient has a mild disc protrusion. Pain that is present at the end of range indicates facet joint hypomobility and pain throughout the range of motion is characteristic of acute inflammation, strain or sprain. A feeling of "slipping" or a moving sensation during range of motion testing is a sign of instability or hypermobility.

Active side bending is examined by first having the patient bend to one side and then the other (Fig. 3-27). Is the patient bending one way as far as the other? An easy way to assess this is to watch how far the patient's fingers reach on the side of his legs. One should see a gentle, smooth and continuous curve from the sacro-lumbar joint through the mid-thoracic spine when the patient actively side bends. Any straight areas indicate hypomobility and any areas of sharp bending indicate hypermobility (Fig. 3-28). One must be careful to keep the patient from shifting the pelvis laterally when examining active side bending. If the sacral base is uneven it is important that it be leveled before checking active side bending.

Active rotation is checked with the patient sitting on the edge of a treatment plinth with his arms held straight out in front with his hands together. A general assessment is made first, followed by a closer examination of the specific area of the patient's complaint (Fig. 3-29). As rotation

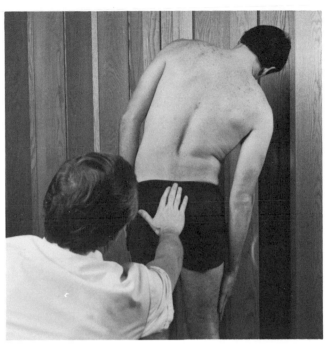

Fig. 3-27. Active side bending of lumbar, mid and lower thoracic spine.

occurs in one direction, side bending will occur in the opposite direction. The spinous processes also move in the opposite direction of the rotation. It is this movement of the spinous processes and the side bending component that the physical therapist observes when he looks for rotation at specific levels (Fig. 3-30).

As a general rule, facet joint restrictions are more noticeable during side bending than in forward or backward bending. Conversely, restrictions due to muscular tightness will be proportionately more noticeable in forward bending.

In summary, facet joint restrictions will be painful at the end of range of motion and will often tend to loosen up with repeated movement. Muscular restrictions will be most painful when the involved muscle is actively contracting, as in the tortuous recovery described earlier. Disc lesions tend to be aggravated by certain repeated movements, especially forward bending, and the pain tends to linger after the movement is stopped. For example, when using the standing forward bending test, if the patient has pain (mostly in the back) at the end of available range of motion and it is relieved as soon as he starts to return to standing and if repeating the movement several times tends to relieve the pain, one would suspect facet joint hypomobility. If the pain felt (mostly in the leg) at the end of range of motion tends to worsen with repeated movements and lingers after the movement is stopped, one would suspect disc involvement. If the pain is felt mostly on returning from the forward bent position, one would suspect muscle involvement.

If all active range of motion appears normal and does not cause pain or other symptoms, the

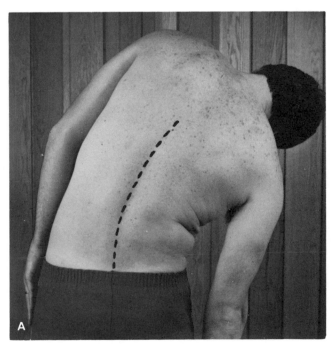

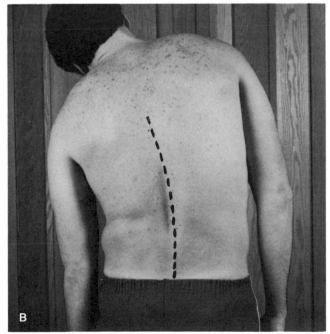

Fig. 3-28. Active side bending. A) Normal mobility to the right; B) Generalized restriction of side bending to the left.

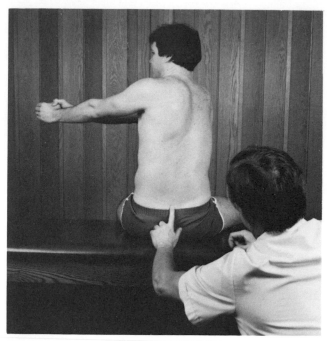

Fig. 3-29. Active rotation of lumbar, mid and lower thoracic spine.

pressure is applied in rotation, the area is considered free of musculoskeletal pathology.

Although **resisted** muscle tests are very helpful when examining other areas, their value in the lumbar and mid and lower thoracic spine is limited because of the difficulty of isolating the muscle contraction without at least some joint movement. Tortuous recovery from the forward bent position, which was described under active movements, is probably the most valid mobility test for muscular involvement in the lumbar and mid and lower thoracic spine.

The **passive** range of motion tests done for the lumbar and mid and lower thoracic spine are forward bending, backward bending and rotation.

During normal forward bending, the spinous processes separate slightly. The therapist passively forward bends the spine while feeling between two spinous processes with his finger. If the therapist feels the spinous processes separate slightly and the supraspinous ligament become taut under his finger, there is movement present at that segmental level. This amount of movement is compared to other levels and the therapist determines if the movement at the involved segment is hyper or hypomobile, or if it is normal. This test is done with the patient lying on his side for the lumbar and lower thoracic spine (Fig. 3-31), and sitting for the mid-thoracic spine (Fig. 3-32).

movements are repeated and passive overpressure is given at the end of rotation. This is done to clear the area being examined. In other words, if the lumbar and mid and lower thoracic spine has full active range of motion with no pain or other symptoms associated with movement, even when passive over-

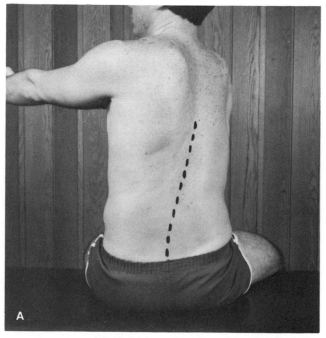

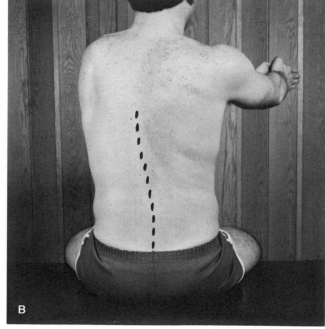

Fig. 3-30. Active rotation of lumbar, mid and lower thoracic spine. A) Normal rotation to the left; B) Restricted rotation to the right in the lower lumbar spine.

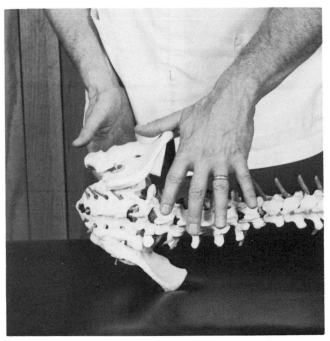

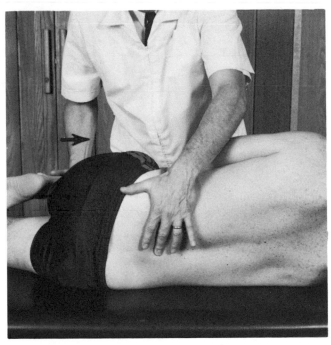

Fig. 3-31. Passive forward bending test, lumbar and lower thoracic spine, showing finger positioning.

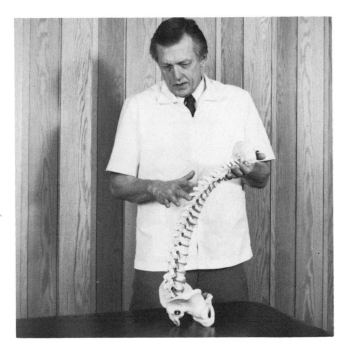

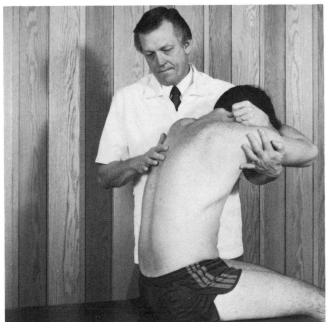

Fig. 3-32. Passive forward bending test, mid-thoracic spine.

Passive forward bending is also checked with the patient lying supine by bringing the knees to the chest. A general assessment of lumbar flexion is made. This test is also compared with standing forward bending to rule out nerve root involvement. It may also be repeated several times to determine if the symptoms change with repeated movement (Fig. 3-33).

Passive lumbar backward bending is checked with the patient lying prone. The patient is asked to press up with his arms while letting his back passively extend. The starting position for the hands should be directly in front of the shoulders. One should observe flattening of the mid and lower thoracic kyphosis and an increase in lumbar lordosis, especially in the lower lumbar area, with

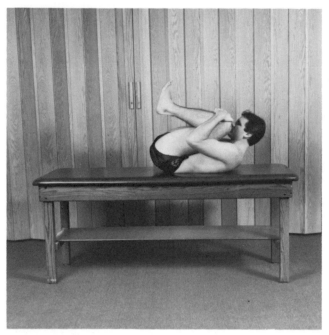

Fig. 3-33. Passive forward bending being tested in a different position to help distinguish between lumbar joint restrictions and spinal nerve root restrictions.

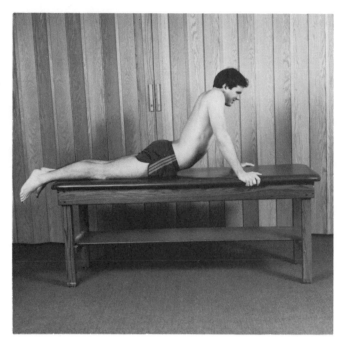

Fig. 3-34. Passive backward bending test.

this test. The distance of the ASIS from the table should be measured (approximately 2″ is considered within normal limits.) Repeated passive lumbar extension is done to determine if the symptoms change with repeated movements (Fig. 3-34).

During normal spinal rotation, each spinous process moves laterally in relation to the spinous process of the vertebrae below. For example, during right rotation, each spinous process moves to the left. During left rotation, each spinous process moves to the right. The therapist, with the patient positioned in the sidelying position, passively rotates the spine while feeling between two spinous processes with his finger (Fig. 3-35). If he feels the

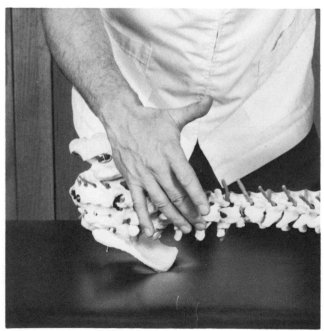

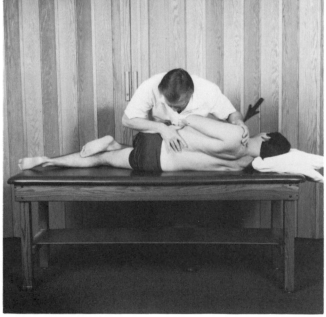

Fig. 3-35. Passive rotation test in the lumbar, mid and lower thoracic spine, showing finger positioning.

superior spinous processes move laterally, as described above, there is movement at that level. This amount of movement is compared to other levels and is graded by the therapist. Right rotation should be tested with the patient lying on his left side, and the patient should lie on his right side to test left rotation.

The anterior spring test is a special mobility test that is done by contacting three spinous processes in a row with the thumbs (Fig. 3-36). The patient is positioned prone. Downward (anterior) pressures are applied with both thumbs. This pressure is applied to the two spinous processes that are directly under each of the thumbs while the one spinous process between, which is being contacted by the tips of both thumbs, receives no direct pressure. If there is normal anterior-posterior movement, the two "outside" spinous processes are felt to move, while the one between is felt to stay in position.

Sacroiliac Joints — Mobility Examination

Active range of motion of the sacroiliac (iliosacral) joints is tested with the patient standing. The therapist places his thumbs on the posterior-superior iliac spines and asks the patient to forward bend. If there is less movement in one sacroiliac, the PSIS on that side will move upward and forward sooner and farther than the PSIS on the opposite side (Fig. 3-37).

Another way to evaluate active range of motion of the SI joint is to strap a two-inch belt around the patient's pelvis and note if any changes are made in his symptoms when he tries to perform certain activities such as stair climbing or sitting with the legs crossed. If the symptoms are relieved it is an indication that the SI joint is hypermobile and excessive movement is taking place with these activities.

Passive movement at the SI joints can be felt by placing the middle finger across the joint in such a way that the volar surface of the proximal interphalangeal joint is in contact with the PSIS and the tip of the finger is on the sacrum (Fig. 3-38). The patient is then positioned supine with the hip and knee flexed and a downward force is applied through the femur to cause anterior rotation of the ilium on the sacrum. The movement is felt as the PSIS moves on the stabilized sacrum (Fig. 3-39). To test passive posterior rotation of the ilium on the fixed sacrum the same position is used, except the patient's thigh is pushed toward his chest to cause the ilium to move in posterior rotation on the fixed sacrum (Fig. 3-40). Because movement at the sacroiliac varies a great deal within the range of normals, the only way an accurate assessment can be made with this test is to compare one side to the other.

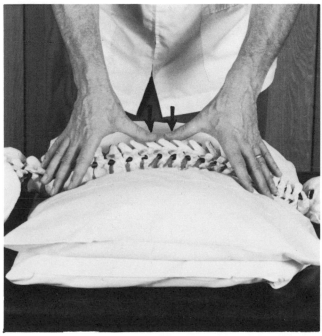
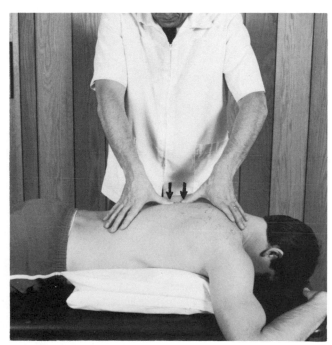

Fig. 3-36. Anterior spring test of lumbar, mid and lower thoracic spine.

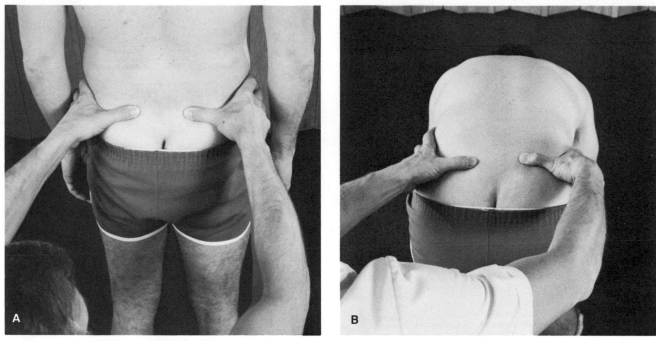

Fig. 3-37. Test to determine active movement of the sacroiliac joints: A) Patient standing — level PSIS's; B) Patient forward bending — PSIS on right is higher. This indicates that the right sacroiliac joint has less mobility than the left.

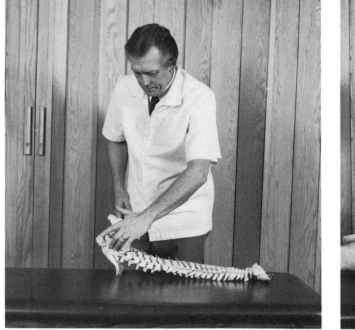
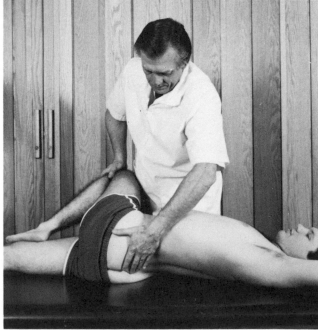

Fig. 3-38. Position of middle finger to feel passive movement at the sacroiliac joint.

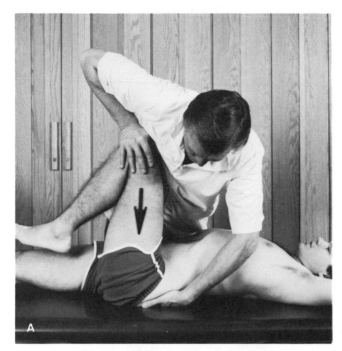
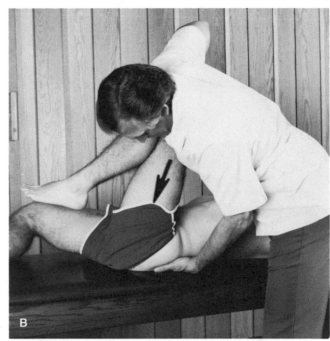

Fig. 3-39. Position to test passive anterior rotation of the ilium on the sacrum: A) Reaching across the patient to test the joint on the opposite side; B) Standing on the same side as the joint being tested. This may be necessary with larger patients.

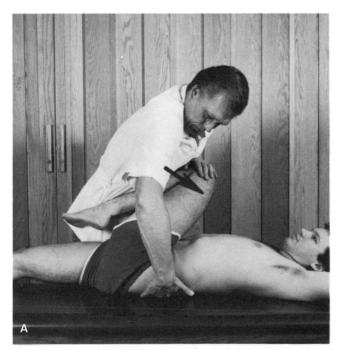
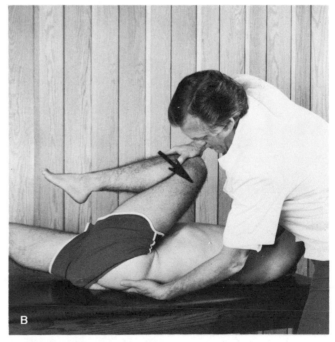

Fig. 3-40. Position to test passive posterior rotation of the ilium on the sacrum: A) Reaching across the patient to test the joint on the opposite side; B) Standing on the same side as the joint being tested. This may be necessary with larger patients.

The sacroiliac spring tests are special mobility tests used to determine if there is pathology in the SI joints. If either of these tests elicits pain, it is an indication that there is pathology in the joint.

The spring test to stress the anterior portion of the SI joint is done with the patient lying supine. The examiner contacts the ASIS's with the heels of both hands. The forearms are crossed, and a postero-lateral spring is given (Fig. 3-41).

The spring test to stress the posterior portion of the SI joint is done with the patient lying on his side with hand contact on the anterolateral rim of the ilium. A downward thrust is given to gap the joint on the top side (Fig. 3-42).

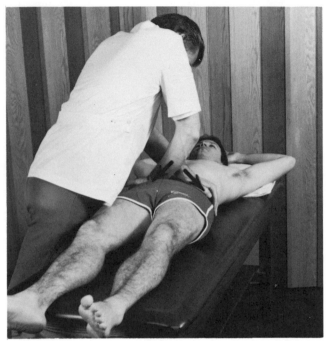

Fig. 3-41. Sacroiliac spring test to stress the anterior portion of the joint.

Sacrococcygeal Joint — Mobility Examination

The sacrococcygeal joint flexes passively while sitting and extends passively when standing. When the sacrococcygeal joint has been injured, it may become hypomobile as it heals. If this occurs, passive flexion may be restricted. This causes the soft tissue around the tip of the coccyx to be irritated when the patient attempts to sit. If, on the other hand, the injury is severe, the sacrococcygeal joint or the coccyx itself may be hypermobile, unstable, subluxed or dislocated. In any case, the patient will have pain in the soft tissue around the coccyx and will be unable to sit comfortably.

To examine passive movement of the sacro-coccygeal joint, a surgical glove is used with the index finger lubricated. The finger is inserted into the rectum as far as possible, in a position so that the volar surface rests against the coccyx. The coccyx is held with the thumb externally and the index finger internally. The coccyx is moved as a unit passively in flexion and extension (Fig. 3-43).

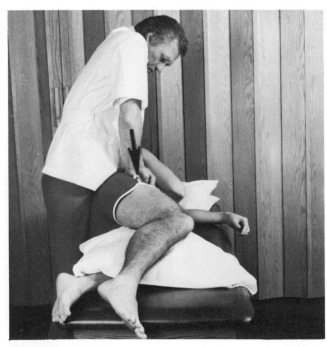

Fig. 3-42. Sacroiliac spring test to stress the posterior portion of the joint.

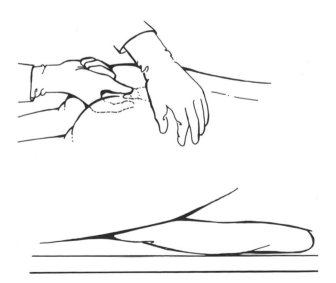

Fig. 3-43. Position to test passive movement of the sacrococcygeal joint.

A complete mobility exam of the lumbar-sacral complex should also include checking for hamstring and hip flexor muscle tightness because of their relation to anterior-posterior pelvic rotation. Tight hamstring muscles can restrict hip joint motion during forward bending, thus causing increased stress on the lumbar spine. Tight hip flexors can contribute to excessive anterior pelvic tilt which can cause an increased lumbar lordosis. The hamstrings are evaluated during the straight leg raise test. The hip flexors are evaluated during the femoral nerve stretch test or by doing a Thomas stretch test.

NEUROLOGICAL EXAMINATION

The neurological portion of a musculoskeletal evaluation consists of a series of tests to determine if there is impingement or encroachment upon a spinal nerve root, entrapment of a peripheral nerve or central nervous system involvement.

Resisted (isometric) muscle tests are done to determine either muscular or neurological involvement. If resisted muscular contraction produces pain, there is pathology within the muscle, tendon or its attachment. When weakness is also present with the painful contraction the therapist cannot be certain if the muscle is weak because of a neurological deficit or because of the pain itself. If pain and/or immobilization has been present for an extended period of time, the muscle can also be weak because of disuse. Specific muscular weakness that is not associated with pain or disuse is considered a positive neurological finding. Resisted muscle tests are done bilaterally at the same time, when possible. This makes it easier to determine slight differences in strength. It also makes it more difficult for the patient to exaggerate a weakness. A true weakness will be smooth and present throughout the range of motion, whereas an exaggerated weakness or weakness caused by pain will often be intermittent through the range of motion.

Muscle stretch reflexes are often helpful in finding neurological deficits. As a general rule, hyperactive reflexes indicate upper motor nerve pathology and hypoactive reflexes indicate impingement, entrapment or injury of a lower motor nerve (spinal nerve root or peripheral nerve.) Normal reflexes vary a great deal from person to person. Occasionally, reflexes appear hypoactive or hyperactive, but are symmetrical. These findings are probably normal for those patients. When a reflex appears hypo or hyperactive when compared to the corresponding reflex on the opposite side, the finding is significant.

The patient is questioned closely during the subjective examination concerning aberration of **sensation.** It should be remembered that patients will confuse paraesthesias with anaesthesias. Paraesthesias are of subjective value and can indicate a certain nerve root level if they follow a given pattern. Anaesthesia of the skin is a positive neurological finding and must be documented. If the patient has indicated there is a sensory deficit, the therapist should determine by pin prick testing the extent and exact location of involvement. An area of numbness that follows a dermatomal pattern or the distribution of a peripheral nerve indicates nerve root impingement or nerve entrapment or injury. If the area of numbness involves the entire circumference of an extremity (glove or stocking effect), a sensory nerve deficit due to a vascular insufficiency or other medical disorder is suspected rather than musculo-skeletal pathology.

Pain that follows a dermatomal, sclerotomal or myotomal pattern does not necessarily indicate nerve root impingement or peripheral nerve entrapment. Pain may be referred from muscles, joints and/or other structures which are innervated by the same spinal nerve level or peripheral nerve. As a general rule, pain is referred distally from the structure that is causing the pain. It is rarely referred proximally. Therefore, it is from the proximal ends of the longer segments that diffuse referred pains usually arise.

Nerve root pain is often felt as a deep burning pain specific to one nerve root segment, whereas referred pain is felt as a diffuse aching pain. Since the sensory nerves supplying pain producing structures of the spine are not specific to one level, referred pain is usually felt in more than one dermatome. Referred pain is usually felt first in the proximal ends of the involved dermatomes and spreads toward the periphery as the pain intensifies.

Referred pain can also facilitate motor activity in the area of referral. This increased muscular activity can inhibit the antagonistic muscle group. For example, pain arising from pathology in any pain producing structure* in the lower lumbar spine

---

*Pain producing structures in the spine are: 1) Paraspinal musculature; 2) Facet joints: 3) Dura mater; 4) Outer layers of the annulus fibrosis and 5) Spinal ligaments[10-12].

can be felt as pain down the posterior aspect of the thigh. This referred pain may cause increased muscular activity in the hamstring muscles which, in turn, may inhibit the quadriceps group. This inhibitory influence on the quadriceps may cause a hypoactive muscle stretch reflex. The implication is that some muscle stretch reflex changes can be caused by referred pain as well as by spinal nerve root impingement or compromise or peripheral nerve entrapment[9].

Cervical Spine — Neurological Examination

As a general rule, neurological involvement of levels C4 through C7 is more indicative of a cervical nerve root disorder such as a herniated disc or encroachment of the nerve root within the intervertebral foramen. Thoracic outlet syndrome is more frequently seen involving levels C8 and T1.

Resisted muscle tests — As noted earlier, if resisted muscle tests are painful or painful and weak, muscular pathology may be involved. If they are painless and weak, however, and disuse atrophy is ruled out, a neurological disorder is indicated. All resisted muscle tests for the cervical spine are done with the patient sitting.

The tests for the cervical spine involve the following muscle groups:

Cervical rotation (C1) is tested with the head and neck held in a neutral, mid-range position. The patient is asked to hold as a rotational force is applied (Fig. 3-44).

To test shoulder elevation (C2, 3, 4), the shoulders are passively elevated and the patient is asked to hold against resistance (Fig. 3-45).

To test shoulder abduction (C5), the shoulders are abducted to 90° and the patient is asked to hold against resistance (Fig. 3-46).

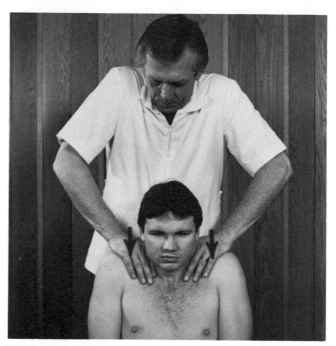

Fig. 3-45. Resisted muscle test — shoulder elevation (C2, 3, 4).

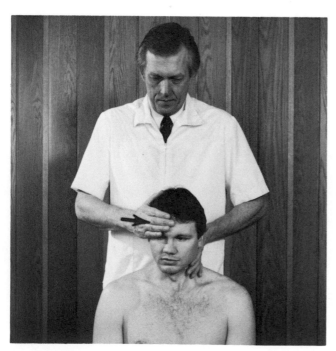

Fig. 3-44. Resisted muscle test — cervical rotation (C1).

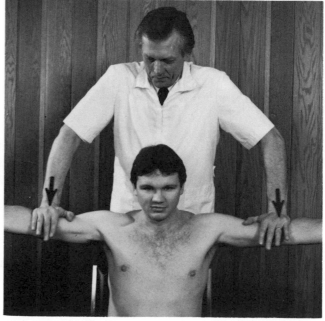

Fig. 3-46. Resisted muscle test — shoulder abduction (C5).

Elbow flexion (C6) is tested with the elbows flexed to 90°. The patient is asked to hold against resistance (Fig. 3-47).

Elbow extension (C7) is tested with the elbows flexed to 45°. The patient is asked to hold against resistance (Fig. 3-48).

Wrist extension (C6) is tested with the wrists held in extension as resistance is applied (Fig. 3-49).

Wrist flexion (C7) is tested with the wrists held in flexion as resistance is applied (Fig. 3-50).

Thumb extension (C8) is tested with the thumbs held in extension as resistance is applied (Fig. 3-51).

Finger abduction (T1) is tested with the fingers held in abduction as resistance is applied (Fig. 3-52).

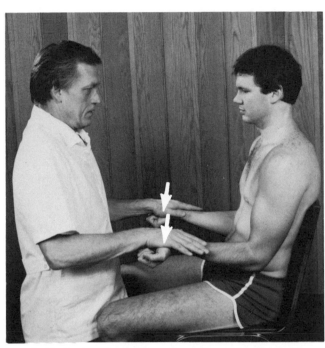

Fig. 3-47. Resisted muscle test — elbow flexion (C6).

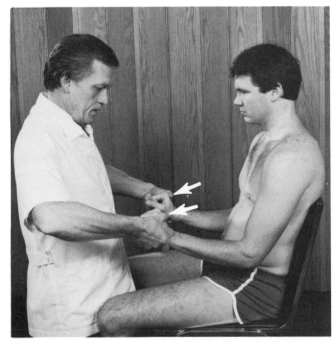

Fig. 3-49. Resisted muscle test — wrist extension (C6).

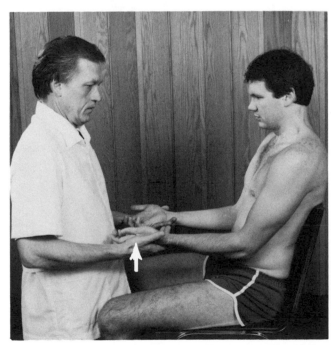

Fig. 3-48. Resisted muscle test — elbow extension (C7).

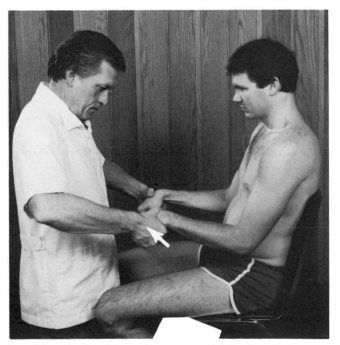

Fig. 3-50. Resisted muscle test — wrist flexion (C7).

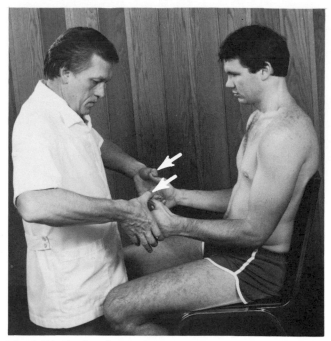

Fig. 3-51. Resisted muscle test — thumb extension (C8).

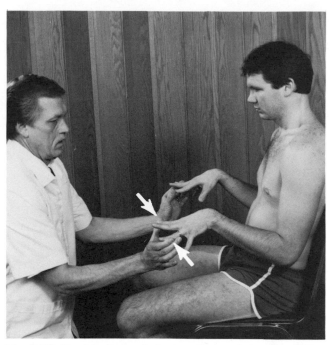

Fig. 3-52. Resisted muscle test — finger abduction (T1).

Muscle stretch reflexes — The biceps (C6) and triceps (C7) muscle stretch reflexes are tested in the sitting position (Fig. 3-53).

Sensation testing — Specific sensation testing is carried out with the patient sitting. The therapist carefully maps out areas of numbness by using the pin prick method (Fig. 3-54). The C5 neurological level supplies sensation to the lateral arm from the shoulder to the elbow. The purest patch (autonomous zone) of C5 innervation lies over the lateral portion of the middle deltoid muscle. C6 supplies sensation to the lateral forearm, the thumb, the index finger and one-half of the middle finger, with the purest patch being on the lateral portion of the

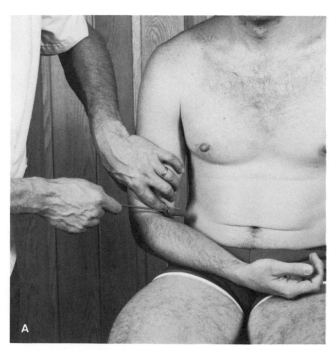

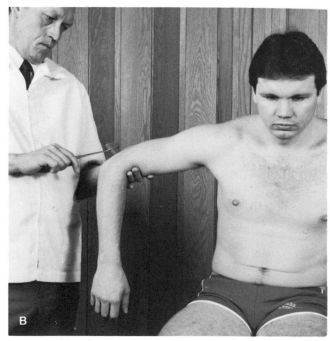

Fig. 3-53. Muscle stretch reflex tests for upper extremity: A) Biceps (C6); B) Triceps (C7).

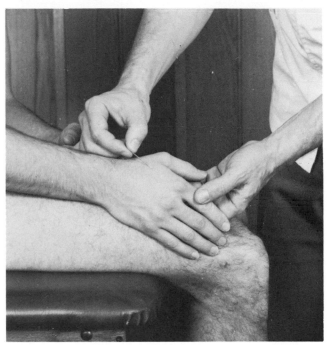

Fig. 3-54. Sensation (pin prick) test, upper extremity.

web space between the thumb and index finger. C7 supplies sensation to the middle finger. Since middle finger sensation is also occasionally supplied by C6 or C8, there is no autonomous zone for C7. C8 supplies sensation to the ring and little finger of the hand and the distal one-half of the ulnar forearm. The ulnar side of the little finger is the purest area for C8 testing. T1 supplies sensation to the upper one-half of the medial forearm and the medial portion of the arm. T2 supplies the axilla[13].

Distraction test — The therapist stands behind the patient if he is seated or at the head of the patient if he is lying supine and applies long axis distraction to the cervical spine through the occiput. This maneuver tends to open the foramina and stretches the joint capsules. If it relieves the patient's symptoms it may indicate that a spinal nerve root is impinged. It should be noted, however, that any facet joint or disc pain may also be relieved with this test and therefore, it is not a completely reliable test for spinal nerve root impingement. The test is most valuable in that it is a good indication as to whether traction will be beneficial as a treatment (Fig. 3-55 A & B).

Compression test — The therapist presses down on top of the patient's head either while he is seated or lying supine. If symptoms increase, it is a good indication of foraminal encroachment or facet joint pressure being the source of pain. (Fig. 3-55C).

Valsalva test — The patient is asked to hold his breath and bear down as if having a bowel movement. If the patient notes an increase in pain or radiation, this may indicate the presence of a space-occupying lesion such as a herniated disc or tumor.

Babinski's test — The neurological exam is completed by doing a Babinski test. The test is done by drawing a blunt instrument across the sole of the foot, starting at the heel, moving along the lateral aspect and crossing the ball of the foot. A positive reaction consists of extension of the great toe, usually associated with fanning (abduction and slight flexion) of the other toes. This indicates an upper motor neuron disorder (Fig. 3-56).

Peripheral nerve entrapment tests — It is often necessary to carry out additional tests to distinguish between spinal nerve root impingement and peripheral nerve entrapment. These will be discussed under the neurological exam of the extremities.

Thoracic Spine — Neurological Examination

Spinal nerve root impingement and peripheral nerve entrapment are rare in the thoracic spine.

Sensation testing involves the dermatome patterns of the thoracic spinal nerves as they pass laterally and slightly inferiorly around the torso of the body.

Neurological involvement in the thoracic spine may cause weakness of the abdominal and/or intercostal muscles, and may also cause dysfunction of certain visceral structures.

Lumbar Spine — Neurological Examination

Resisted muscle tests — Resisted muscle tests for the neurological exam of the lumbar spine involve the following muscle groups:

Hip flexion (L1,2) is done with the patient lying supine with the hip and knee flexed to 90° (Fig. 3-57). The patient is asked to hold the position as resistance is applied. As noted earlier, increased pain with resisted muscle tests indicates muscular pathology. There is often an exception in this case. Increased pain with this test can also mean joint pathology in the lumbar spine and/or hip. The attachment of the iliopsoas muscle on the anterior portion of the lumbar vertebral bodies causes an anterior pull on the lumbar spine as the iliopsoas

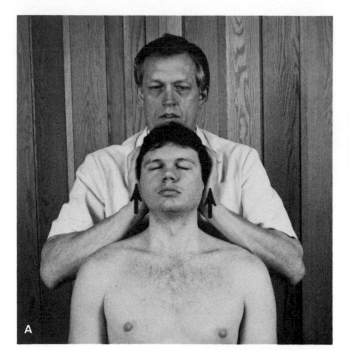

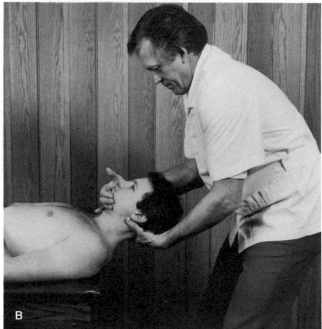

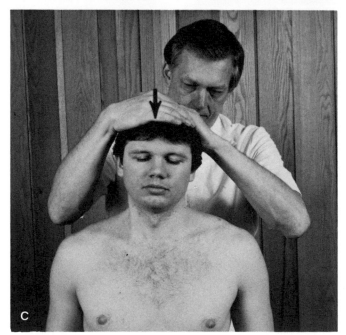

Fig. 3-55. Traction/compression tests for cervical spine.

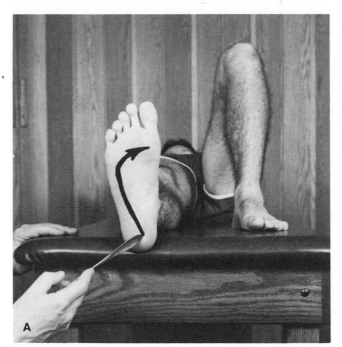
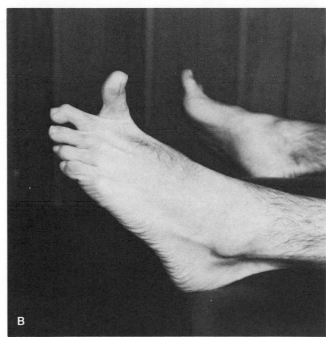

Fig. 3-56. A) Babinski's test. B) Positive reaction.

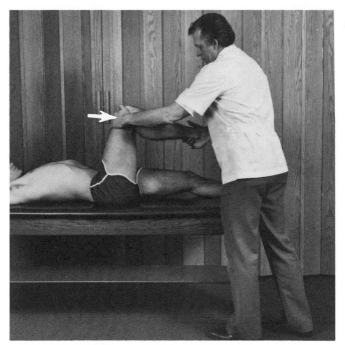

Fig. 3-57. Resisted muscle test — hip flexion (L1, 2).

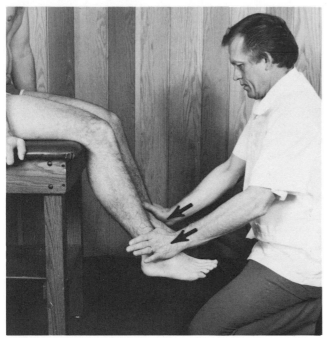

Fig. 3-58. Resisted muscle test — knee extension (L3, 4).

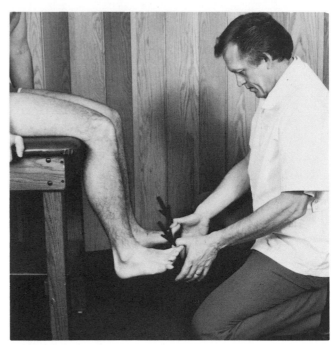

Fig. 3-60. Resisted muscle test — great toe extension (L5).

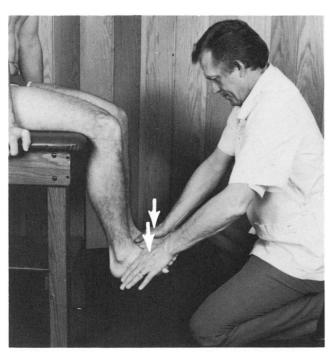

Fig. 3-59. Resisted muscle test — ankle dorsiflexion (L4).

Knee extension (L3,4) is tested with the patient sitting with the knees slightly flexed (Fig. 3-58). This test is done bilaterally at the same time whenever possible.

Ankle dorsiflexion (anterior tibialis muscle, L4) is tested bilaterally with the patient sitting. The patient is asked to hold the position as resistance is applied (Fig. 3-59). Heel walking is an alternate way of testing ankle dorsiflexion.

Great toe extension (L5) is tested bilaterally with the patient sitting. The patient is asked to hold the position as resistance is applied (Fig. 3-60).

Ankle plantar flexion (S1) is tested with the patient standing or walking on his toes. Since the gastrocnemius and soleus muscle group is quite strong, it is often necessary to test plantar flexion by having the patient repeat 10 to 20 repetitions of rising on his toe, first with the uninvolved side then with the involved side, before a true comparison can be made (Fig. 3-61).

Knee flexion (S1,2) is tested bilaterally with the patient lying prone or sitting (Fig. 3-62).

Muscle stretch reflexes — The quadriceps (L3,4) and gastrocnemius-soleus (S1,2) muscle stretch reflexes are tested in the sitting position (Fig. 3-63). The "ankle jerk" is sometimes elicited better with the patient in a prone position with the knees flexed. The examiner may passively dorsiflex the ankles with one hand and quickly alternate a tap on

contracts, often causing increased pain if there is pathology in the spinal segments. Tumors or metastatic lesions should always be suspected if a true neurological deficit is found in the upper lumbar spine since spinal nerve root impingement or peripheral nerve root entrapment or injury at this level is very rare.

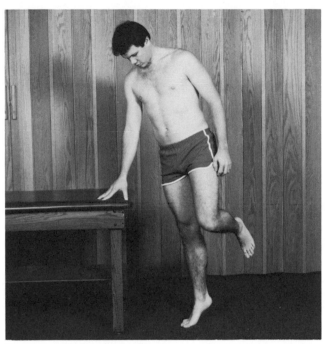

Fig. 3-61. Resisted muscle test — ankle plantar flexion (S1).

each heel cord to pick up subtle changes in muscle stretch reflexes. There is no muscle stretch reflex for the L5 nerve root, and the L4,5 intervertebral disc is sometimes known as the "silent disc".

Sensation testing — If specific sensation testing is indicated, it is carried out with the patient standing, sitting or lying in a position that is

convenient to check the specific areas involved. The pin prick tests are done to map out the areas of numbness. The exact area is measured and described in detail in the evaluation report (Fig. 3-64). Neurological levels L1 through L3 provide sensation in oblique bands over the general area of the anterior thigh between the inguinal ligament to the knee. The L4 dermatome covers the medial side of the leg and foot. Neurological level L5 covers the lateral leg and dorsum of the foot with the crest of the tibia being the dividing line between L4 and L5 (all that is lateral to the crest including the dorsum of the foot is L5.) The S1 dermatome covers the lateral side and a portion of the plantar surface of the foot. The dermatomes around the anus are arranged in three concentric rings (S2 outermost, S3 middle and S4-S5 innermost[13].)

Straight leg raise test — Straight leg raise is a test to determine if there is compromise of the nerve roots or irritation of the sciatic nerve. It is a good idea to test the uninvolved extremity first. The patient is positioned supine for this test. The examiner raises the leg by lifting the leg under the heel and passively extending the knee with the opposite hand. As the straight leg is raised, progressive tension is applied to the sciatic nerve, which in turn places tension on the nerve roots. If compromise or irritation exists, the symptoms will be exacerbated by this maneuver. Straight leg raising also stretches the hamstring muscles. If the test

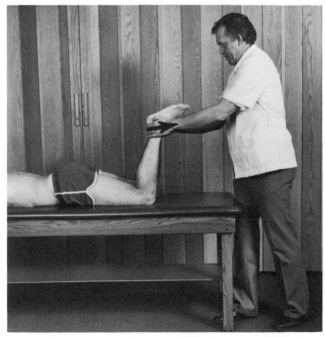

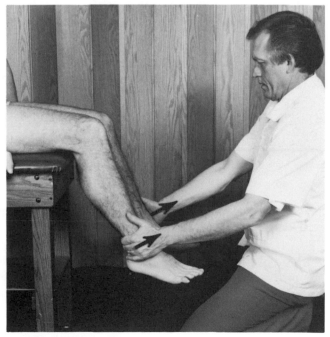

Fig. 3-62. Resisted muscle test — knee flexion (S1, 2).

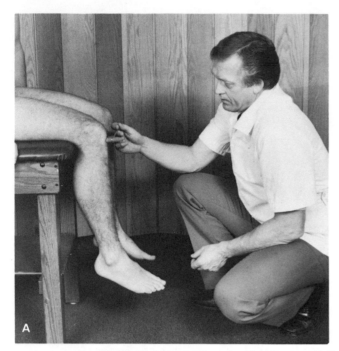 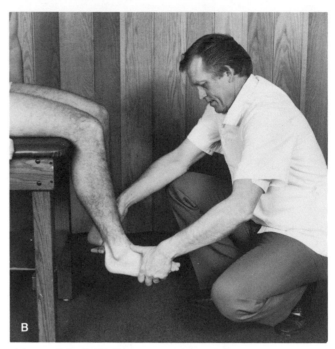

Fig. 3-63. Muscle stretch reflex test — A) Quadriceps (L3, 4); B) Gastrocnemius-soleus (S1,2).

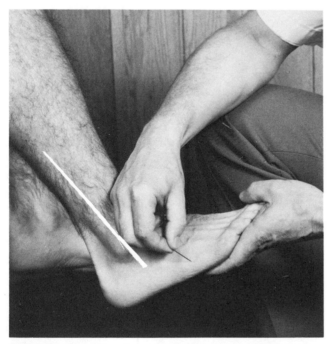

Fig. 3-64. Sensation (pin prick) test, lower extremity.

this point that the hamstrings have engaged the pelvis, causing such movement to occur. By comparing both sides, the examiner can determine the degree of hamstring tightness of that patient. When doing the straight leg raise test, if the only sign is increased pain in the posterior thigh, it is probably hamstring tightness rather than a spinal nerve root impingement. If the pain produced extends into the lower back this may also be a neurological sign. It is also helpful to do hold-relax muscle stretching of the hamstring if there is some doubt. If the hold-relax stretching seems to increase the range of motion, the pain and restriction is probably in the hamstring. If, on the other hand, the hold-relax technique does not seem to change the pain or restriction, spinal nerve root impingement or irritation is probably involved. Another useful variation of the straight leg raise test is to do it with and without having the patient raise his head. When the head is raised, the dura is pulled superiorly, putting an added tension on the spinal nerve root, which increases any positive sign of straight leg raise. Dorsiflexion of the ankle also adds tension to the sciatic nerve and, when added to the straight leg raise test, will often increase the positive sign if true nerve root impingement or irritation is involved.

increases pain in the posterior thigh, one must determine if the pain is caused by tightness of the hamstrings or if it is truly a positive neurological sign.

The examiner should palpate the ASIS for the first sign of movement into posterior rotation. It is at

The bowstring test is another useful variation of the SLR test. The therapist flexes the patient's hip and knee, each to 90°. With one hand, he palpates the sciatic nerve in the popliteal fossa. When the nerve is located, the therapist extends the knee to the point of hamstring tightness and then presses the sciatic nerve with the other hand. If pain is produced proximally, this is a sign of nerve root irritation.

One must be aware that any acute, painful condition in the lumbar spine or sacroiliac may be aggravated by the straight leg raising test. Piriformis syndrome can also be affected by the straight leg raise test. Therefore, considering all of the variables associated with this test, one must by careful when determining if there is nerve root involvement if the only evidence is a positive straight leg raise test.

Normally, the positive straight leg raise test indicates more severe pathology when positive at 20° to 40° of hip flexion and less severe pathology if positive at 50° to 70°. It is difficult to interpret a straight leg raise as being positive at ranges over 70°. The degree of flexion present when the symptoms occur should be recorded so comparison can be made later to determine if there is progress.

Occasionally, symptoms are aggravated as the opposite leg is raised. This may indicate a disc herniation with protrusion medial to the nerve root. If symptoms are relieved as the opposite leg is raised, a bulge lateral to the nerve root may be present.

A sitting straight leg raise test may be done to determine if the patient's reaction to the supine straight leg raise test is genuine. The supine SLR is one test that the malingering patient will be familiar with and he may exaggerate his pain when the test is done. However, he may not be aware that the same action is being done while sitting and will not know to exaggerate his pain. The therapist should do the sitting SLR as he is doing the resisted muscle tests at the knee but should not call attention to it. A combined maneuver of SLR and dural stretch may be done in sitting by having the patient slump and bend the neck forward while the leg is extended. If the sitting SLR is pain free or causes very little reaction and the supine straight leg raise causes considerably more reaction, the patient is probably exaggerating his symptoms. If, on the other hand, the straight leg signs and symptoms are more pronounced in the sitting position than the supine, the sitting test is regarded as being more accurate because the spine is weight bearing in the sitting position and, under certain circumstances, the sitting position may be the only position where certain positive signs and symptoms are evident (Fig. 3-65).

Femoral nerve stretch — If the patient is complaining of pain or other symptoms in the upper lumbar spine and/or in the L1-3 dermatomal region, a femoral nerve stretch test should be done. The femoral nerve stretch is done with the patient lying prone. As the femoral nerve is stretched by flexing the knee and hyperextending the hip, the nerve roots L1, 2 and 3 are stretched across their respective intervertebral foramen. If there is impingement of one of these spinal nerve roots, the symptoms will be increased as this test is done. One must be careful to distinguish between a painful quadriceps muscle and a true nerve root sign. If nerve root impingement is present, the symptoms will extend into the lateral aspect of the hip and into the upper lumbar spine as well as into the anterior thigh (Fig. 3-66).

Distraction test — The distraction test is a neurological test as well as a mobility test. As traction is applied to the spine, certain symptoms may be altered indicating a possible spinal nerve root impingement. For example, if traction relieves the patient's symptoms it may indicate that a spinal nerve root is impinged. Actually, any facet joint or disc pain may also be relieved with this test and therefore, it is not a completely reliable indication of spinal nerve root impingement. The test is valuable in that it gives the therapist an indication when traction might be an effective treatment or when it might aggravate the patient's condition (Fig. 3-67).

Babinski's test — The Babinski test, as described under the neurological exam, cervical spine, completes the neurological exam of the lumbar spine.

PALPATION EXAMINATION

The palpation portion of the evaluative procedure can give valuable information to the examiner about the condition of the structures and tissues in question. During the palpation exam, an inexperienced examiner uses a single palpation procedure to gain information concerning tenderness, muscle tone and position of the bone. A better approach is to study each element of the palpation exam as a separate procedure. The elements considered are the skin, subcutaneous, muscle, ligament and bone.

The **skin** is palpated and examined for tenderness, color, temperature, moisture and texture. Because pain is often referred, the site of the primary disorder may not be the same place that the patient describes the symptoms[1]. Tenderness to palpation is

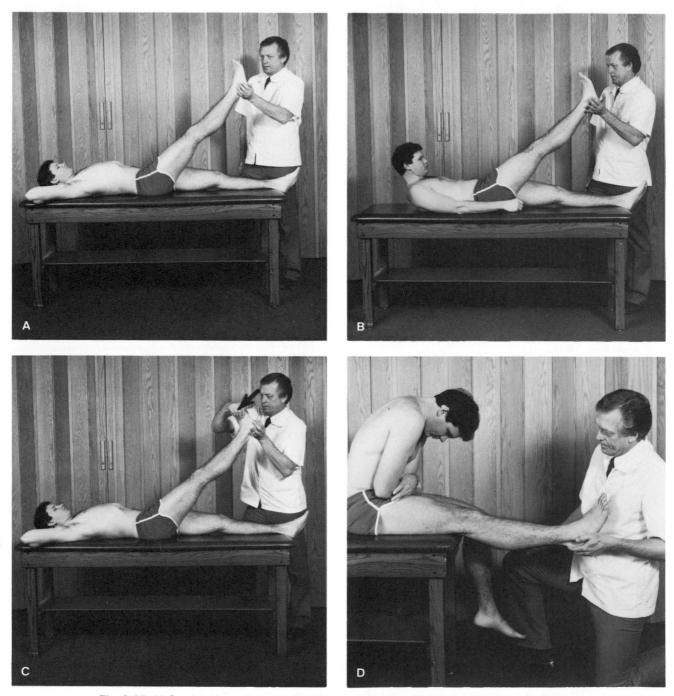

Fig. 3-65. A) Straight leg raise test; B) With neck flexion; C) With ankle dorsiflexion; D) Sitting.

a more reliable indication of the site of the primary pathology, but prolonged muscle guarding and spasm in response to referred pain can fool the inexperienced examiner. Temperature changes are helpful in finding areas of pathology. A warm area may indicate acute inflammation or a cool area may mean chronic pathology such as joint hypomobility. Dry, smooth, shiny skin is indicative of a chronic condition, whereas a slight rise in moisture may mean an acute condition.

The **subcutaneous tissue** is palpated for abnormal amounts of fat, tissue fluid, tension, localized swelling and nodules. Normally the skin can be rolled over the spine freely and painlessly. If there are pathological changes in the subcutaneous tissue, there will be tightness and pain when the skin

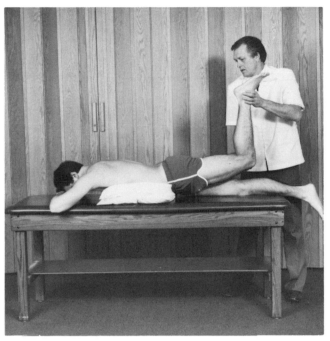

Fig. 3-66. Femoral nerve stretch (note pillow to flex lumbar spine.)

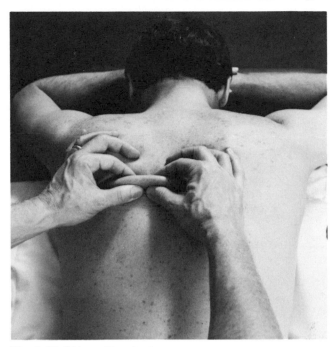

Fig. 3-68. Skin rolling test.

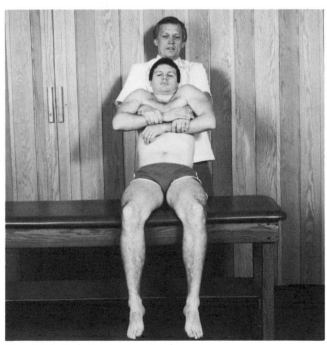

Fig. 3-67. Traction test — lumbar spine.

rolling test is done (Fig. 3-68). Any moles on the skin are examined to determine whether they are superficial or deep.

Muscle tenderness is examined and careful interpretation is given to any positive findings. Muscle guarding and/or spasm is noted.

Next, the condition of the palpable **ligaments** is noted. They may be tender if the joint is sprained or inflamed. They may be thickened and coarse if joint hypomobility is present.

The position of the **bone** is felt to rule out dislocation, subluxation or positional changes such as seen with facet joint impingement. The examiner must not assume that all bony abnormalities are pathological. Some may be congenital and may be unrelated to the patient's present complaint.

Cervical and Upper Thoracic Spine — Palpation Examination

The palpation exam of the cervical and upper thoracic spine involves inspection of the skin and subcutaneous tissue as described above. When palpating the muscles, the examiner must pay close attention to the suboccipital, upper trapezius and rhomboid muscles. Muscle guarding and spasm in these muscles is often associated with various syndromes in the cervical spine. It is often necessary to treat muscle guarding and spasm in these muscles even though they are not the primary disorders. Injury or prolonged muscle guarding of the rhomboid muscles often causes a coarseness or crepitus which can be palpated. Muscle guarding and spasm of the suboccipital muscles are often associated with headaches. Trigger points can often be palpated along the occipital line and in the belly of the upper trapezius muscles.

The supraspinous ligament and spinous processes of the lower cervical and upper thoracic spine can be palpated. In the mid and upper cervical spine, the spinous processes usually cannot be palpated. The facet joint lines of the mid-cervical spine (articular pillar) can be palpated during passive range of motion testing.

Lumbar, Mid and Lower Thoracic Spine — Palpation Examination

Due to the depth of many of the structures of the lumbar, mid and lower thoracic spine, palpation of the skin may not reveal temperature or color changes even though inflammation may be present.

A useful test to assess muscle guarding and/or spasm in the lumbar spine is the weight shift test. With the patient standing, the examiner places his thumbs on the patient's lumbar paraspinals. The patient is then asked to shift his weight from one foot to the other (Fig. 3-69). Normally, the paraspinals on the side of the stance foot will relax, but if muscle guarding and/or spasm is present, the muscle will not be felt to relax.

When palpating the lumbar, mid and lower thoracic spinal joints (ligament and bone), the spinous processes and the supraspinous ligament are all that the examiner can feel. What can be felt through these structures is surprisingly valuable. The supraspinous ligament is normally springy and supple. If it is thick and hardened, the segment may be hypomobile. When palpation between the spinous processes elicits pain, it may be an indication that the spinal segment (facet joints and/or intervertebral disc) is involved.

The position of the spinous processes is felt to determine alignment of the spine. If one spinous process is lateral to the one below it, the segment may be locked in rotation or side bending. When the spinous processes are close together the segment may be locked in backward bending, or if they are far apart the segment may be locked in forward bending or a compression fracture may be present. These changes in position of the bone are called "positional changes" and suggest the presence of facet joint impingement or facet joint hypomobility (Fig. 5-3). Positional changes may also be congenital in nature and when seen by themselves they do not necessarily mean a joint is locked or hypomobile. Mobility testing must confirm that a segment is locked or hypomobile before the final assessment is made.

Positional changes are usually felt with one finger placed between two spinous processes. The "pinch test" may also be useful in finding rotational positional changes. The pinch test is done by

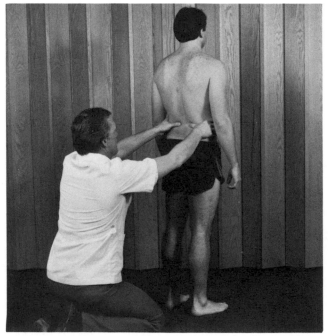
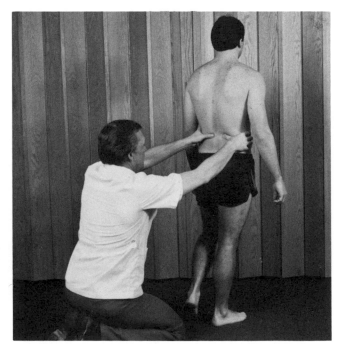

Fig. 3-69. Weight shift test to assess muscle guarding and/or spasm.

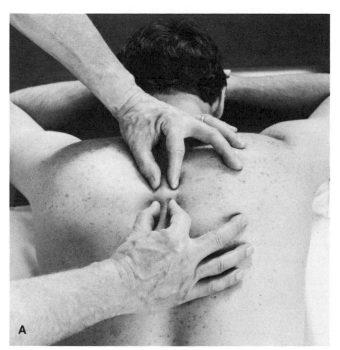 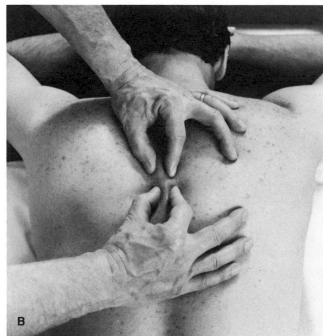

Fig. 3-70. Pinch test to assess positional changes in rotation: A) Normal alignment; B) Positional change in right rotation.

pinching the spinous processes of two adjacent vertebrae between the thumb and index finger of each hand and looking to see if they are properly aligned (Fig. 3-70).

Sacroiliac — Palpation Examination

The position of the sacrum may be palpated to determine if one side of the sacrum has moved in an anterior-posterior or superior-inferior direction. The sacroiliac ligaments may be palpated medial to

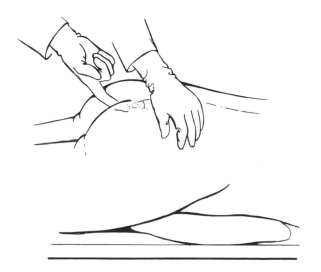

Fig. 3-71. Palpation of coccyx and sacrococcygeal joint.

the posterior-superior iliac spines. Pain with palpation of this area often indicates sacroiliac pathology and is a major clue in determining whether the patient's complaint is primarily of sacroiliac origin rather than related to lumbar spine dysfunction.

Coccyx — Palpation Examination

The position for examination is shown in Fig. 3-71. The coccyx and sacrococcygeal joints are palpated for tenderness both externally and internally. The piriformis muscle can also be palpated internally. The internal contours of the anus should be smooth and the piriformis muscle should feel relaxed. If it is "cordlike" and/or tender to palpate, pathology is indicated. Externally, the coccyx and surrounding soft tissue is palpated. Special attention is directed to the tip of the coccyx to determine if it is tender.

EXTREMITIES

Structural Examination

Inspection involves the observation of bony, joint and muscular structures in the areas involved. In most cases, the examiner has an advantage when examining the extremities because there is a normal side to use for comparison.

The size of the specific muscles should be inspected. A muscle or muscle group that appears smaller may be a clue to peripheral nerve injury or atrophy. The musculature around the scapula, shoulder, hand, thigh and calf is most often subject to atrophy which can readily be seen during inspection. Muscular spasm and guarding can also be seen during visual inspection. A muscle or tendon rupture can be seen as a knot or lump in the soft tissue.

Obvious joint deformities of the lower extremities include genu valgus, genu recurvatum, genu varus, valgus heel, pronated foot, fallen arches and hammer toes. The sole of the foot should be examined for callous formation, a clue to abnormal gait patterns. Other foot problems such as a depressed metatarsal head should be noted.

Each joint should be inspected and any deviations from normal surface anatomy should be noted. Clues to degenerative joint disease can be observed in the sternoclavicular joints and in the elbows, fingers, knees and toes. If the acromioclavicular joint is separated, this can often be seen by visual inspection. A subluxation of the glenohumeral joint can also be seen in many cases. The classical deformities of rheumatoid arthritis such as ulnar drift of the fingers and enlarged proximal interphalangeal joints, should be noted during the structural examination.

The patient's gait should be observed to find muscular weakness such as that found in the gluteus medius when the patient has a Trendelenburg gait. Also, abnormal gait patterns are often clues to stiff or painful joints. The patient lacking full extension of the knee will often walk on his tiptoe. The patient with painful metatarsal heads will walk with the knees extended and the hips flexed. Whether or not the patient should use a cane or crutches is often determined at this time.

MOBILITY EXAMINATION

The mobility exam consists of active, passive, resisted and special mobility tests. It is done to determine which joints and muscles are involved and to what extent they are involved. During the mobility exam, the therapist is looking for either hyper or hypomobility, or is trying to see if movement or joint position causes a change in the patient's symptoms. The examination must include all tissues from which the patient's symptoms might arise. Stresses must be selectively applied to each of these tissues to note which movements provoke or change the patient's symptoms or are otherwise abnormal.

For purposes of examination, the tissues may be divided into two groups: noncontractile (inert) and contractile. The noncontractile group includes capsules, ligaments, bursae, nerves and their sheaths and cartilages. These structures can have tension applied to them by passive stretching (passive movements.) The contractile group includes muscles, tendons and their attachments. These structures may have tension applied to them by passive stretching also, but it is much more effective to test them actively or by utilizing resisted movements.

In the extremities, bilateral musculoskeletal problems are the exception. Therefore, testing the uninvolved extremity for comparative purposes is essential to the mobility examination. Such comparison not only gives the physical therapist an assessment of the patient's normal mobility, but also provides a good method of demonstrating the test or procedure to the patient, putting him at ease prior to examining the involved extremity. This is especially important when examining joint play movements as the patient will most likely be unfamiliar with these tests and may be apprehensive if they are done to the involved joint before adequate demonstration and explanation is given.

Active movements — Active movements combine joint range of motion and muscular contraction. If a patient has pain or other symptoms with active movements, the therapist cannot determine if the joint, the muscle or both are at fault. Active movements test the patient's willingness to move. If a patient is symptom free with both passive and resisted movement testing but has symptoms with active movements there may be a question concerning the patient's willingness to perform the movement. In such cases consideration should be given to psychogenic causes for the patient's complaint.

Resisted (isometric) tests — Resisted movements are strong static contractions done in a comfortable neutral position within the available range of motion. No movement should be allowed at the joint when performing resisted movement tests. If pain is produced with resisted tests, there is probably a disorder within the muscle, tendon or tendinous attachment (contractile group.) A disorder within the contractile group may be a result of injury (muscle strain, contusion or strain of the tendon insertion) or inflammation (myositis or tendinitis.) Prolonged muscle guarding and spasm may cause circulatory stasis and retention of metabolites which will in turn cause the muscle to be tender to palpation and the resisted tests to be painful. This must be considered when determining whether muscular dysfunction is the primary problem.

If a resisted muscle contraction is strong and painless, there is nothing wrong with the muscle, tendon or the tendinous attachment. If the contraction is strong and painful, there is a minor disorder in the contractile group. If the contraction is weak and painless, there is a neurological deficit or the muscle is weak from disuse. If the contraction is weak and painful, there is a dysfunction in the contractile group but it is sometimes difficult to determine by this test alone if the weakness is a result of the pain or if a neurological deficit is present[1].

Passive movements — Passive range of motion is done to test the noncontractile (inert) structures around a joint. Passive movements are done with the patient as relaxed as possible, presumably in the supine position. The passive movement is carried through full functional range, gently if necessary, to determine if there is a limitation of range and, if so, whether it is painful. The examiner should attempt to assess the joint's end feel. If a noncontractile tissue is stressed during passive movement, pain will be produced and hyper or hypomobility may be present.

Although passive movement tests are primarily done to find joint (noncontractile tissue) involvement, they also passively stretch the muscles (contractile tissue) that surround the joint. If pain is found with passive movements, it must not be assumed that in all cases the pain is arising from the joint. The location of the pain will often help the therapist determine which structure is involved. Comparison of the active and passive ranges of motion and those findings of the resisted muscle tests should determine which structures are implicated. The value of assessing active vs. passive vs. resisted movement testing can be summarized by the following examples:

1. If active and passive movements are painful in the same direction, the pain appears toward the limit of range of motion and resisted movements are not painful, noncontractile tissue is at fault.

2. If passive movement is painful in one direction and active movement is painful in the opposite direction, contractile tissue is at fault.

3. If resisted movement is painful or weak, contractile tissue is at fault[1].

Although these distinctions can be made, there are certain exceptions. For example, certain bursal problems are diagnosed on the basis of painful active movements and a mixed reaction to passive movements.

Restriction of joint movement, both actively and passively, may be in a capsular or a noncapsular pattern. If the restriction is in a **capsular** pattern, it indicates that the restriction is in the joint capsule (joint hypomobility, joint contracture, joint inflammation or adhesive capsulitis.) If such is the case, there will be a predictable, proportionate limitation in certain motions. The reason certain directions will be more restricted is largely due to the normal rest position that the joint assumes during the immobilization that usually precedes the restriction and/or the mechanism of injury to which that particular joint is vulnerable. Fig. 3-72 lists capsular patterns which are commonly seen in the extremity joints[1].

Limitation of motion in a **noncapsular** pattern follows no predictable pattern. The restriction is usually found in one or two directions while all other directions will be unrestricted. Restrictions in a noncapsular pattern may be caused by muscle tightness, bursitis, tendinitis, tendon injuries or mechanical defects within the joint, such as loose bodies, calcific changes and cartilage tears.

SHOULDER = External Rotation — Abduction —Internal Rotation — Flexion
ELBOW = Flexion — Extension (Pronation and Supination — full range)
DISTAL RADIOULNAR = Pronation — Supination
RADIO ULNA-CARPAL = Flexion — Extension
MID-CARPAL = Extension — Flexion
THUMB CARPALMETACARPAL = Abduction — Extension
METACARPOPHALANGEAL = Flexion — Extension
INTERPHALANGEAL = Flexion — Extension
HIP = Internal Rotation — Abduction — Flexion — Extension — Adduction — External Rotation
KNEE = Flexion (great) — Extension (slight)
ANKLE = Dorsiflexion — Plantar flexion
METATARSOPHALANGEAL = Flexion — Extension
INTERPHALANGEAL = Flexion — Extension

Fig. 3-72. Capsular patterns, listed in order of greatest restriction[1].

During passive movement testing it is important to check **end feel** to determine if the movement being tested has an end feel that is normal for that joint movement. Fig. 3-73 lists the types of joint motion end feels and gives an example of each. For example, if a bone-on-bone end feel is found for a particular joint movement after an interarticular fracture has healed, the therapist should not expect to greatly improve that range of movement. However, if a capsular end feel is found, the therapist could reasonably expect to gain range of movement with stretching and mobilization.

Another important consideration during passive movement testing is if a **sequence of pain** develops during passive range of motion. This observation determines when in the range of motion the patient experiences pain in relation to restriction of joint motion. Pain that is experienced before any restriction can be felt indicates an active lesion such as an acute sprain, strain or inflammation. If the pain and restriction are felt to occur at approximately the same time, the inference is that the lesion is in a subacute stage. If the restriction is felt and there is little or no pain until the joint is moved into the restriction, a joint contracture or long-standing joint hypomobility is indicated. A painful arc (no pain-pain-no pain sequence) indicates that a tender structure is being pinched or irritated as it is moved through the range of motion. A subdeltoid bursitis or supraspinatus tendinitis may cause a painful arc. Determination of the pain sequence during passive

range of motion is also helpful during treatment planning. For example, an acute lesion should be treated with caution, anti-inflammatories, ice and rest. Mild mobilization exercises and heat may be started for the subacute patient, and the patient with a long-standing joint contracture may be ready for more vigorous mobilization, exercise and ultrasound treatments (Fig. 3-74).

Special mobility tests — Joint play tests — Normal range of joint movement is that movement which is available to a normal joint as a result of normal muscle action. These voluntary movements cannot be achieved unless certain well-defined movements of joint play exist, independent of the action of voluntary muscles. Painless, full, voluntary range of motion is dependent upon the presence of these very small, precise joint play movements[14].

In order to properly assess joint play movements, it is essential that the patient and examiner be relaxed. At no time should the examiner's grip be painful to the patient. One joint and one joint play movement is examined at a time for each joint. There should be one stabilizing force and one mobilizing force exerted when the joint is being examined. No forceful or abnormal movement should ever be used and the examining movement should be stopped at any point at which pain is elicited. In the presence of obvious clinical signs of joint inflammation or disease, no examining movements need be or should be undertaken[14].

The joint play examining techniques should be

CAPSULAR (Like stretching a piece of leather. Slow with a building up of resistance. Example: external rotation of shoulder.)

LIGAMENTOUS (Like capsular, but a little harder. Example: knee extension.)

SOFT TISSUE APPROXIMATION (Painless squeeze. Example: flexing elbow.)

BONE ON BONE (Hard sudden stop. Example: elbow extension.)

MUSCLE TIGHTENING OR SPASM (Can feel muscle reaction similar to other soft tissue, but hold-relax will alter it. Example: straight leg raises.)

SPRINGY (Example: block of meniscus.)

EMPTY (Pain reaction, patient won't let you determine an end feel.)

Fig. 3-73. Common end feels found with passive range of motion[1].

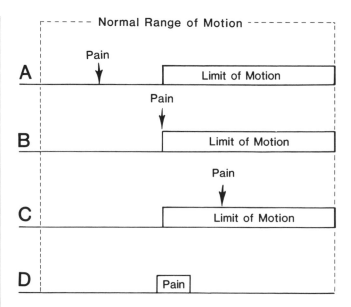

Fig. 3-74. Sequence of pain during range of motion. A) Acute lesion; B) Subacute lesion; C) Joint hypomobility (contracture); D) Painful arc.

done with the joint in a neutral, mid-range position. The mobilizing force should be concentrated as close to the joint line as possible to avoid long lever arms which might cause excessive force. Joint play mobility may be graded 0-6 as described earlier. The therapist should remember to compare movements bilaterally.

Muscle strength testing — Specific muscle strength testing may be done if weakness is suspected. It is important that muscle strength testing be measured as objectively as possible using accepted manual muscle testing procedures. More elaborate procedures such as isokinetic muscle testing are also available to aid in diagnosis and to establish a more accurate data base.

Ligament stress tests — In many cases, joint play tests also examine the integrity of the ligaments as well as the joint capsule; however, in a few cases, the joint play tests will not accurately test certain ligaments. The most obvious example is in the knee. The joint play tests of medial and lateral tilting (varus or valgus) are done in 15° of flexion, whereas the tests for medial and lateral collateral ligament stability are done in a similar fashion, but with the knee in full extension. The examiner should see some slight medial and lateral tilting when testing for joint play with the knee flexed to 15° but should appreciate no movement when testing in full extension. Therefore, if the examiner is particularly interested in testing a certain ligament, the joint should be carried to the position within the range of motion that brings that ligament taut, then the therapist should perform the testing movement. These positions are usually in full extension, flexion or rotation of the joint and the test is usually a tilt, shear or traction movement. Specific joint play and ligament stress tests are shown in Chapter 8.

NEUROLOGICAL EXAMINATION (Fig. 3-75)

Although many neurological tests are performed on the extremities, they are usually done to determine if there is impingement upon the nerve roots which innervate them. Resisted muscle tests, muscle stretch reflexes and sensory testing, as described earlier, will provide much information concerning peripheral nerve injuries and entrapments. However, there are special tests to determine specific peripheral nerve entrapment syndromes. Some of the more common are:

Thoracic outlet syndromes — The three common thoracic outlet syndromes are shown in Fig. 6-3. They are described as follows:

1) Scalenus-anticus and cervical rib syndromes. The subclavian artery and brachial plexus pass over the first rib through a normally occurring space between the anterior and middle scalene muscles. Occasionally, due to an accessory cervical rib or its fibrous extension, or a congenital or acquired abnormality of the scalene muscles, the neurovascular bundle becomes entrapped, causing neurological and/or circulatory changes in the upper extremity. Adson's maneuver is a test to determine if one of these disorders is present. The patient is instructed to take and hold a deep breath, extend his neck fully and turn his chin toward the side being examined. At the same time, the examiner is taking the patient's radial pulse. In theory, this maneuver should traction the neurovascular bundle over the accessory rib, or cause the scaleni to "scissor" against the bundle. If the pulse disappears and the pain and other symptoms are reproduced, the test is positive. A diminished pulse alone is not a true positive finding. In some subjects, a greater effect upon the neurovascular bundle is exerted by turning the head to the opposite side. Therefore, both positions should be tested (Fig. 3-76).

2) Costoclavicular syndrome — The subclavian artery and lateral cord of the brachial plexus can also be entrapped as they pass between the clavicle and the first rib. The test to determine this syndrome requires the patient to take and hold a deep breath as he retracts and depresses his shoulders. Again, the examiner determines if the radial pulse disappears and if there is reproduction of pain and other symptoms in the arm (Fig. 3-77). The patient with this condition will tend to experience his symptoms when carrying objects such as suitcases or briefcases. Backpackers or women carrying heavy shoulder bags also experience symptoms.

3) Hyperabduction syndrome — The subclavian vessels and brachial plexus can also be entrapped beneath the tendon of the pectoralis minor muscle and under the coracoid process. The arm is held in a hyperabducted, externally rotated position while the examiner palpates for disappearance of the radial pulse and a reproduction of pain and other symptoms in the arm. The patient suffering from this syndrome will often complain that the symptoms come on while he is sleeping on his back or stomach with his arm overhead (Fig. 3-78).

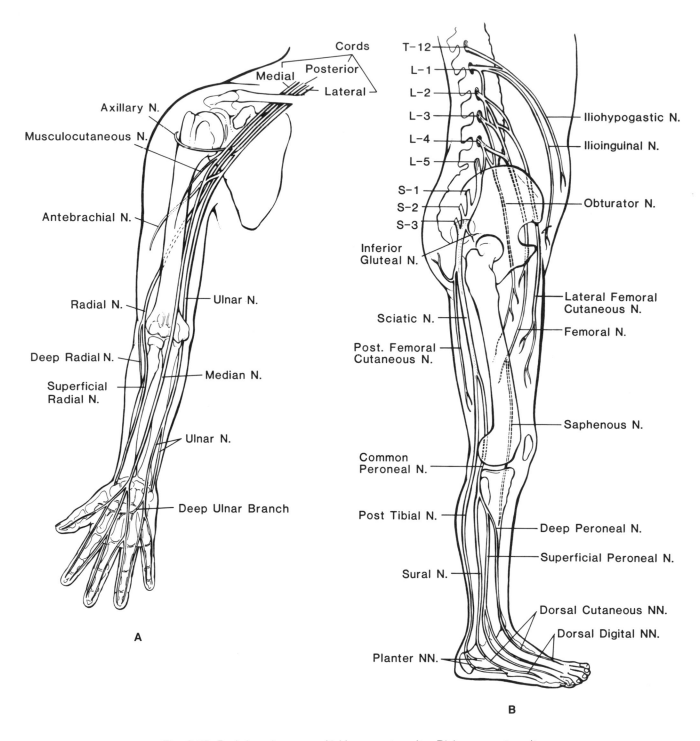

Fig. 3-75. Peripheral nerves: A) Upper extremity; B) Lower extremity.

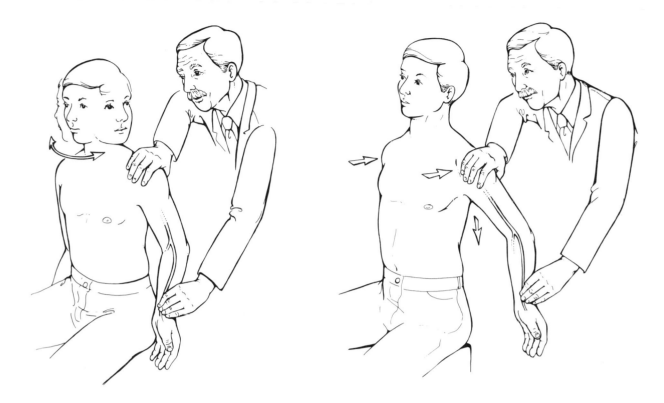

Fig. 3-76. Adson's test.

Fig. 3-77. Wright's test.

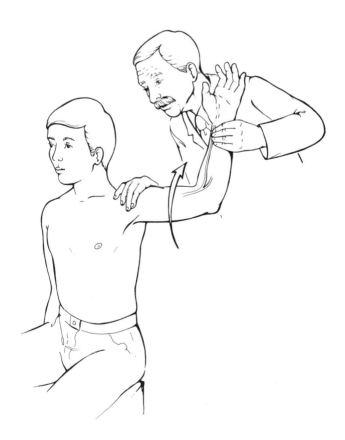

Fig. 3-78. Hyperabduction test.

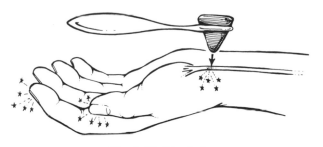

Fig. 3-79. Tinel sign.

Carpal tunnel syndrome — Diagnosis of this syndrome is almost always established by noting the presence of one or more of the three major clinical signs: 1) Hyposthesia restricted to median nerve distribution in the hand; 2) Tinel sign — a tingling sensation radiating into the hand on percussing the median nerve at the wrist (Fig. 3-79) or 3) Phelan's test — reproduction or exaggeration of symptoms after holding the wrist in complete flexion or extension for 30 to 60 seconds (Fig. 3-80). One must keep in mind that the source of compromise can occur anywhere along the nerve pathway. Just because a patient complains of symptoms in the median nerve distribution, the problem is not necessarily carpal tunnel syndrome. The therapist must remember to correlate signs and symptoms and must not jump to conclusions with this and with other peripheral nerve syndromes.

Ulnar groove entrapment — The most common site of entrapment of the ulnar nerve is at the ulnar groove of the elbow. Symptoms will initially be of paraesthesia in the ulnar distribution and discomfort in the epicondylar area.

Piriformis syndrome — The sciatic nerve and buttock musculature often become tender, secondary to referred pain from a lower back disorder. During palpation, a particularly tender spot is often found at the point inferior to the piriformis muscle where the sciatic nerve emerges from beneath the muscle. It is this author's belief that this tenderness often leads to a diagnosis of piriformis syndrome when it should be interpreted as simply referred pain and inflammation secondary to a lower back disorder.

A true piriformis syndrome is characterized by reproduction of symptoms with resisted external rotation of the hip and reproduction of symptoms

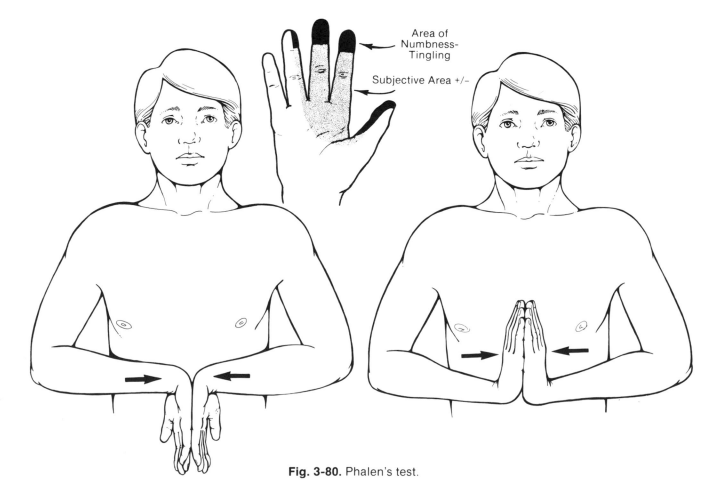

Area of
Numbness-
Tingling

Subjective Area +/-

Fig. 3-80. Phalen's test.

upon straight leg raising but relief upon passively externally rotating the leg while it is still in the straight leg raised position. Also, other lower back and/or hip joint signs and symptoms are absent.

Common peroneal syndrome — Signs and symptoms (pain, paraethesia and weakness) may be present in the structures supplied by the common peroneal nerve because of scar tissue resulting from a fracture of the fibular head, surgery for Baker's cyst, sprain of the superior tibio-fibular joint or from direct nerve injury. One often sees restriction of joint play movements at the superior tibio-fibular joint and loss of complete knee extension with this syndrome.

It is not within the scope of this text to explore all of the peripheral nerve entrapment syndromes or neurological diseases. Sometimes, electrodiagnostic studies and sophisticated neurological testing are required when symptoms suggest a neurological basis that cannot be explained by a musculoskeletal examination.

PALPATION EXAMINATION

During the palpation examination, an inexperienced examiner frequently uses a single palpation procedure to gain information concerning tenderness, muscle tone and position of the bone. A better approach is to study each element of the palpation examination as a separate procedure. The elements considered should be the skin, subcutaneous tissue, peripheral circulation, muscles, ligaments and bone.

The **skin** is palpated and examined for tenderness, color, temperature, moisture and texture. Because pain is often referred, the site of the primary disorder may not be the same place that the patient describes the symptoms. Tenderness to palpation is a more reliable indication of the site of a primary disorder, but prolonged muscle guarding and spasm in response to referred pain can fool the inexperienced examiner. Temperature changes are helpful in finding areas of dysfunction. For instance, a warm area may indicate acute inflammation or a cool area may mean a chronic disorder such as joint hypomobility. A dry, smooth, shiny skin is indicative of a chronic condition, whereas a slight rise in moisture may mean an acute condition.

The **subcutaneous** tissue is palpated for abnormal amounts of fat, tissue fluid, tension, localized swelling and nodules. Normally the skin can be rolled over the underlying structures freely and painlessly. If there are pathological changes in the subcutaneous tissue there will be tightness and pain when the skin rolling test is done. Any moles on the skin are examined to determine if they are superficial or deep in nature.

The dorsalis pedis and posterior tibial pulses are felt in the foot to assess **peripheral circulation** (Fig. 3-81).

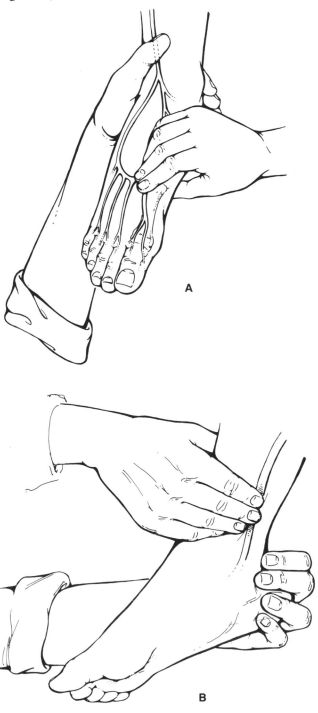

Fig. 3-81. A) Dorsalis pedis pulse; B) Posterior tibialis pulse.

Muscle tenderness is examined and careful interpretation is given to any positive findings. Muscle guarding and/or spasm is noted. Specific muscles and tendons are identified and palpated for tenderness, edema, tension and other muscular pathologies such as myositis ossificans, rupture or fibrositis. If there is pathology within the muscle structures, the muscles will be tender to palpation. The examiner must remember, however, that muscle tenderness if often a secondary condition due to prolonged muscle guarding, spasm or referral from other areas.

Next, the condition of the palpable **ligaments** is noted. They may be tender if the joint is injured, inflamed or thickened, and coarse if joint hypomobility is present. Bursae and other joint structures are also palpated. If there is pathology within the joint, the ligaments and joint capsule will be tender to palpation.

The position of the **bones** is felt to rule out dislocation, subluxation or joint locking. The examiner must not assume that all bony abnormalities are pathological, as some may be congenital and unrelated to the patient's present complaint.

Palpation is an especially valuable evaluation tool when examining the extremities. Many of the joint structures, muscles and tendons are more superficial and easier to identify in the extremities than in the spine.

Shoulder (Fig. 3-82)

Shoulder pathology rarely involves the glenohumeral joint alone. For this reason, examination of the shoulder must involve the entire shoulder girdle. This includes the sternoclavicular, acromioclavicular and scapulothoracic structures as well as the glenohumeral joint and its surrounding tissues and muscles.

Acute subacromial and subdeltoid bursitis' are often accompanied by skin redness and warmth and swelling on the lateral aspect of the shoulder just inferior to the acromion. Acute glenohumeral joint sprain and/or inflammation may show skin redness and warmth along the joint line.

The musculature of the shoulder girdle should be palpated systematically, starting with the upper trapezius and moving counter-clockwise around the scapula to feel the rhomboids, middle and lower trapezius, latissimus dorsi, teres major and minor, infraspinatus and supraspinatus. Special attention should be directed toward the insertions of the posterior rotator cuff muscles (teres minor and infraspinatus) which actually lie beneath the acromion, but can be palpated for tenderness just posterior and inferior to the acromion when the glenohumeral joint is externally rotated. The supraspinatus muscle insertion can be palpated just anterior and inferior to the acromion when the glenohumeral joint is fully extended and internally rotated. Special attention should also be paid to the upper trapezius and rhomboid muscles, as they are often involved with painful conditions of the neck and shoulder. A thickened, coarse, grating sensation is often felt when the rhomboid muscles are palpated. The posterior, middle and anterior deltoids are palpated with the examiner paying particular attention to the common insertion of the muscles as it is often tender. The tendon of the long head of the biceps is felt within the bicipital groove. The serratus anterior muscle can be palpated against the rib cage inferior to the axilla. The triceps, biceps, pectoralis major and sternocleidomastoid muscles are also palpated.

The subacromial and subdeltoid bursae can be palpated just anterior and lateral to the acromion when the glenohumeral joint is held in hyperextension. The subdeltoid bursa can also be palpated lateral to the acromion with the arm held in its normal resting position at the side of the body.

Next, the sternoclavicular and acromioclavicular joints are palpated for tenderness. The glenohumeral joint is palpated around the joint line for tenderness. Occasionally, effusion can be felt along the joint line. The position of the bones is also noted. Subluxation of the sternoclavicular joint is easily palpated, as is a separation of the acromioclavicular joint. The glenohumeral joint is examined for passive subluxation with the arm hanging in a dependent position. The examiner can appreciate a space between the tip of the acromion and the greater tuberosity of the humerus. Passive subluxation of the glenohumeral joint indicates dysfunction of the rotator cuff musculature. Dislocation of the glenohumeral joint is also easily palpated and can be distinguished from passive subluxation by the fact that it does not reduce when the arm is supported.

Elbow (Fig. 3-83)

Skin redness and warmth at the elbow is usually associated with acute sprain and/or inflammation of the radioulnar joint, acute capsulitis of the

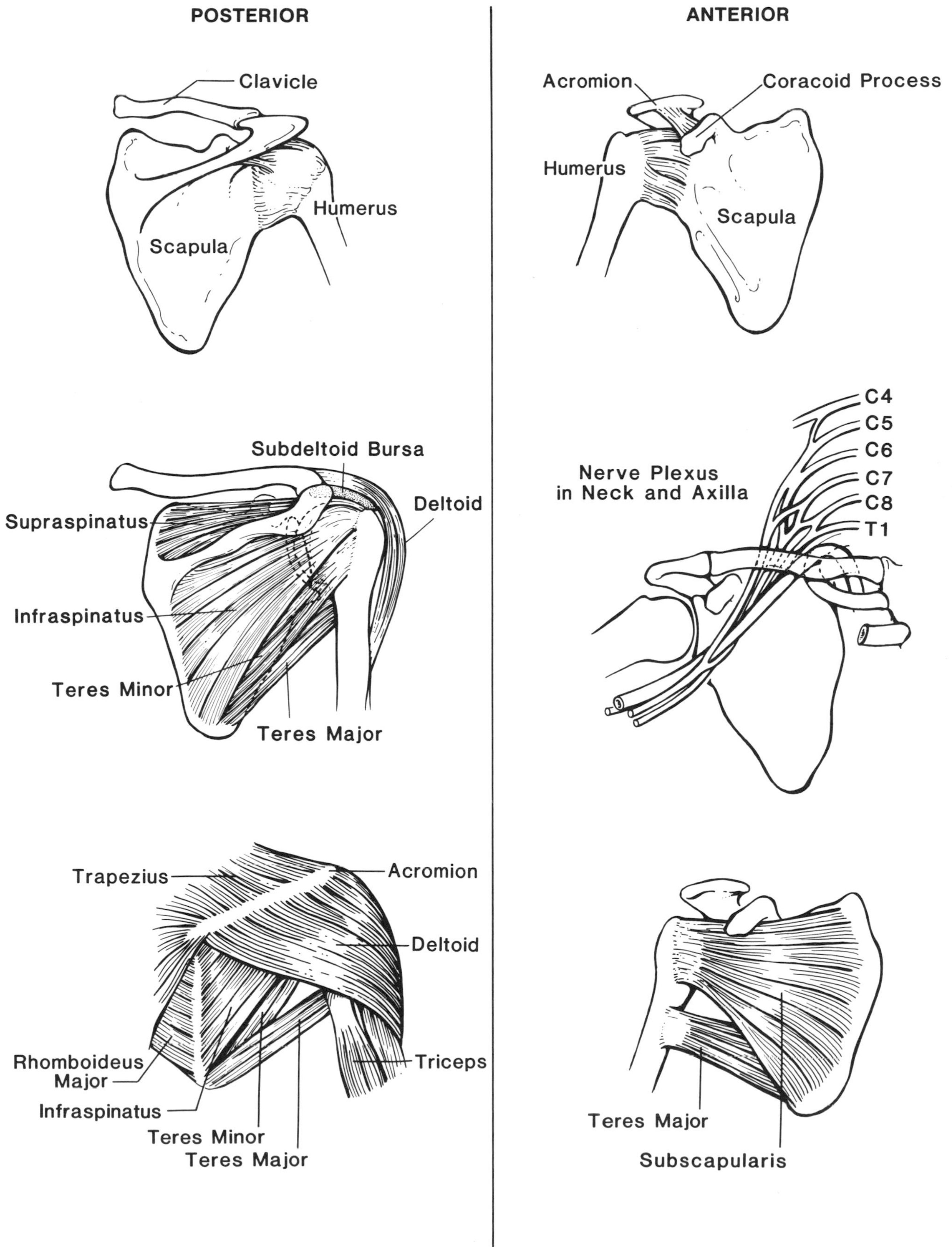

Fig. 3-82. Shoulder.

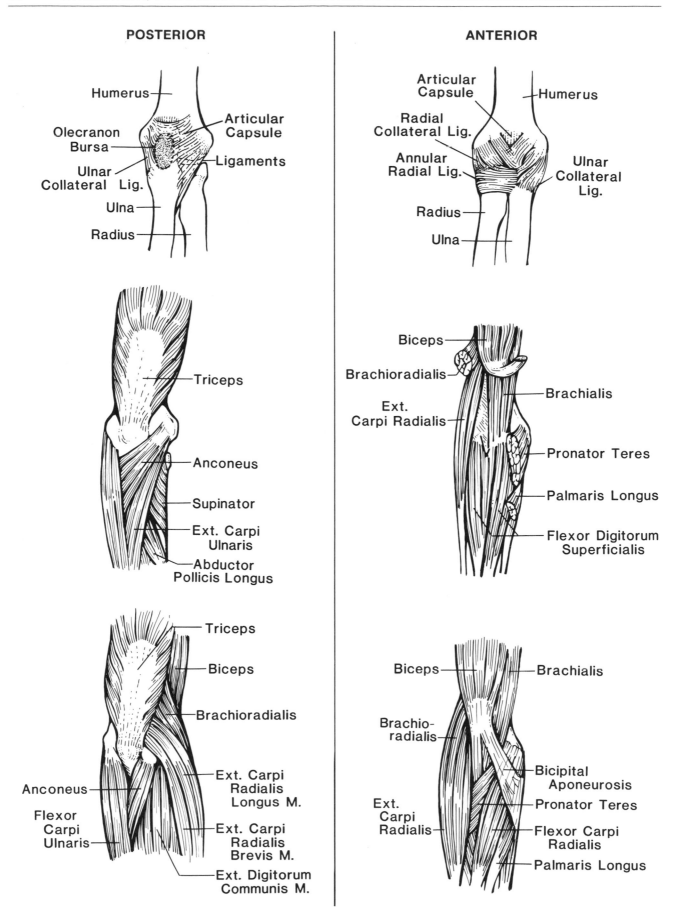

Fig. 3-83. Elbow.

humeroulnar joint or acute medial or lateral epicondylitis.

Swelling may be of a local or a diffuse nature. Localized swelling may involve the olecranon bursa or the joint capsule. In both cases, the swelling is confined to the limits of the structure involved, whereas diffuse swelling is widespread and involves the entire elbow region. The muscles of the arm and forearm are palpated on the dorsum of the forearm and near their origin on the epicondyles. Strain and inflammation of these muscle groups is known as "tennis elbow".

Other especially important points to palpate at the elbow are: 1) The ulnar nerve as it passes posterior to the medial epicondyle; 2) The median nerve as it passes beneath the pronator teres muscle on the volar surface of the forearm; 3) The head of the radius and 4) The medial epicondyle.

The ulnohumeral joint capsule lies beneath the biceps tendon anteriorly and the triceps tendon posteriorly. It is not palpable unless there is effusion of the joint.

Wrist and Hand (Fig. 3-84)

The palpation examination of the hand must include the muscles of the forearm and the flexor and extensor tendons of the wrist, fingers and thumb. Particular attention is directed to the palm of the hand to determine if there is a Dupuytren's contracture. Each joint in the wrist, thumb and fingers should be palpated individually to detect tenderness or swelling.

Hip (Fig. 3-85)

Although patients often feel pain in the hips it is seldom the sight of the true pathology. Frequently hip pain is referred from the lumbar spine or sacroiliac joint(s). The hip, primarily innervated by L2,3, will usually refer pain to the anterior thigh or knee. Localized pain in the groin area can arise from the capsule, iliopectinial bursa and origin of the short head of the rectus femoris. If the patient says "hip" but points to lateral or posterolateral areas, the problem is probably lumbosacral in origin.

Skin temperature and color changes or swelling are seldom associated with hip joint pathology because of the depth of the soft tissue around the joint.

The sciatic nerve is palpated as it passes through the buttocks midway between the greater trochanter and the ischial tuberosity through the sciatic notch. When the hip is extended, the sciatic nerve is covered by the gluteus maximus muscle, but when it is flexed, the gluteus maximus tends to move out of the way. Therefore, the patient should be positioned lying on his side with the hip flexed for this examination. Tenderness of the sciatic nerve may be due to nerve root impingement or direct trauma and/or inflammation of the nerve itself.

Tenderness elicited during palpation of the ischial tuberosity may result from ischial bursitis, but this is rare. The trochanteric area is palpated with the patient lying on his side. Tenderness may indicate bursitis. The bursa itself is not palpable unless it is distended or inflamed.

The hip and pelvic muscles are palpated in a systematic order according to their positions and functions. The four groupings are the flexors, abductors, extensors and adductors.

The piriformis muscle, an external rotator of the hip, arises from the anterior sacrum and ilium and passes laterally out of the sciatic notch to insert upon the greater trochanter of the femur. The belly of the muscle usually passes over the sciatic nerve and may entrap the nerve if the muscle is in spasm. In a small population of patients, the sciatic nerve may actually pass through the substance of the muscle. The piriformis can be palpated internally by way of rectal examination. It can also be palpated through the gluteus maximus muscle at a point just lateral to the sciatic notch. The examiner cannot be certain from which of three structures (piriformis, sciatic nerve or gluteus maximus) pain is arising if tenderness is found in this area. Correlation with resisted muscle tests will be helpful in determining piriformis muscle involvement.

Knee (Fig. 3-86)

During the palpation exam of the knee, the patient is sitting or lying supine in such a manner that the examiner can easily see and palpate all sides of the joint. Swelling at the knee may be of a local or a diffuse nature. Localized swelling may involve the superficial or deep infrapatellar bursa, the pre-patellar bursa or the joint capsule. If this is the case, the swelling will be confined to the limits of the structure involved, whereas diffuse swelling is widespread and may involve the entire knee structure. If the joint capsule is palpable along the medial or lateral joint line, it is a sign of swelling within the joint capsule because the normal joint capsule is not

PALMAR

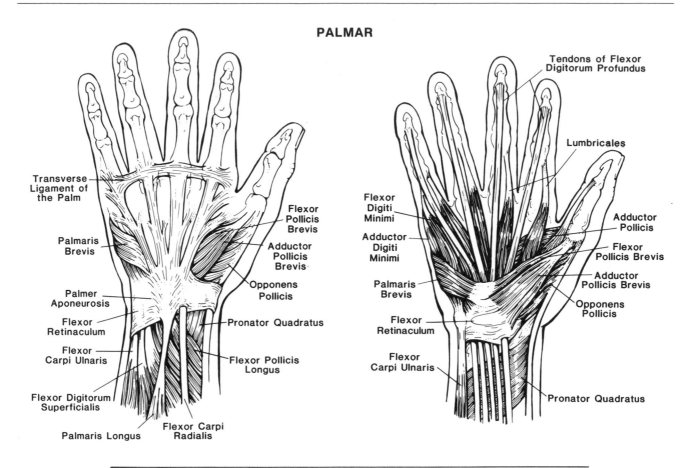

DORSAL

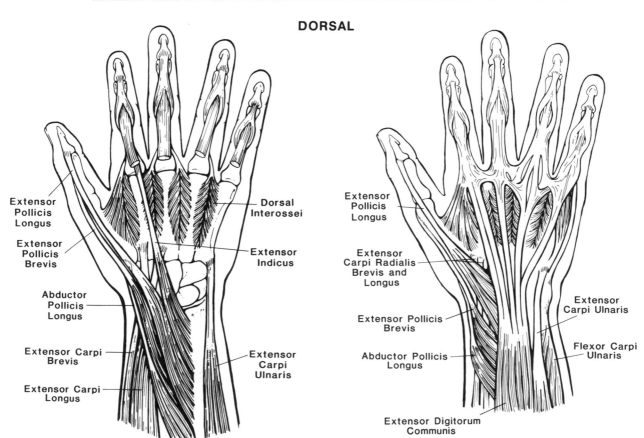

Fig. 3-84. Wrist and Hand.

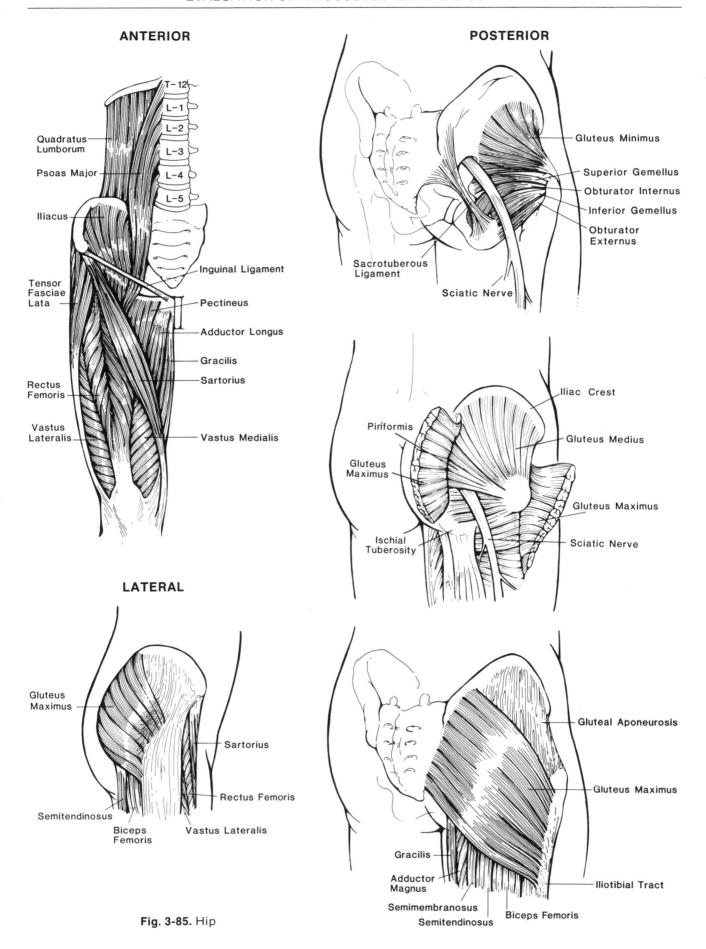

ANTERIOR

Quadratus Lumborum
Psoas Major
Iliacus
Tensor Fasciae Lata
Rectus Femoris
Vastus Lateralis

T-12
L-1
L-2
L-3
L-4
L-5

Inguinal Ligament
Pectineus
Adductor Longus
Gracilis
Sartorius
Vastus Medialis

POSTERIOR

Gluteus Minimus
Superior Gemellus
Obturator Internus
Inferior Gemellus
Obturator Externus
Sacrotuberous Ligament
Sciatic Nerve

Piriformis
Gluteus Maximus
Ischial Tuberosity
Iliac Crest
Gluteus Medius
Gluteus Maximus
Sciatic Nerve

LATERAL

Gluteus Maximus
Semitendinosus
Biceps Femoris
Sartorius
Rectus Femoris
Vastus Lateralis

Gluteal Aponeurosis
Gluteus Maximus
Gracilis
Adductor Magnus
Semimembranosus
Semitendinosus
Biceps Femoris
Iliotibial Tract

Fig. 3-85. Hip

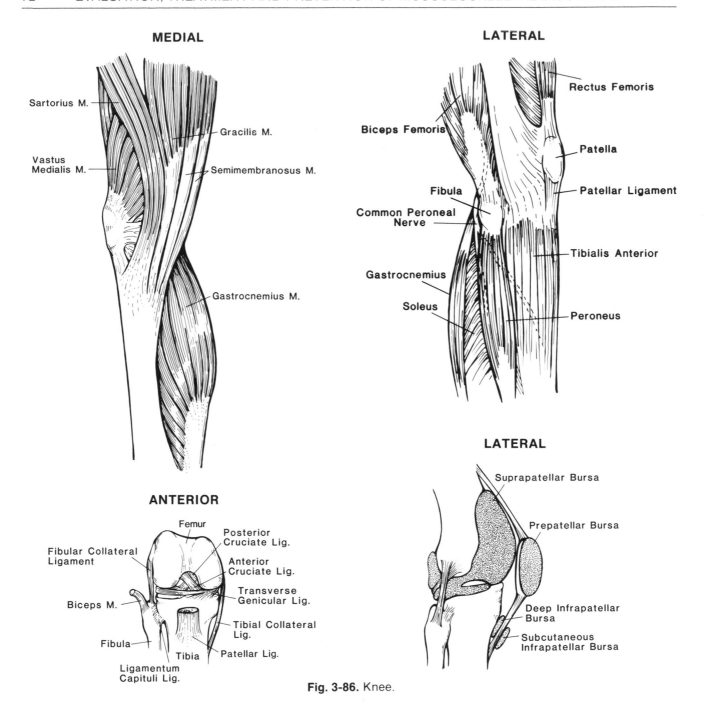

Fig. 3-86. Knee.

palpable. The posterior compartment of the joint is carefully palpated for tenderness and swelling to detect a Baker's cyst.

The muscles which cross the knee joint are palpated in a systematic order. Special attention is paid to the insertion of the patellar and hamstring tendons. Tenderness and swelling at the site of the patellar tendon insertion is a possible indicator of Osgood-Schlatter's syndrome.

The collateral ligaments are carefully palpated along the medial and lateral aspects of the knee. Tenderness the length of the collateral ligament as opposed to pin point tenderness at the joint line is important to differentiate because the former indicates collateral ligament pathology whereas the latter indicates meniscus injury.

The common peroneal nerve is palpated as it passes lateral and inferior to the fibular head.

Ankle and Foot (Fig. 3-87)

All of the muscles of the foot and ankle are palpated. Particular attention is paid to the Achille's tendon and the tendons of the anterior tibialis, peroneus longus and brevis and posterior tibialis.

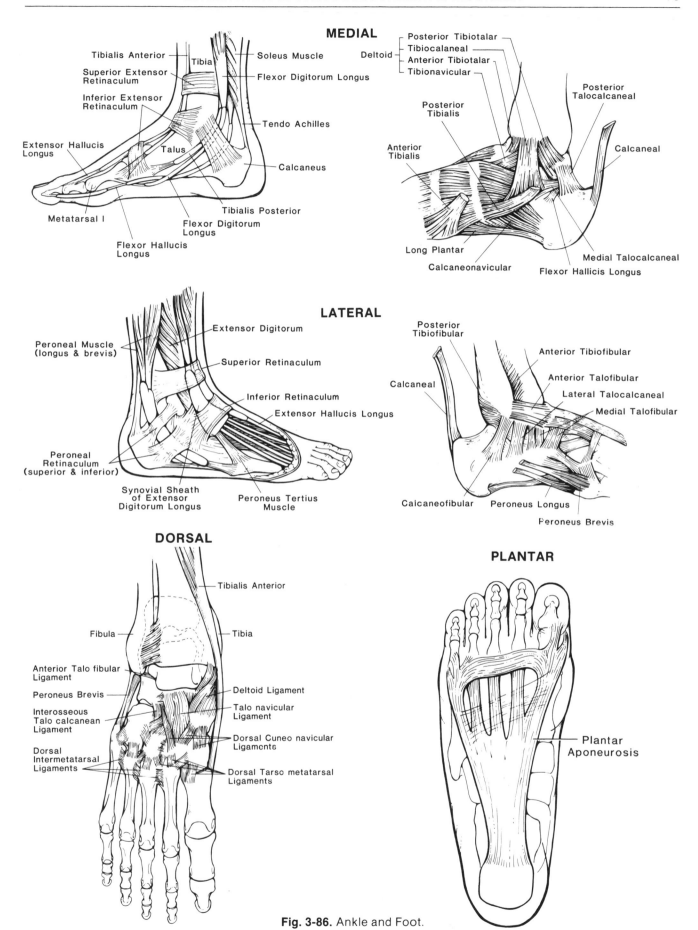

Fig. 3-86. Ankle and Foot.

An inversion sprain is characterized by swelling inferior and anterior to the lateral melleolus and tenderness of one or more of the three ligaments on the lateral aspect of the ankle. A less common injury, an eversion sprain, is characterized by swelling inferior to the medial malleolus and tenderness of the medial ligaments of the ankle. Tenderness on or above the medial or lateral melleoli indicates a bone bruise or fracture. Generalized swelling of the entire foot is an indication of severe trauma or a circulatory deficiency.

Pain associated with pronation of the foot can be felt inferior to the lateral malleolus due to a mechanical pinching of the soft tissue, or can be felt inferior to the medial malleolus due to a stretching of the ligamentous structures and/or direct pressure on the head of the talus in association with shoe wearing.

Pain elicited upon palpation of the medial tubercle of the calcaneus and/or the plantar aponeurosis may indicate the presence of a heel spur. A heel spur is usually secondary to plantar fasciitis, which is often associated with a fallen longitudinal arch.

Pain elicited upon palpation directly upon the plantar surface of the calcaneus indicates a bruised heel or a subcalcaneal bursitis usually associated with direct trauma to the heel. The heads of the metatarsals are palpated for tenderness, a callus or a depression. Pain proximal to the metatarsal heads, usually between the third and fourth metatarsals, may indicate Morton's neuroma or a possible stress fracture.

Because of the high incidence of circulatory problems in the feet, the palpation exam is not complete until the arterial pulses are checked. The posterior tibial artery, the main blood supply to the foot, is felt just posterior and superior to the medial malleolus. The dorsal pedal artery is palpable between the extensor hallucis longus and the extensor digitorum longus tendons. This artery provides a secondary blood supply to the foot.

CORRELATION WITH OTHER REPORTS AND TESTS

Upon completion of the evaluation, the therapist correlates his findings with other information that is available such as medical diagnosis, physician's reports, x-rays, lab and other tests. In order that the evaluation be done without bias, this correlation should be done at the conclusion of the evaluation rather than at the beginning.

It should be noted that physical therapists as a group, perhaps because of their inate desire to help and make their patients feel better, somtimes fall victim to manipulative patients who have secondary gain, conversion syndromes or other psychophysiologic reasons for their complaints. While no one can deny the fact that psychological and emotional factors can significantly influence a patient's perception of pain and actually increase muscular tension, one needs to be attuned to the possibility of these factors for the patient's total management picture.

The following mneumonic "M-A-D-I-S-O-N" is provided as a guide for Psychophysiologic Conversion syndrome:

M — Multiplicity of symptoms. When one goes, another one comes. The patient presents a past history of bizarre or non-organic symptoms in multiplicity.

A — Authenticity. The patient seems more concerned with convincing the therapist that his symptoms are real than with the symptoms themselves.

D — Denial. The patient refuses to even consider the possibility that these symptoms may be psychogenic.

I — Interpersonal variation. Symptoms get better when the patient is enjoying himself and worse when a professional is around.

S — No one else has ever had anything exactly like this patient has.

O — Only you can help! Patients are setting the therapist up for a fall. "All those other doc's before you were dumb, but you'll figure out what it is."

N — Never varies. Symptoms are always terrible and are theatrically described with superlatives.

References:

1. Cyriax, J: Textbook of Orthopaedic Medicine; Diagnosis of Soft Tissue Lesions. Vol 1, 8th ed, Bailliere-Tindall, London 1982.
2. Spangford, E: Personal Communication, Orthopaedic Surgeon, Huddinge, Sweden 1982.
3. Kendall, F, McCreary, E: Muscles: Testing and Function, Williams & Wilkins, Baltimore, 1983.
4. Waitz, E: The Lateral Bending Sign. Spine 6:388-397, 1981.
5. McKenzie, R: The Lumbar Spine. Spinal Publications, Waikanae, New Zealand 1981.
6. Finneson, B: Low Back Pain. Lippincott, Philadelphia, 1973.

References: (Continued)

7. Maitland, G: Vertebral Manipulation. 2nd ed, Butterworth, London 1968.
8. Mennell, J: Back Pain. Little-Brown, Boston 1964.
9. Mooney, V and Robertson, J: The Facet Syndrome. Clinical Orthopaedics and Related Research 115:149-156, March-April 1976.
10. Hirsch, C; Ingelmark, B and Miller, M: The Anatomical Basis for Low Back Pain. Acta Ortho Scanda 33:1-17, 1963.
11. Jackson, H; Winkelmann, R and Bickel, W: Nerve Endings in the Lumbar Spinal Column. J Bone Joint Surg 48A:1272-1281, 1966.
12. Roofe, P: Innervation of the Annulus Fibrosis and Posterior Longitudinal Ligament: Fourth and Fifth Lumbar Level. Arch Neurol Psych 44:100-103, 1940.
13. Hoppenfeld, S: Orthopaedic Neurology. Lippencott, Philadelphia 1977.
14. Mennell, J: Joint Pain. Little-Brown, Boston 1964.

CHAPTER 4

BASIC SPINAL BIOMECHANICS

The purpose of this chapter is not to provide the reader with an academic or detailed picture of the biomechanics or applied anatomy of the spine. Some areas are controversial and some speculations and findings vary greatly among the various researchers. The complexity of the spine and its relative inaccessibility compared to the extremities has made its study very difficult until quite recently. Therefore, in keeping with the philosophy of this text as a basic reference, this chapter will present what is considered to be the essential material on this topic which has direct clinical application.

TENSEGRITY

Kapandji makes a good comparison of the vertebral column to the mast of a ship in the

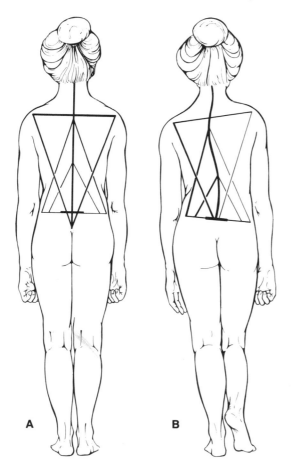

Fig. 4-1. Tensegrity: A) rigidity and B) plasticity (adapted from Kapandji[1].)

mechanical requirements of rigidity and plasticity in that the spine must be able to rigidly support the trunk on the pelvis, yet provide flexibility and movement[1]. This dual role of the spine has sometimes been referred to as "tensegrity." The spine accomplishes these contradictory requirements through a system of muscular and ligamentous tighteners at all levels which link the shoulder girdle to the pelvis (much like the main yard and the guy ropes on a sailing ship.) When these forces are in balance, the spine is straight and the pelvis and shoulders are level (rigidity) (Fig. 4-1A). However, when the pelvis is not level, as when the body rests on one limb, the vertebral column is forced to bend (plasticity) (Fig. 4-1A). Since the spine is made of multiple components superimposed on one another, it will first bend in the lumbar region (convex toward the resting limb), then in an attempt to compensate, the spine bends concavely in the thoracic region and again convexly in the cervical area. The muscular/ligamentous tighteners will actively adapt to these changes automatically in order to maintain rigidity, shortening on one side and lengthening on the other. This automatic postural accomodation is under the influence of the extrapyramidal system and is geared to maintaining the eyes in the horizontal plane.

PHYSIOLOGICAL CURVES

Viewed from the front or back, the spine is straight. However, viewed from the side, the spine has four curves: 1) sacral — the fused sacrum is convex posteriorly; 2) lumbar — concave posteriorly; 3) thoracic — convex posteriorly and 4) cervical — concave posteriorly (Fig. 4-2). These curves reciprocate and balance one another in such a way that in the normal spine if a plumb line were dropped from the atlanto/occipital joint at the top of the column, it would intersect the center of motion at the lumbosacral junction at the bottom. If dropped further, the plumb line would intersect the hip joint. These curves not only provide balance, they provide added strength for the vertebral column to withstand axial compressive loads. Engineers have calculated that the presence of the three curves in the spine (excluding the sacrum)

ANATOMY

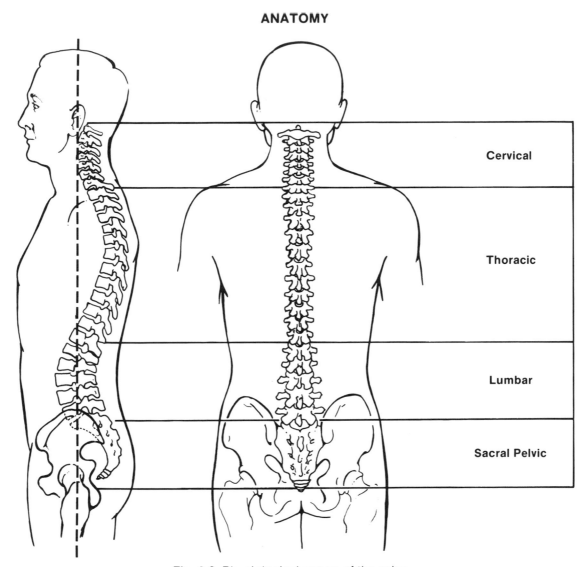

Cervical

Thoracic

Lumbar

Sacral Pelvic

Fig. 4-2. Physiological curves of the spine.

increases the resistance of the spine to compression ten times compared to one with no curves at all. These curves can also be shown to influence the function of the spine as a whole. Spines with exaggerated curves tend to be more dynamic and spines with reduced or flattened curves tend to be more static[1] (Fig. 4-3).

FUNCTIONAL COMPONENTS OF THE VERTEBRAL COLUMN

Each spinal segment (i.e. two adjacent vertebrae with the intervertebral disc between) may be divided into an active portion and a passive portion. The vertebral bodies are the passive portion while the disc, the intervertebral foramen, articular

processes, ligaments and muscles are the active portion[1] (Fig. 4-4). Each segment, through the vertebral arches, forms a first class lever system where the articular processes are the fulcrum. Axial compressive loads are applied through the vertebral column with direct and passive absorption of some of the force at the disc and indirect and active absorption by the ligaments and muscles (Fig. 4-4).

INTERVERTEBRAL DISC

The intervertebral disc consists of two portions: an inner gelatinous center called the nucleus pulposus, and an outer structure made up of layers of concentric fibers called the annulus fibrosis (Fig. 4-5). The nucleus, which tends to be spherical in shape, is basically water with a muccopolysac-

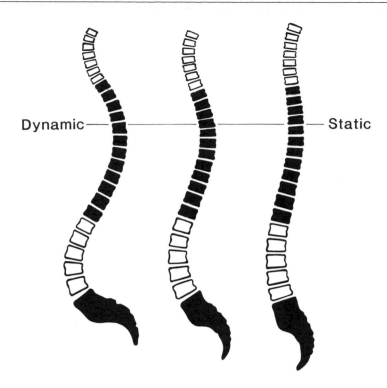

Fig. 4-3. Dynamic and static spines. An increase in the normal curves tends to make the spine more flexible or dynamic. A spine with flattened curves tends to be less flexible or static.

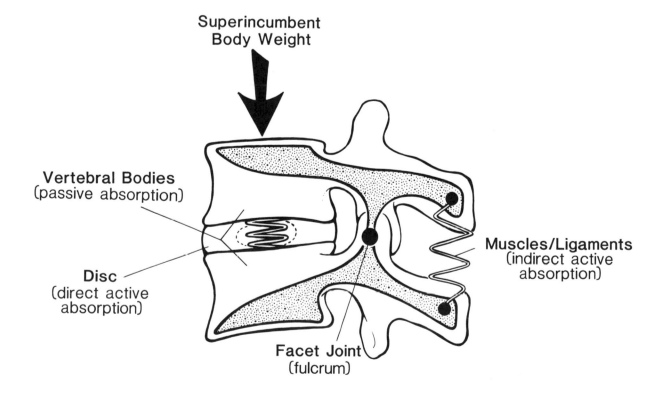

Fig. 4-4. The spinal segment as a first class lever system, showing active and passive portions (adapted from Kapandji[1].)

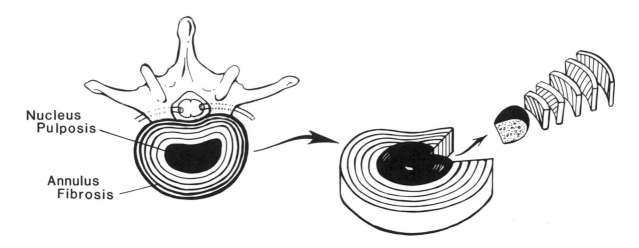

Fig. 4-5. Intervertebral disc.

charide matrix and is hydrophilic; that is, it has the ability to imbibe water. During the day, the compressional forces of the upright position cause water to be lost from the nucleus. This is why one tends to be shorter at the end of the day than when first arising in the morning. It is during the recumbent, non-weight bearing position overnight when the nucleus imbibes water, thus increasing its height. The aging process diminishes the ability of the nucleus to imbibe fluid. There is a transitional area between the nucleus and the innermost of the annular rings where the gel of the nucleus is interspaced between these first few rings [1,2].

The fibers of the annulus are oriented diagonally and alternate their direction between layers in a criss-cross (X) fashion. The inner fibers are more obliquely oriented and the outer fibers are more vertical (Fig. 4-5). This arrangement is very much like a bias-ply tire where the criss-cross pattern allows for strength and flexibility. The inner fibers of the annulus are quite weak in comparison to the outer. The annular rings are firmly attached superiorly and inferiorly to adjacent vertebral bodies and the vertebral endplates and serve to maintain the nucleus under constant pressure and in a central position. In the adult, the disc is considered to be both avascular and aneural except for some sensory innervation in the outermost layers of the annulus[2].

The disc is flexible, allowing motion in all directions, and serves to dissipate forces and stresses transmitted to it, especially vertical or compressive loads. The disc may thus be likened to a shock absorber. Forward bending (flexion) of the spine causes compressive forces to be placed upon the anterior portion of the vertebral body and the disc, thus exerting a posterior force on the nucleus pulposus. This action is analogous to the squeezing of a water-filled balloon on one end, observing that the fluid moves away from the compressive force. Backward bending of the spine (extension) produces the opposite effect on the disc [2,3]. Side bending produces a force which is opposite to the direction of the side bend (Fig. 4-6). In the healthy disc, the annular rings tend to resist displacement of the nuclear gel, thus maintaining the nucleus in its proper shape and location. In the unhealthy disc where the annular fibers have torn, usually in a radial manner, the nuclear gel is permitted to migrate, thus setting the stage for the clinical manifestations of the herniated disc.

Rotation, a compressive force, causes an increase in intradiscal pressure and tends to narrow the joint space. When rotation occurs, the annular fibers which are oriented in the direction of the rotatory movement become taut while the fibers which are oriented in the opposite direction tend to slacken. This situation puts the disc in a vulnerable position for injury, particularly if it is also under a load (Fig. 4-7). Intradiscal pressure is greatly affected by body position and activities. Nachemsom has published important data concerning intradiscal pressures in various body positions and under various loads[4] (Fig. 4-8). Knowledge of these pressures is of importance to the physical therapist when designing activity and exercise programs for patients with disc problems. Note that sitting and forward bending (flexion) of the spine tend to cause greater intradiscal pressures than the upright standing posture.

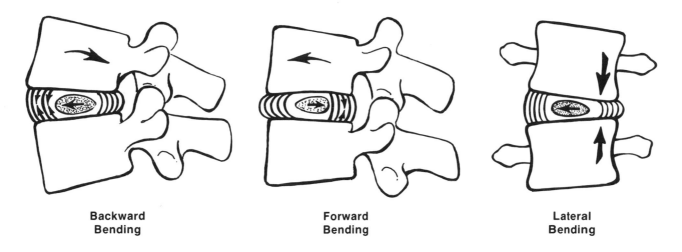

Backward Bending

Forward Bending

Lateral Bending

Fig. 4-6. Effects of forward, backward and side bending on the nucleus pulposus (adapted from Kapandji[1].)

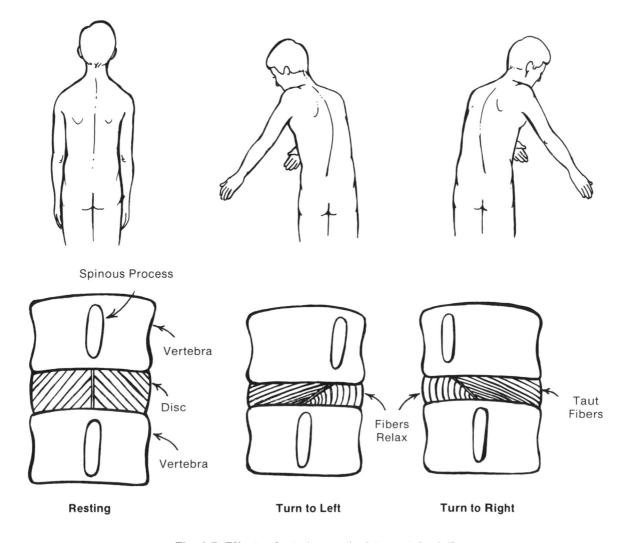

Spinous Process

Vertebra

Disc

Vertebra

Resting

Fibers Relax

Turn to Left

Taut Fibers

Turn to Right

Fig. 4-7. Effects of rotation on the intervertebral disc.

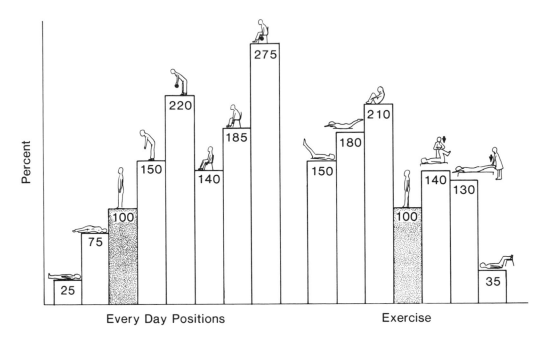

Fig. 4-8. Intradiscal pressures as they relate to body positions and activities (adapted from Nachemson[4].)

SPINAL MOVEMENTS

Movement takes place in the spine generally about an axis situated slightly posterior to the center of the intervertebral disc. This axis moves slightly anteriorly with spinal flexion and slightly posteriorly with spinal extension[1]. The facet joints, sometimes referred to as zygoapophyseal or apophyseal joints, act to guide and limit these motions. The facet joints are diarthrodial joints complete with synovial membrane and joint capsule, and are highly innervated. The plane of the facet joint determines the direction and amount of movement possible between segments. These movements may generally be thought of as gliding movements. The nucleus, due to its spherical shape, functions like a ball-bearing or a swivel. This capacity facilitates the gliding of the facets. Thus, in three-dimensional space, the spinal segment has six degrees of freedom (Fig. 4-9). In other words, a vertebral body can move in the following six ways:

1. In the longitudinal axis of the spine, e.g. under compression or distraction effects.

2. Forward or backward in the sagittal plane, e.g. a degree of gliding or translation motion.

3. Forward and backward tilting around a frontal axis, i.e. flexion and extension.

4. Lateral glide in a frontal plane, e.g. a degree of gliding or translation motion.

5. Lateral tilting or rotation around a sagittal axis, i.e. movement in the frontal plane.

6. Rotation in the horizontal plane around a vertical axis.

It must be recognized that spinal movement is complex and intricate and normal physiological movement occurs through the coupling of two or more of these possible movements simultaneously.

Before looking at spinal movement by region, certain laws of movement must be appreciated.

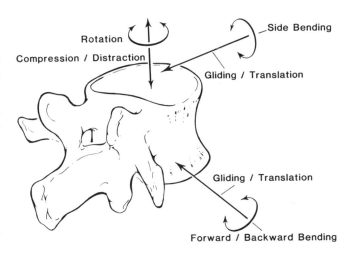

Fig. 4-9. Six degrees of freedom of movement of a spinal segment (adapted from Grieve[5].)

These laws were first described by Fryette in the early part of this century[6].

Law I: If the segments are in "neutral" (or Easy Normal), without locking of the facets (erect standing posture), rotation is to the *opposite* side of side bending. Simply stated, if one side bends to the right, rotation of the spine occurs to the left. This law is true for the lumbar and thoracic regions (Fig. 4-10).

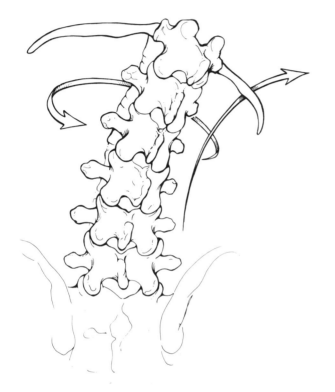

Fig. 4-10. Fryette's Law I: Sidebending and rotation occur in opposite directions.

Law II: If the segments are in full flexion or extension with the facets engaged (or locked), rotation and side bending occur to the *same* side. Thus, if one bends forward (flexes) and side bends to the right, rotation of the spine will also occur to the right. This law is true for the lumbar and thoracic regions. Law II always applies to the cervical area, regardless of the position of the neck.

Law III: If motion is introduced into a segment in any plane, motion in all other planes is *reduced*. This means that since vertebral movements are usually coupled (concomitant), movement into one plane lessens the range of movement available in the other two planes.

Depending on whether the trunk movement is primarily one of side bending or of rotation, the concomitant movements will involve greater or lesser degrees of forward/backward bending vs. compression/distraction of the facets. For example, in the lumbar spine, if one rotates left, distraction (widening of the joint space) occurs on the left and compression (squeezing together) occurs on the right. If one side bends left, the left facet will glide inferiorly (close) while the right facet will glide superiorly (open). Thus, if the left facet should become restricted, the loss of motion would be most noticeable in rotation left and side bending right. Cyriax calls this the capsular pattern of motion restriction for the spine[7].

The importance of understanding the normal physiological motions of the spine comes with the realization that one can override these movements voluntarily. One can make the spine move in ways opposite to its natural tendency for motion. This fact has great implications in the mechanics of injury and for subsequent treatment.

Generally speaking, spinal joints oriented in the sagittal plane and moving about a frontal axis produce the gross motions of flexion and extension; joints oriented in the horizontal plane moving about a vertical axis produce rotation; and the joints oriented in the frontal plane moving about an anterior-posterior axis produce side bending. It should be remembered that any movement of the spine is described as the superior portion of the segment moving relative to the inferior portion of the segment.

Atlanto-Occipital Joint — The A/O joints, which are condyloid in nature, are oriented in the horizontal plane and move primarily about a frontal axis producing motion in the sagittal plane. Nodding of the head on the cervical spine is the most free movement with approximately 10° occurring in flexion and 25° in extension. Only small amounts of side bending and rotation take place at the A/O joints due to the concave-convex relationships of the joint surfaces. This small rotational movement is of clinical significance and can be easily palpated at the end of range.

During flexion of the head and neck all cervical vertebrae move simultaneously. The atlas may be thought of a performing a "meniscus-like" function during movements of the head on the neck. If the cervical spine is stabilized, either through pathological processes or by voluntary action, the occipital condyles **glide backward** on the atlas while the atlas moves slightly forward and cranially, moving the odontoid with it. Thus, the occiput and posterior arch of the atlas tend to move apart in this situation. In the more normal physiological flexion motion where the cervical spine is free to move, the occipital condyles **roll forward** on the atlas while the atlas itself glides backward, tilting upward slightly so that the atlas and occiput approximate[5].

Atlanto-Axial Joint — The A/A joint (C1-C2) is a plane joint whose surfaces are oriented in the horizontal plane with a vertical axis as its primary axis of movement. The presence of the odontoid process of the axis which projects through the ring of the atlas provides a pivot joint which further facilitates rotation at this level. Nearly one-half of the entire range of cervical rotation occurs at the A/A joints, approximately 40° to either side with 50° or so recruited in the lower segments. There are only small amounts of motion available in the sagittal (flexion-extension) and frontal (side bending) planes.

C2-C6 Segments — The facet joint planes of these segments are oriented between the horizontal and frontal planes. These surfaces tend to separate during forward bending, approximate during backward bending and move asymmetrically in rotation and side bending. For example, in side bending to the right, the right facet joints will close and the left facet joints will open. Remembering that Fryette's Law II is true for the cervical spine, the segmental action of side bending right will occur in rotation to the right. According to Kapandji, this combined movement of side bending and rotation totals 50°. The total range of motion in flexion and extension for these segments is 100-110°. When combined with the movement of the upper cervical spine, the total range of motion is 130°[1].

Uncovertebral Joints — The uncovertebral joints (Joints of Von Lushka) are formed by the articulations of the uncinate processes of the inferior vertebral body (superolateral plateau) and the semi-lunar facets of the superior vertebral body (inferolateral plateau). These joints are cartilagenous and encapsulated. During flexion and extension, these joints slide relative to each other, guiding the vertebral bodies in this A-P movement. During side bending and rotation, the contralateral joint tends to open while the ipsilateral joint tends to close. These joints can be of significance in cervical pathology, especially spinal stenosis and degenerative joint disease [1, 2].

C7-T3 Segments — This is a transitional zone between the cervical lordosis and the thoracic kyphosis. Forward and backward bending are not great and all ranges are diminished (not necessarily in a graduated manner.) The facet joints become somewhat more vertically oriented into the frontal plane.

T3-T10 Segments — The thoracic spine is characterized by narrow disc spaces and elongated spinous processes. These spinous processes gradually become nearly vertical in their frontal plane orientation throughout the spine. This elongation of the spinous processes limits the amount of extension possible at each segment. In forward bending, the nearly vertical facets separate superiorly, but this is somewhat restricted. Side bending and rotation occur in much the same manner as in the cervical spine. Both side bending and rotation are limited by the bony thorax. It should be noted that all thoracic vertebrae (except T12) have three demi-facets on each side for the articulations of the ribs.

T11-L1 Segments — This is a transitional zone between the thoracic kyphosis and the lumbar lordosis. While the facet joints remain vertically oriented, they begin to change from the frontal to the sagittal plane. Thus, the T12 vertebrae has its superior facets in the frontal plane and its inferior facets in the sagittal plane to match those of L1. The discs in this area are also beginning to increase in height and general mobility is somewhat greater in comparison to the rest of the thoracic spine.

L1-L4 Segments — The lumbar facet joints are vertically oriented in the sagittal plane. Thus flexion/extension is facilitated while side bending and rotation is limited by apposition of the facets.

Lumbosacral Junction (L5-S1) — The facet joints abruptly change their orientation from the sagittal plane somewhat obliquely into the frontal plane. This tight apposition of the facet surfaces limits side bending and rotation to one or two degrees but does not similarly restrict flexion/extension. Cailliet states that 75% of the total amount of lumbar flexion/extension takes place at the lumbosacral junction with 20% at L4-L5 and the remaining 5% of motion at the remaining segments L1-L3 (Fig. 4-11). Farfan, however, believes that the greatest flexion/extension range occurs at L4-L5 (10° extension and 12° flexion) with slightly less at the lumbosacral junction[9].

Regardless of the amount of motion which exists at this segment, the tight apposition of the facet surfaces provides the main counterbalance to the tremendous shear forces which are present at the lumbosacral junction. The normal lumbosacral angle is 140° with a sacral inclination angle of 30°.

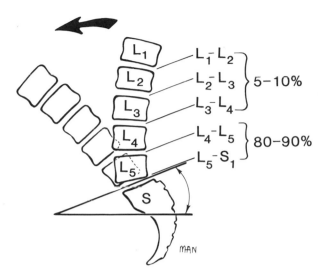

Fig. 4-11. Percentage of total flexion of the lumbar spine by segment (adapted from Cailliet[8].)

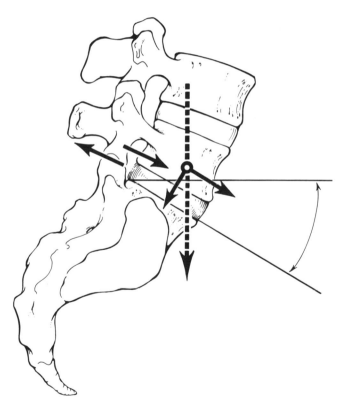

Fig. 4-12. Resistance of L5-S1 facet joints to shear forces at the lumbosacral junction (adapted from Kapandji[1].)

The arrangement produces shear forces of 50% of the superincumbent body weight. If the sacral inclination angle increases to 40° (Fig. 4-12) the shear increases to 65%. An increase to 50° produces a 75% shear force. It should also be remembered that the orientation of the auricular surfaces of the sacroiliac joint will influence this angle. Should the posterior arch become fractured at the pars interarticularis, the condition of *spondylolysis* results. Should the spondylolysis be bilateral and the anterior elements begin to separate from the posterior elements, the condition of *spondylolisthesis* results. Thus, the integrity of this joint is of primary importance.

The total range of motion of the spine is summarized in Fig. 4-13. The values given are for the normal adult [1, 5]. One should keep in mind that motion will vary by age with the greatest amounts available in the 2-13 year age group, progressively declining to the least available in the 65-77 year age group[10].

LUMBO-PELVIC RHYTHM

There is an interconnection of movement between the spine and the pelvis. This is especially true in the total forward bending of the spine: there is a synchronous movement in a rhythmic ratio of the lumbar spine to that of pelvic rotation about the hips.

During forward bending, the lumbar curve reverses itself from concave to flat to convex. At the same time, there is a proportionate degree of pelvic rotation about the hips. While the amount of movement at each lumbar level is different (more at L5-S1 and L4-5 and less at the other levels), the rhythm between levels should be so smooth and precise that at every point in the forward bending arc, there will be balance between lumbar reversal and pelvic rotation[8] (Fig. 4-14). Obviously, the ability of a person to forward bend will thus be influenced by this balance or lack of it. Many factors

	Rotation	Sidebending	Flexion	Extension
Upper Cervical C1-2	40°	5 – 8°	10°	10 – 20°
Cervical C3-7	50°	35 – 45°	40°	75°
Thoracic T1-12	35°	20°	24 – 48°	12 – 24°
Lumbar L1-5	5°	20°	40 – 43°	30 – 40°

Fig. 4-13. Spinal range of motion by region.

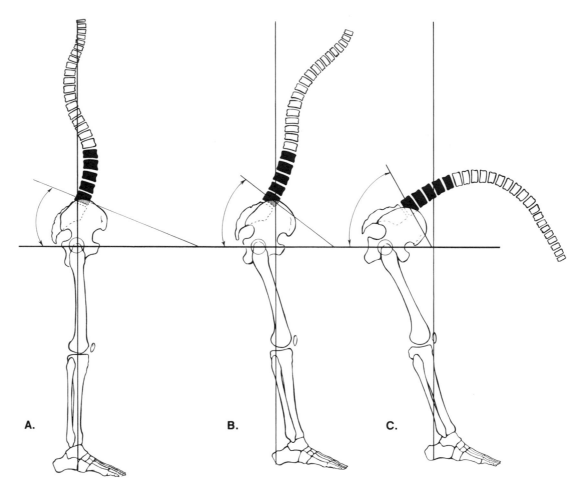

Fig. 4-14. Lumbo-pelvic rhythm: A) Normal standing posture with lumbar concavity; body weight superimposed directly over the hip joints; normal pelvic inclination angle with respect to horizontal. B) Flattening of the lumbar spine; pelvis begins to rotate anteriorly around the hips; hips and pelvis move posteriorly in the horizontal plane. C) Reversal of the lumbar spine into lumbar convexity; pelvis rotates anteriorly to the fullest extent; hips and pelvis are posteriorly displaced in the horizontal plane.

such as facet restriction, degenerative joint disease or tight hamstring muscles can influence this balance. Thus, in order to achieve full forward bending, the lumbar spine must fully reverse itself and the pelvis must rotate to its full extent. The sacrum is also moving within the ilia during this action of forward bending. Initially, the sacrum nutates (flexes). As motion in the lumbar spine is recruited and the pelvis is rotating anteriorly over the hips, the sacrum begins to counternutate (extend) within the ilia (see discussion of the sacroiliac joint.)

At the same time as these movements are occurring in the sagittal plane, there is a backward movement of the pelvis on the hips in the horizontal plane. This represents a shift in the pelvic fulcrum so that the center of gravity is maintained over the feet,

otherwise the person would fall forward onto his head.

As the person returns to the standing position, just the converse occurs: the lumbar spine becomes concave, the pelvis derotates and also shifts forward. The same degree of smoothness and rhythm should be achieved for this movement with extension as well as with forward bending.

SACROILIAC MOVEMENT

The fact that the sacroiliac joints move is not a matter of speculation. Adequate documentation exists in a variety of literature to demonstrate the certainty of their movement both in vivo and in vitro. As to how much they actually do move varies

according to the sample studied and the metho-
dology of the researchers [11-15].

The sacroiliac joint (SI) will be considered as
being two joints: iliosacral (IS) — the innominates
moving on the sacrum; and sacroiliac (SI) — the
sacrum moving within the ilia. Functionally and
from a treatment standpoint, these descriptions hold
true although they are one in the same articulation[6].

The sacrum itself is wedge shaped and fits
vertically between the wings of the two iliac bones. It
is suspended between the ilia by strong, dense
ligaments. The wedge shape of the sacrum facilitates
a self-locking mechanism of the sacrum within the
ilia with the ligaments tightening as heavier weight
may be imposed on it from above[1].

With the possible exception of the piriformis,
movement of the SI joint is not directly produced by
muscular action. Motion of the SI joint is indirectly
imposed by actions, movements and stresses of
other and adjacent body parts[3] (Fig. 4-15).

The SI joint is auricular (ear-like) in shape with
corresponding parts between the sacrum and the

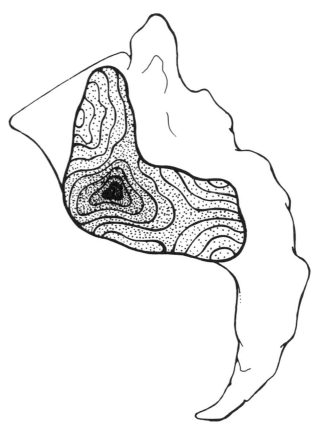

Fig. 4-16. Irregular auricular surfaces with central depression of left sacral articulation. There will be a corresponding surface on the left ilium (adapted from Kapandji[1].)

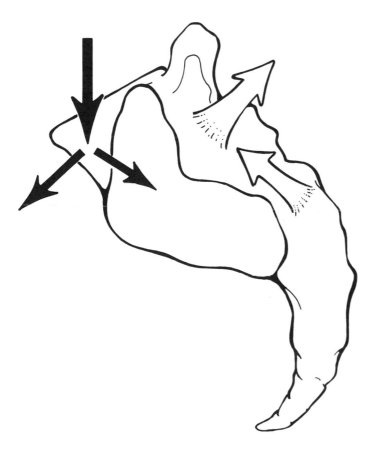

Fig. 4-15. Posterior ligaments (white arrows) resist the
superincumbent forces of body weight imposed by the
sacroiliac joint (adapted from Kapandji[1].)

iliac portions of the joint. The joint surfaces are
irregular and characterized by peaks and valleys.
Generally, there is a long crest running through the
center of the iliac portion of the joint and a
corresponding trough on the sacral portion[1]. According to Weisel, the cranial portion of the sacral
articular facet is longer and narrower than its caudal
portion. He reports that there is a central depression
at the junction of these segments and an elevation at
the edge of each segment[14] (Fig. 4-15).

Kapandji describes the movements of nutation
and counternutation (flexion and extension) of the
sacrum within the ilia about a transverse axis
posterior to the joint at the sacral tuberosity at the
insertion of the sacroiliac ligaments[1]. During
nutation (flexion), movement of the sacral promontory is anterior and inferior (the coccyx moves
posteriorly), the iliacs approximate and the ischial
tuberosities move apart. Conversely, during counternutation (extension), the sacral promontory moves
posterior and superior (the coccyx moves
anteriorly), the iliacs move apart and the ischial
tuberosities approximate. These movements occur

naturally during forward bending and backward bending as part of the lumbo-pelvic rhythm.

Other movements of the sacrum and ilia are possible about any of several other axes. Mitchell, Moran and Pruzzo[6] describe the following axes and movements (Fig. 4-17):

1) Superior Transverse Axis — runs through the second sacral segment horizontally. This is the respiratory axis about which the movements of flexion and extension occur.

2) Middle Transverse Axis — located at the second sacral body, it is the principle axis of normal sacroiliac flexion and extension.

3) Inferior Transverse Axis — runs transversely through the inferior pole of the sacral articulation and extends laterally through the PSIS. It is the principle axis of normal iliosacral motion.

4) Right and Left Lateral Oblique Axes — these axes run from the superior end of the articular surface of the sacrum obliquely to the opposite inferior lateral angle (ILA). Each axis is named for its site of origin at the sacral base.

5) Transverse Pelvic Axis — runs transversely through the symphysis about which the pubes rotate allowing movement of the ilia in an anterior-posterior direction about the symphysis pubis during locomotion[6].

Thus, one can see that multiple actions of the sacrum and ilia are possible given the number of axes of motion described above, and it is simplistic to think only in terms of SI joint anteroposterior rotation.

Normal iliosacral (IS) movements are usually anteroposterior rotations of one innominate with respect to the other about the inferior transverse axis and the transverse pelvic axis described above. Other movements of the ilia on the sacrum are possible, but do not normally occur except as seen in dysfunctional states. These uncommon movements are described as up/down slips and in/out flares of the ilia. Cyriax considers SI joint problems to be more common in females than in males[7].

The following anatomical considerations affect the SI joint in function and stability: 1) the lateral distance of the pelvic outlet is larger in females; 2) the bone density in the female pelvis is lesser; 3) the SI joint is located farther from the hip joints, creating a longer lever arm in females; 4) females have smaller SI joint surfaces; 5) females have flatter SI joint surfaces; 6) the iliac crests are farther apart in the female and 7) the vertical dimension of the pelvis is smaller in females [1, 2, 5, 7, 11]. Some other factors contributing to the functioning of the rest of the spine include the horizontal/vertical orientation of the sacrum within the ilia. A more vertical sacrum usually results in a flattened lumbar spine which increases compression forces on it. A more horizontally oriented sacrum increases lumbar curving and also increases shear forces at the lumbosacral junction. The vertical sacrum is associated with the static spine and the horizontal sacrum with the dynamic spine previously described (Fig. 4-18).

The iliolumbar ligaments deserve special notice as they can influence both the lower lumbar spine

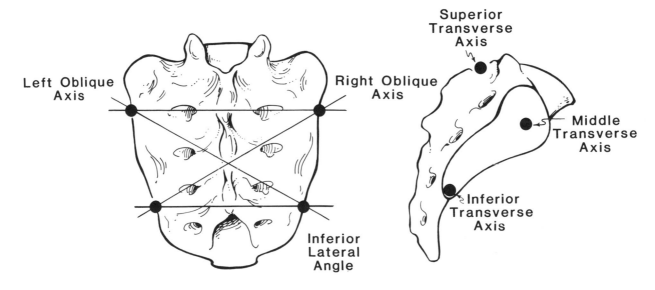

Fig. 4-17. Multiple axes of the sacroiliac joint (adapted from Mitchell, Moran and Pruzzo[6].)

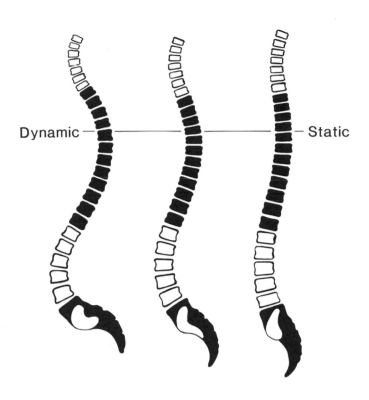

Dynamic — — — Static

Fig. 4-18. Orientation of the sacroiliac joint and subsequent effect on the spine, producing dynamic or static types of function and posture (adapted from Kapandji[1].)

and the sacrum. That is to say, movements of L4 and L5 can influence sacral and iliac position and movement. Conversely, movement of the sacrum and ilia can influence the movements and positions of L4 and L5.

The iliolumbar ligaments have two bands: the superior band runs from the transverse process of L4 to the iliac crest; the inferior band runs from the transverse process of L5 to the iliac crest, the anterior surface of the SI joint and the lateral sacral ala (Fig. 4-19). During side bending of the spine, these ligaments tighten contralaterally and slacken ipsilaterally. During flexion, the superior band tightens and the inferior band slackens. During extension, the reverse takes place[1].

Because of this direct ligamentous influence between the L4 and L5 segments and the SI joint, these areas must be adequately examined when dysfunction exists in order to institute proper treatment. For example, a posteriorly rotated innominate on the left will tighten the iliolumbar ligaments ipsilaterally and tend to side bend L4 and L5 to the left and also rotate them to the right. Thus, restriction of lumbar movement in side bending right and rotation left may be observed with this dysfunction.

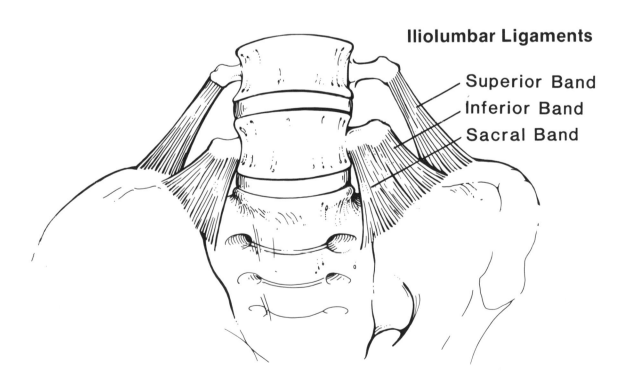

Iliolumbar Ligaments

Superior Band
Inferior Band
Sacral Band

Fig. 4-19. Iliolumbar ligaments.

GAIT AND SACROILIAC JOINT FUNCTION

Understanding the position of the sacrum and ilia during gait and various body positions will help give the clinician an appreciation of SI joint pain which may occur with locomotion. In standing, the base of the sacrum moves anteriorly. At heel strike, the ipsilateral ilium is in a posteriorly rotated position. As one steps onto that side, sacral torsion occurs to that side. At mid-stance, increased tension of the iliopsoas encourages the ilium to move toward anterior rotation. Running merely accelerates this process. However, at heel strike with the increased impact forces, upslipping of the ilium can occur. Additionally, rotation is increased on the side of the unsupported leg and inflaring may occur on the non-weight bearing side[17].

References:

1. Kapandji, I: The Physiology of the Joints. The Trunk and the Vertebral Column, Vol 3, 2nd ed. Churchill-Livingstone, New York 1974.
2. Warwick, R and Williams, P (eds): Gray's Anatomy. British ed 35. W.B. Saunders, Co. Philadelphia 1973.
3. Shah, J: Structure, Morphology and Mechanics of the Lumbar Spine. The Lumbar Spine and Low Back Pain, Jayson, M, ed., Pitman Medical, London, 1980.
4. Nachemson, A: The Lumbar Spine, An Orthopaedic Challenge. Spine 1:50-71, 1976.
5. Grieve, G: Common Vertebral Joint Problems. Churchill-Livingstone, New York 1981.
6. Mitchell, F; Moran, P and Pruzzo, N: An Evaluation and Treatment Manual of Osteopathic Muscle Energy Procedures. Mitchell, Moran and Pruzzo Associates, Valley Park, MI, 1979.
7. Cyriax, J: Textbook of Orthopaedic Medicine. Vol I, Diagnosis of Soft Tissue Lesions, 8th ed. Bailliere-Tindall, London 1978.
8. Cailliet, R: Low Back Pain Syndrome. 2nd ed. FA Davis, Co., Philadelphia 1982.
9. Farfan, H: Mechanical Disorders of the Low Back. Lea & Febiger, Philadelphia 1973.
10. Gregerson, G and Lucas D: An In Vivo Study of Axial Rotation of the Human Thoracolumbar Spine. JBJS 49A, 1967.
11. Beal, M: The Sacroiliac Problems: Review of Anatomy, Mechanics and Diagnosis. JAOA 81(10):667-679, June 1982.
12. Colachis, S; Warden, R et al: Movement of the Sacroiliac Joint in the Adult Male. Arch Phys Med Rehab 44:490, 1963.
13. Solonen, K: The Sacroiliac Joint in the Light of Anatomical, Roentgenological and Clinical Studies. Acta Ortho Scand (Suppl 27):1-115, May 1957.
14. Weisel, H: Movements of the Sacro-Iliac Joint. Acta Anat 23:80-91, 1955.
15. Frigeria, N; Stowe, R and Howe, J: Movement of the Sacroiliac Joint. Clin Orthop and Rel Res 100:370, 1974.
16. Stratton, S: Evaluation and Treatment of the Sacroiliac Joint. Course Notes and Personal Communication, Sept 84.
17. Tanz, S: Motion of the Lumbar Spine. Amer J Roentgen 69:399, 1953.

CHAPTER 5

PATHOLOGY AND TREATMENT CONCEPTS — SPINE

The physical therapist is becoming increasingly interested in and involved with the evaluation and assessment of the patient with musculoskeletal disorders. An understanding of the causes of these disorders is essential before an accurate assessment can be made. Assessment and treatment planning are cognitive processes. The assessment must be based on correlation of the patient's comparable signs and symptoms in a "rule out" process. This chapter is not intended to provide "cookbook" answers to difficult problems. Rather, it is intended to be a guide to intelligent decision making for appropriate treatment. Remember that it is not always possible to fully evaluate a patient on the first visit or to determine a specific pathological entity, in which case the therapist must determine signs and symptoms which can be treated (see discussion in Chapter 2).

A problem encountered in preparing a text of this sort is the wide differences of opinions and placement of emphasis found in available literature. All theories postulated concerning musculoskeletal disorders cannot possibly be discussed, but the object is to present the major "schools of thought" and some of the more recent trends in this area.

Many questions remain unanswered concerning spinal pathology. Consider the following two cases. In one instance, a disc protrusion is identified by myelography and is determined to be the cause of the patient's complaint. The disc protrusion is surgically removed but the patient's signs and symptoms remain unchanged. Or, in the other instance, a disc protrusion is identified by CAT scan, appropriate physical therapy measures or another form of treatment is applied, and the patient's signs and symptoms disappear. Yet on a follow-up CAT scan, the disc protrusion remains unchanged. The point is that there is often no clear cut cause and effect relationship between what we see, or think we see, and what may be actually causing the patient's problem. Certainly many of the things we observe, especially radiographic findings, are difficult to assess and are probably, in many cases, unrelated to the actual problem. With good reason, questions arise as to just what exactly is taking place when one patient with a documented nerve root syndrome secondary to foraminal encroachment improves with spinal traction and another patient, with presumably the same disorder, does not improve. Or, what is really happening to the disc when a lateral shift correction maneuver is done and followed by extension exercises? While there is some scientific evidence to support such techniques, much of what we as physical therapists practice has its base in the theoretical realm. We must use caution in making the assumption that a certain pathology actually exists based, at least partially, on theoretical evidence. The same caution applies in making the assumption that anything which shows up on the patient's radiographic examination is the cause of the patient's complaint.

This is not to suggest or imply that just because we do not have all the answers, we should not discuss what we think may be happening. We certainly should not stop using effective treatment methods just because at this point in time we do not understand everything concerning spinal pathology. However, because specific etiologies may not be fully understood or recognized, and because much of our treatment **is** based in theory, we must be cautious in our approach to a patient's problem. We must work our way through the problem with each patient, individualizing treatment appropriately.

Musculoskeletal disorders are of primary importance because they represent the largest group of complaints that are most often seen by health care practitioners and the physical therapist in particular. However, the therapist should also be capable of recognizing systemic and visceral problems that can mimic musculoskeletal disorders and also appreciate that musculoskeletal disorders can produce visceral responses as well.

MUSCLE DISORDERS

Spinal disorders primarily of muscular origin are uncommon. While it is true that muscle guarding and/or intrinsic muscle spasm usually accompanies spinal pain regardless of the underlying cause, there is no neurophysiological reason for a normal muscle to spontaneously go into spasm. Also, the paraspinal musculature will adaptively shorten to abnormal postures. Therefore, without a thorough evaluation and assessment, it is often an easy "cop-out" to incriminate the muscles as the source of the patient's complaint. Primary muscular disorders may be classified as strains, contusions and inflammations.

ADAPTIVE MUSCLE CHANGES

Any skeletal muscle has a given number of sarcomeres at its normal resting length. The muscle can adaptively add or subtract sarcomeres at the musculotendinous junction, thus increasing or decreasing length according to the stresses placed upon it. This is a normal, nonpathological response that begins to take place shortly after the new position is introduced. For example, the biceps will adaptively shorten when the elbow is casted for a fracture (sarcomere subtraction.) Additionally, within one to two weeks, the collagen fibers of the connective tissue will adaptively shorten and thicken. Following cast removal, the biceps must lengthen (add sarcomeres) and the collagen fibers must be stretched in order for it to regain normal resting length[1,2].

Similarly, postural and structural changes that can lead to adaptive changes in the muscle often occur in response to injury, working position or habits. For example, one usually sees the forward head, slumped posture develop secondary to cervical injuries (whiplash) or in relation to an occupation which requires prolonged sitting (CRT operator.) The muscles in the upper back, chest and neck soon adapt to the new posture. Another example is adaptive shortening of the lumbar spinal muscles secondary to hyperlordosis or sway back. Adaptive shortening of muscles may also occur if normal range of joint mobility is lost. Thus, the physical therapist must always take into account the possibility of adaptive muscle shortening when treating patients with postural changes or restricted joint motion.

Treatment of adaptive length changes is most effectively accomplished by emphasizing normal physiological function (active exercises) rather than passive stretching or other techniques[3]. Of course, one should also treat the joint hypomobility and any structural or postural changes which may be present. This is one reason why it is important to get the patient on an active exercise program as soon as possible in the treatment program, and why emphasis on return to activities of daily living such as walking, return to work and general fitness exercises is so important. Active exercises can be done in short arcs of motion or isometrically if the patient's primary disorder is aggravated by exercising through the entire range of motion. At any rate, muscles need to be exercised functionally as soon as the condition of the primary disorder allows.

MUSCLE GUARDING AND INTRINSIC MUSCLE SPASM

Muscle guarding nearly always accompanies pain, regardless of the underlying cause. Muscle guarding may develop wherever pain is felt, even if it is referred from elsewhere in the body. Prolonged muscle guarding leads to a circulatory stasis and the retention of metabolites. The muscle then may become inflamed (myositis) and a localized tenderness develops in the muscle. This intrinsic muscle spasm adds additional pain and discomfort (Fig. 5-1).

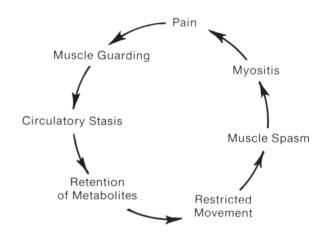

Fig. 5-1. This painful cycle often occurs with musculoskeletal disorders.

Muscle guarding and intrinsic muscle spasm may be noted during the palpation exam by the tension and tenderness of the muscles. A positive weight shift test indicates muscle spasm. Prolonged intrinsic muscle spasm tends to generalize up and down the spine and may aggravate areas of degenerative joint and disc disease.

Without a thorough evaluation, it is easy to incriminate muscle guarding and the resulting intrinsic muscle spasm as the primary cause of the patient's problem. It is unwise to make this assumption as there is always an underlying cause of the muscle guarding. It is, however, often necessary to treat muscle guarding and intrinsic muscle spasm first in order to deal with the underlying problem.

Treatment is necessary to reduce the pain and stiffness caused by the muscle guarding and spasm; this will enable the physical therapist to complete the evaluation, assessment and treatment of the primary disorder, which ultimately is the answer to reducing the muscle guarding and spasm. Effective treatment includes medication, heat, cold, massage, electrical stimulation, rest, active and stretching exercises and relaxation techniques.

MUSCLE STRAINS AND CONTUSIONS

Musculotendinous strains and contusions have a definite history of trauma such as a blow to the back, a tearing sensation while lifting or another traumatic event, or a more subtle history of aggravation such as constant repetition of a new activity. With rest, the patient will claim relief of pain but will complain of "stiffening". He will usually report that, although movement initially hurts, activity will often "loosen up" the stiffness. In the spine, there are no particular positions or activities, such as standing or sitting, that stand out as being especially painful; rather, it is a general, vague loss of active and passive movements accompanied by pain which the patient will describe. Mennell describes these patients as having a tortuous recovery from the forward bent position[4]. One of the most significant findings will be pain upon palpation of the muscle but no pain upon palpation of the joint or upon spring testing the spinal segment passively. Pain is usually referred over several spinal levels and the patient has difficulty "pinpointing" the pain. The neurological exam will reveal no true positive findings. The patient may have radicular pain following the sensory distribution of the associated nerve root[5].

Treatment – See Muscle Inflammation (Myositis)

MUSCLE INFLAMMATION (MYOSITIS)

Muscle inflammation, or myositis, occurs by itself only on rare occasions. The patient may describe the onset after sleeping in a draft or sitting too close to an air conditioner. Muscle inflamma-tion more commonly follows muscle strain or contusion or develops secondary to prolonged muscle guarding or chronic stress. It essentially has the same characteristics as a muscle strain except that myositis will be of insidious onset and may show temperature and color changes over the involved musculature.

Treatment of primary muscular disorders should initially include rest with gentle activity within the pain free range. One may progress to mild activities and mobilization in the subacute stage. Ice massage, cold packs and electrical stimulation are usually preferred in the acute stage, changing to moist heat and electrical stimulation in the subacute stage. Massage is also a useful modality for treatment of muscular disorders, especially those of the chronic strain variety. A particularly helpful technique is to use high voltage electrical stimulation with the active pads coupled to the therapist's hands while he massages the soft tissue. This technique also helps identify trigger points. As the patient progresses, the activity and mobilization treatment should also progress. **Restoration of full function (strength and mobility) and normal posture should be the most important aspects of treatment.** Primary muscle disorders will probably heal in spite of the care given to them, but stiffness, weakness and postural changes may take place while healing is occurring. These losses of function and adaptive postural changes can lead to more serious chronic problems and, therefore, should be of primary concern to the therapist treating these disorders.

JOINT DISORDERS

For classification purposes, the following structures are considered to be a part of the vertebral three-joint complex (two facet joints and the intervertebral disc): 1) disc; 2) cartilaginous endplate; 3) hyaline cartilage; 4) subchondral bone; 5) meniscoid bodies; 6) synovial lining; 7) joint capsule and 8) ligament. Joint disorders considered in this text are impingement, sprain, inflammation, hypomobility, hypermobility, degenerative disease, postural strain and herniated nucleus pulposus.

FACET IMPINGEMENT

Facet blockage, subluxation, fixation, locking and acute cervical torticollis are all terms sometimes used to describe facet joint impingement. Impingement is one of the disorders that has made chiropractors popular because manipulation is usually an effective treatment. The mechanism of injury is usually a sudden, unguarded movement involving backward bending, side bending and/or rotation with little or no trauma. Kos and Wolf describe it as a nipping of the intervertebral menisci[6]. Kraft and Levinthal, in their article "Facet Synovial Impingement," describe a mechanism in which the synovial and capsular tissue which line the facet joint capsule become impinged between the joint surfaces[7] (Fig. 5-2). Maitland[8] and Sprague[9] have accurately described cervical joint locking, its signs and symptoms and its treatment.

The patient with a facet impingement will report that rest relieves, movement hurts and certain **specific** passive and active movements will be restricted and/or painful. The patient will often be "locked" into a scoliotic posture. The scoliosis will involve side bending and rotation to the same side in the cervical spine and side bending and rotation in opposite directions in the thoracic and lumbar spine. The rotary component may not be readily observable but occurs according to the laws of spinal motion (see Chapter 4.)

Pain and/or restriction of movement will be present when the patient attempts movement in the direction opposite the position in which he is locked. For example, in acute cervical torticollis, if the patient is in left side bending and left rotation, he will have pain and/or restriction of movement in

side bending and rotation to the right. Further movement to the left is usually free and painless. An example of facet locking in the thoracic or lumbar spine, however, will involve a patient locked in a position of side bending to the left and rotation to the right and the pain and/or restriction will be noticed when the patient side bends to the right and rotates to the left. Pain may follow the corresponding dermatomal distribution[5]. Cailliet states that pain arising from the facet joint may be felt as pain in the entire sensory distribution of the corresponding spinal nerve root[10].

Facet joint impingement and other facet disorders should not present true positive neurological signs. However, considering the findings of Mooney and Robertson, the definition of "true" neurological signs must be discussed. They found that injection of hypertonic saline solution into a lower lumbar facet joint not only produced local pain, but also pain that radiated distally in a pattern corresponding to the dermatomal distribution of the adjacent spinal nerve roots (posterior buttock and thigh[5].) Similar pain patterns have been demonstrated by injecting irritants into spinal muscles, interspinous ligaments and the intervertebral disc [11-17] (refer to the classic work of Travell and Rinzler [18] for more studies on referred pain patterns.) However, perhaps of even greater significance, Mooney and Robertson also found increased myoelectrical activity in the hamstring muscles, painful straight leg raising and depressed quadriceps muscle stretch reflexes to be associated with the referred pain stimuli. These so-

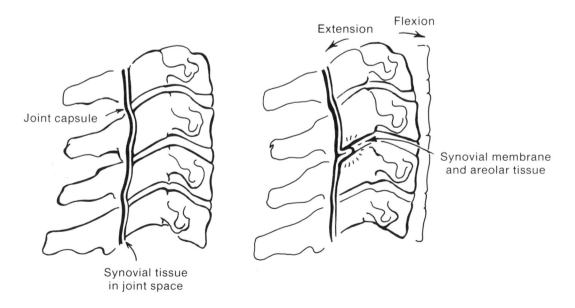

Fig. 5-2. Mechanism of facet impingement.

called "positive" neurological findings were found in a group of patients diagnosed as having herniated nucleus pulposus (HNP). However, upon injection of a local anaesthetic into the appropriate soft tissue or facet joints, these "positive" findings returned to normal. Based on this preliminary experience, these researchers no longer consider painful straight leg raising or reflex changes of the quadriceps group to necessarily implicate nerve root compromise. The only true neurological signs which they will now accept are specific motor weakness or specific dermatomal sensory loss[5].

As with muscle problems, one of the keys to finding joint involvement is the palpatory exam. When the examiner palpates between the spinous processes or along the articular pillars (cervical), the single involved segment will be tender. Good judgement is necessary with palpation because of muscle guarding and spasm. If the patient has had pain for more than one or two days, the muscles may also be tender from guarding and spasm alone. As previously pointed out, this reflexive guarding and spasm may sometimes be incorrectly interpreted as being the primary disorder.

The positional changes previously discussed can occasionally be felt by palpating the spinous processes (Fig. 5-3). For example, if the segment is locked in rotation and side bending, the superior spinous process will not be in alignment with the adjacent inferior spinous process. If the segment is locked in forward bending, the space between the spinous processes will be wider at that level. If the segment is locked in backward bending, the space will be narrower. However, if the segment is locked in mid-range, a positional fault may not be evident upon palpation.

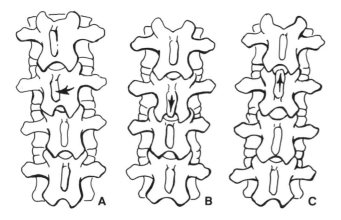

Fig. 5-3. Positional changes related to facet joint impingement: A) rotation; B) backward bending; C) forward bending.

Lab findings and routine radiographs will be negative. Mobility x-rays, which are special techniques that show spinal motion and position, may be helpful in demonstrating a locked or immobile segment. However, such procedures seem unnecessary since the clinical exam will also demonstrate this loss of mobility and/or positional change. Clinical confirmation of the other signs and symptoms must also be made before the diagnosis is clear.

Treatment: Facet joint impingements respond well to mobilization therapy and manual or mechanical traction (see Chapters 8 and 9.) If it is often wise to precede the mobilization or traction with ice or heat and massage in order to relieve the muscle guarding and spasm which may be accompanying the facet disorder. Treatment for cervical facet impingement (acute torticollis) involves manual traction and gentle rotation and side bending, first in the pain free direction, then gradually working toward the painful directions while the traction is being maintained.

FACET JOINT SPRAIN

It is necessary to distinguish between facet joint impingement and facet joint sprain because the treatment for these two disorders differs. The two disorders are, of course, quite different, but their objective signs and symptoms are often hard to distinguish during the musculoskeletal examination. The key to separating them is found in the patient's history. With facet joint sprain, the patient has a history of moderate to severe trauma, enough so that the examiner must consider the possibility of joint sprain with effusion in and around the joint. Facet joint impingement can be treated with mobilization as soon as the disorder is confirmed. Facet joint sprain, on the other hand, must be treated with a more conservative approach using physical therapy modalities, pain free movements, support and rest. The joint sprain needs time to heal. It is possible for facet joint impingement to occur with trauma also, but in this case, the examiner must assume that the soft tissue around the joint has also been injured and must take a more conservative approach to treatment. Mobility tests, palpation and other signs and symptoms of joint sprain will be similar to those found with facet joint impingement, except that movement may be generally more restricted and may involve more than one specific segment. Positional faults are not as common.

Treatment: If the patient gradually increases activities as the joint sprain heals or is treated with mild to moderate mobilization and range of motion during the subacute stage, the joint is likely to have normal mobility by the time complete healing occurs. If the patient has been immobile during the subacute stage and/or there has been a great deal of muscle guarding, the joint(s) is likely to become hypomobile (stiff) as it heals. If, on the other hand, the joint capsule and/or supportive ligaments are actually torn or over-stretched during injury, the joint may be hypermobile (unstable) when healing is complete.

One must especially guard against the development of postural changes such as forward head in a cervical sprain or slumped sitting in a lumbar sprain. During the acute and subacute stages, it may be painful to sit or stand erect or hold the head and neck in normal postures because the spinal muscles are in a painful state. Thus, the patient may tend to stand and sit slumped or develop a forward head posture. As healing occurs and as the muscles and ligaments adapt to their new positions and the faulty posture is maintained, the muscles weaken and a chronic postural strain develops. Supports such as a soft cervical collar, lumbosacral corset or lumbar pillow are often helpful to prevent these postural changes. Modalities and medications may help relieve the pain, making normal posture possible. Above all, patient awareness that long term postural problems can develop is imperative.

JOINT INFLAMMATION

Joint inflammation will have a history of insidious onset, frequently following acute joint sprain or chronic postural sprain. It will also occur secondary to aggravation or overuse in the presence of degenerative joint/disc disease. As in all joint disorders, movement will hurt but it is characteristic of inflammatory disorders to also have some pain and stiffness at rest. The involved segments will be tender to palpation. Active and passive movement will generally be restricted. Joint inflammation often presents bilateral symptoms. The color and temperature changes characteristic of inflammation may not be noticable because of the depth of the joints in the spine. Rheumatoid arthritis is not a consideration here since it is classified as a systemic disease and requires specialized management.

Treatment consists of modality therapy (ice, electrical stimulation), pain free movement and rest to promote healing. This is followed by gradual reconditioning to restore strength, mobility and normal posture.

Generally, treatment in the acute and subacute stages of muscular strain, joint sprain and inflammation is directed to: 1) relieve pain; 2) promote healing; 3) prevent joint stiffness; 4) prevent muscle weakness and 5) prevent postural changes. Often, too much attention is focused on relief of pain (medication, rest and modalities such as TENS) with little or no attention directed toward prevention of joint stiffness, muscle weakness and adaptive postural changes and the resulting disabilities that these disorders will ultimately produce. One should realize that pain is only a symptom of underlying pathology and that healing, in most instances, will eventually take place in spite of any treatment. **Therefore, the emphasis of treatment of muscular strain, joint sprain and inflammation should be the restoration of full joint mobility, muscular strength and flexibility and normal posture rather than the overuse of modality treatments that is sometimes seen.**

JOINT HYPOMOBILITY (DYSFUNCTION/CONTRACTURE)

Joint hypomobility is a disorder that generally involves the entire spinal segment and is the result of prolonged immobilization, usually secondary to injury or poor posture. The facet joint capsule, the disc, the supporting ligaments or any combination of the above may be the primary site of restriction. Joint hypomobility may be due to molecular binding of the collagen fibers within the joint capsule, adhesions or scarring of the surrounding soft tissue following injury[19]. It may result following acute facet joint sprain if normal mobility and posture is not restored as healing occurs. Hypomobility may occur during and following episodes of disc herniation when certain movements are restricted and when scar tissue is laid down to repair the annular defect, or may simply be the result of prolonged poor posture and faulty working positions (Fig. 5-4).

Mobility tests will reveal a limitation of active and passive movement at the involved segments. The involved levels will be tender to palpation. Pain may be referred and is usually unilateral. As with all

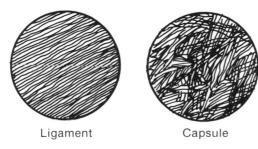

Ligament   Capsule

Fig. 5-4. Collagen fibers are arranged in parallel in ligaments and irregularly in joint capsules. The irregular arrangement allows greater mobility because the fibers can slide (play) on each other. This tissue mobility is soon lost if the joint is immobilized because the fibers bind together easily if mobility is not maintained[19].

joint problems, pain is associated with movement and is noticed especially at the end of available range. Lab findings and routine x-rays will initially be normal. Prolonged segmental hypomobility may lead to degeneration of both the disc and the facets with pathology becoming evident on x-ray[20]. As with other joint problems, there will be no true neurological signs.

Treatment: Mobilization, stretching exercises and traction are the preferred modes of treatment. Ultrasound is especially effective in breaking down the molecular binding of the collagen fibers as well as in "warming" the joint[21]. Both of these effects greatly enhance the effectiveness of the mobilization, stretching or traction. It must be emphasized that ultrasound alone will probably be ineffective unless it is followed by mobilization, stretching or traction.

JOINT HYPERMOBILITY (JOINT INSTABILITY)

Joint hypermobility usually involves the entire spinal segment and may be the end result of postural problems, congenital defects, severe trauma such as whiplash, overtreatment by manipulation or excessive stretching related to certain sports (gymnastics, dancing.) Spondylolisthesis is sometimes hypermobile. Hypermobility can also develop in areas adjacent to a hypomobile segment. Sacroiliac hypermobility often develops with pregnancy.

Patients complain of general soreness in the spine with referred pain down one or both extremities. They cannot maintain any position for more than a few minutes without pain and this pain usually worsens following increased physical activity. They will often describe a "slipping" sensation

or feeling of instability associated with movement.

If joint hypermobility is present, the mobility exam will reveal increased active and passive movement at the involved levels. The segments involved will be tender to palpation. Mobility x-rays may be helpful in revealing an unstable joint. The patient will not have any true neurological signs unless the condition is so severe that the bony structure is impinging upon a nerve root.

There is evidence that joint hypermobility can lead to joint/disc degeneration due to changes in biomechanical stresses and the increased stress and wear and tear placed upon the joint during activity.

Treatment: Hypermobile joints should be treated with postural training, muscle strengthening and/or support (i.e. soft collar or corset.) The patient must be taught to avoid activities and positions that aggravate the condition or cause the "slipping" sensation or feeling of instability to occur.

DEGENERATIVE JOINT/DISC DISEASE (OSTEOARTHRITIS, SPONDYLOSIS)

Degenerative joint/disc disease is a chronic and commonly progressive degeneration of the facet joints and/or the intervertebral disc. There is frequently an associated osteophytosis of the adjacent vertebrae. Degenerative joint/disc disease also occurs with neurological complications which will be discussed later in this chapter. The term spondylosis is also used to describe various degenerative disorders of the spine. The term osteoarthritis is commonly applied to a degenerative disorder of synovial joints only. Degenerative joint/disc disease is more common in the cervical spine than in the lumbar spine.

There are four characteristics of degenerative joint disease in synovial joints: 1) proliferation of calcific deposits in, and especially around, the periphery of the joint; 2) wearing away of the hyaline cartilage; 3) thickening of the synovial lining and joint capsule and 4) thickening of the subchondral bone. Degenerative disc disease is characterized by: 1) dehydration of the nucleus pulposus; 2) narrowing of the intervertebral space; 3) weakening and degeneration of the annular rings and 4) approximation of the facet joints.

Although degenerative joint/disc disease is a natural process of aging and is often asymptomatic, it sometimes develops as the result of hypomobility (loss of joint/disc nutrition.) The intervertebral discs and the hyaline cartilage surfaces of synovial joints do not have a blood supply. The movement of body fluids is necessary for these structures to receive their normal nutritional supply[22-26]. Therefore, loss of mobility contributes to early development of joint/disc degeneration. Joint hypermobility or instability also leads to early joint/disc degeneration because of the increased wear and tear that the disc and joints are subjected to when hypermobility exists. **Thus, both joint hypomobility and joint hypermobility can contribute to the development of degenerative joint/disc disease.** When degenerative disease develops, the joint/disc is vulnerable to increased aggravation and strain, thus a progressive cycle develops as the disorder worsens.

The patient with degenerative joint/disc disease usually presents a history of joint injury with episodes of joint pain and/or stiffness. X-ray will reveal the degenerative process and/or a narrowing of the disc space. The patient will have tenderness at the segmental levels involved. Often, a thickened supraspinous ligament can be palpated. Active and passive movements are usually restricted; however, since degenerative joint/disc disease can also develop because of hypermobility or instability of the joint, active and passive movements are sometimes excessive. In advanced stages, pain is present with any movement. However, it should be emphasized that in other stages, this disorder is often asymptomatic. The joint is more vulnerable to facet impingement, sprain and inflammation when degenerative joint disease is present. The disc can also be injured (disc herniation) more easily. Many factors are thought to contribute to joint/disc degeneration, thus, the etiology is sometimes obscured. As previously stated, joints which are hypomobile or hypermobile, as well as joints continually subjected to repeated trauma, are susceptible to early development of degenerative joint disease.

Many paradoxical situations exist in regard to patients who have suspected degenerative joint/disc disease. Some individuals remain asymptomatic (except for hypomobility) despite radiographic evidence of advanced degenerative joint/disc disease. On the other hand, physical therapists must often deal with those patients who have no radiographic evidence of disease but who have both mobility problems and pain. Obviously, psychological/emotional factors and pain tolerance levels of the individual must be considered, but in such cases what is the source of the pain? Since the hyaline cartilage of the joint surfaces is aneural, the most obvious structure incriminated is the joint capsule.

Discogenic pain related to degenerative joint/disc disease is difficult to assess clinically, but also seems to be intermittent in nature and is related to certain stressful activities. When evaluating a patient, it is often difficult, if not impossible, to determine if the pain the patient is experiencing is coming from the disc or from the facet joints. If the pain is discogenic, it must be because of mechanical irritation or inflammation of the outer wall of the annulus. The mechanism of aggravation and/or analysis of the most painful positions (flexion versus extension) may give the most reliable clues. If flexion (sitting and forward bending) is more painful and/or is the mechanism of aggravation, the disc is probably the irritated structure. If the reverse is true and extension (standing and walking) is most aggravating, the facets are most likely involved.

Treatment in the mild to moderate stages may involve ultrasound, mobilization, manual or mechanical traction and flexibility exercises if the patient has joint hypomobility or support if there is joint hypermobility. Muscle strengthening and postural training may be indicated in either case, and modality therapy and medication may be necessary for relief of pain and inflammation. In the lumbar spine, flexion and extension exercises are indicated when joint hypomobility is present. Usually, the patient should exercise in the direction opposite that of the aggravation. In other words, if flexion aggravates, extension exercises are indicated. Conversely, if extension aggravates, flexion exercises are indicated. The amount of lordosis will also help determine which exercises are appropriate with each patient. If the patient is hyperlordotic, flexion exercises are indicated and extension exercises are indicated if hypolordosis exists. When the patient with *severe* degenerative joint/disc disease also has joint hypomobility, it is usually beneficial to mobilize the involved segments. If this can be done without aggravating the patient's pain, it is probably the treatment of choice. If, on the other hand, any attempt to increase mobility or activity results in increased pain and/or increased inflammatory responses, another approach should be considered. This approach involves bracing or support in an attempt to reduce movement, thus reducing irritation. This approach should not be used unless the patient has rather advanced degenerative joint/disc disease and suffers from frequent episodes of aggravation due to an activity.

POSTURAL SPINAL PAIN

Poor posture contributes to many types of spinal disorders. In some cases, postural correction will be a primary treatment consideration. True postural strain syndromes fall into three categories: 1) lumbar flexion; 2) lumbar extension and 3) forward head.

The **lumbar flexion syndrome** (flat back) is characterized by the patient who slumps with a flattened lumbar spine while sitting or standing. Working postures often contribute to this disorder. Consider, for example, the secretary who slumps over the desk, or the bench worker who stands slightly bent forward at his work. Tight hamstring muscles may also contribute to this syndrome. Pain is intermittent and only comes on after being in this postural position for a length of time. Coming to the standing position after prolonged sitting is especially painful and difficult. Changing posture or position usually brings relief. Ligaments maintained under prolonged tension will adaptively lengthen. Thus, the ligaments which stabilize the spine in flexion (posterior longitudinal ligament, supraspinous and interspinous ligaments) are all subject to stretch. If once stretched beyond normal resting lengths, support for the facet joints and disc is lessened. Pain arising from the ligaments or posterior annulus is often bilateral and may produce referral of symptoms to the extremities. Patients with lumbar flexion syndrome are usually pain free after resting at night. Bilateral backache is the chief complaint but leg ache may also be present. Initially, full mobility is present but prolonged maintenance of these postures will eventually lead to a loss of lumbar extension. This situation often leads to disc herniation because of increased intradiscal pressure resulting from the flexed posture and the tendency for flexion to displace the nucleus posteriorly[27-30].

Treatment consists of avoiding prolonged sitting and standing unless maintaining a lumbar lordosis. A roll placed against the lumbar spine will help maintain the lumbar lordosis while sitting (Fig. 5-5). Hamstring stretching and exercises as shown in Fig. 5-6 and Fig. 5-7 are often necessary to maintain full range of motion in extension and to strengthen the back muscles. If the poor posture is work related, it may be necessary to raise the work area to a higher level so that the patient can stand or sit with a normal lordosis as he works. **Since one cannot always completely eliminate stressful postural positions from daily routines, it is essential that the stressful positions be interrupted or changed frequently when they are a necessary part of one's daily activities.**

The **lumbar extension syndrome** (hyperlordosis) is characterized by the complaint of a dull backache that comes on after prolonged standing. The pain often covers a large non-specific area. There is often a leg ache in one or both legs. The patient actually slumps into lumbar extension while standing by "hanging" on the anterior ligaments. He will often have tight hip flexor muscles and have weak abdominal muscles. In cases of prolonged excessive

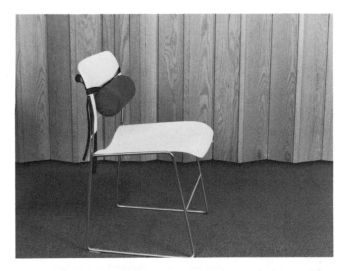

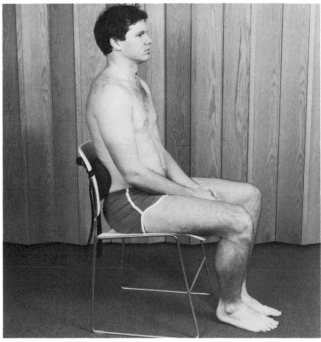

Fig. 5-5. Lumbar roll used to support lumbar lordosis while sitting. If ties are not supplied with the roll it can be slipped inside of a piece of four-inch stockinette and tied to the back of the seat or chair.

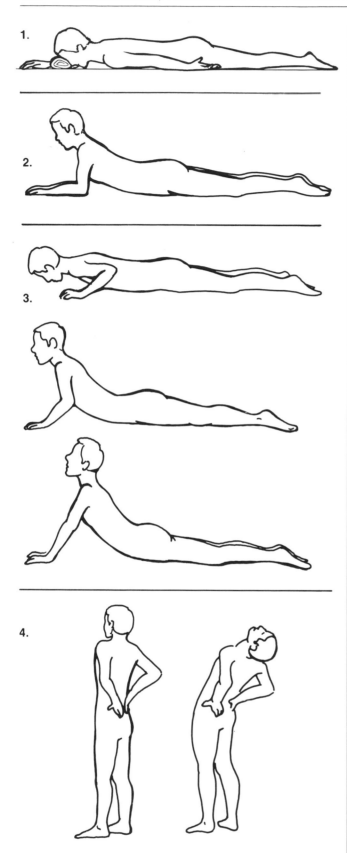

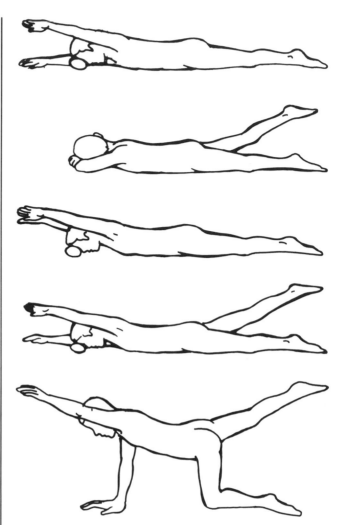

Fig. 5-7. Active back strengthening exercises. These exercises are usually done once or twice daily, starting mildly and increasing as tolerated. Small (two to three pound) weights may be added to ankles and wrists as the patient progresses.

Fig. 5-6. Passive spinal extension exercises which are done to compensate for prolonged periods of forward bending and/or sitting. These exercises increase spinal extension mobility, help correct flat back posture and, in certain cases, correct a mild disc protrusion.

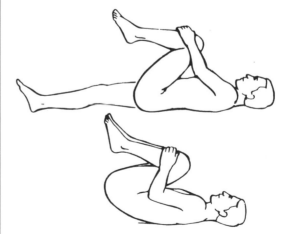

Fig. 5-8. Single and double knee-to-chest exercises. These exercises are done to stretch the posterior elements of the spine to increase spinal flexion mobility and to help correct sway back posture. They are done occasionally as needed to compensate for prolonged periods of standing.

lordosis, adaptive shortening of the posterior spinal musculature and ligaments occurs and flexion may become restricted. As with other postural problems, the patient will get relief by changing the poor postural position. Rest and recumbency will relieve and the patient is usually asymptomatic in the morning with a gradual return of symptoms during the day. This patient is often younger and hypermobile. The level of physical fitness seen in this type of patient may vary from very athletic to very sedentary. The pregnant woman often suffers from this syndrome.

Treatment consists of postural correction, exercises to stretch the hip flexor muscles and the posterior aspects of the spinal segment (Fig. 5-8) and abdominal muscle strengthening (Fig. 5-9). Severe cases may require a corrective support. If prolonged standing is necessary, resting one foot on a small stool may be helpful. Frequently changing the stressful postural position is essential when it cannot be eliminated from one's daily activities.

In either the flexion or extension syndrome, it is the extreme, often prolonged posture that creates difficulty. It is a sad fact that many medical practitioners have prescribed the routine use of one set of exercises (i.e. Williams' flexion) or one often ineffective method of postural correction (i.e. pelvic tilt) to treat essentially opposite postural syndromes. If one is to avoid this type of "cook book" approach, it is essential that the problem first be properly assessed and those principles of treatment applicable to the situation be knowledgably applied.

As previously discussed, it is often difficult to determine the exact pathological process one is dealing with when treating a patient with spinal pain. This is especially true with cervical and upper thoracic problems. Postural change is often the only objective evidence that one has to base treatment upon. Clinical experience teaches that almost every patient seen with neck pain has poor posture and it is usually some degree of the **forward head posture syndrome.** Experience also teaches that when the poor posture is corrected with patient education and exercise, the patient usually experiences relief of his symptoms. In this case, the treatment is correct and the patient gets well, yet the therapist never knows what the exact pathology was. As previously mentioned, there is nothing wrong with this approach to treatment. In fact, it may be the only reasonable approach available in some cases.

In the forward head postural syndrome the upper cervical spine is held in extension while the lower cervical and upper thoracic spine is held in flexion. Protraction and depression of the shoulder girdle results. There are four instances when the forward head posture is seen:

1) The forward head posture may result secondary to either the lumbar flexion or the lumbar extension syndromes.

Treatment: In such cases, treatment of the primary lumbar problem, appropriate spinal strengthening (Fig. 5-7) and general physical fitness exercises are all indicated.

2) In the second instance, the forward head posture results from the development of joint and/or muscular tightness in the upper cervical spine due to injury or muscular tension. As the restriction develops, the upper cervical spine is tilted more and more into extension. As this occurs, the lower cervical and upper thoracic spine is flexed in order to keep the eyes level.

Treatment for this disorder consists of mobilization and stretching (traction) of the upper cervical spine and postural training.

3) In the third instance, the forward head posture results from weakness of the lower cervical and upper thoracic spinal muscles.

Treatment for this problem consists of spinal strengthening exercises and postural training.

4) The fourth and most common instance of forward head posture results secondarily to cervical sprain/strain. Because of pain in the acute and subacute stages of cervical sprain/strain, the patient is likely to let the cervical spine slump into flexion. If he attempts to sit or stand straight with his head held erect, the injured muscles and joints become painful. In time, the muscles become weak and the joints of the lower cervical spine lose extension mobility. At the same time, the upper cervical spine is held in extension in order to keep the head and eyes level. By the time healing of the precipitating injury occurs, the patient is fixed in the new posture.

When the head is held in the forward position, there is considerably more weight and tension exerted at the base of the cervical spine. This occurs mechanically as the neck is now acting as a lever arm, causing a torque force at the base of the cervical spine. Normally, the bony structures of the neck should act as a weight bearing column and simply transfer the weight of the head to the base of the cervical spine as they do when the patient assumes an upright posture (Fig. 5-10).

Chronic forward head posture causes a strain on the ligaments and muscles in the posterior lower

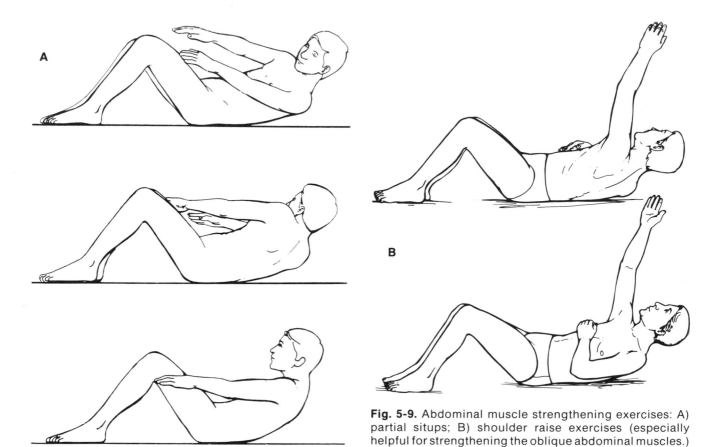

Fig. 5-9. Abdominal muscle strengthening exercises: A) partial situps; B) shoulder raise exercises (especially helpful for strengthening the oblique abdominal muscles.)

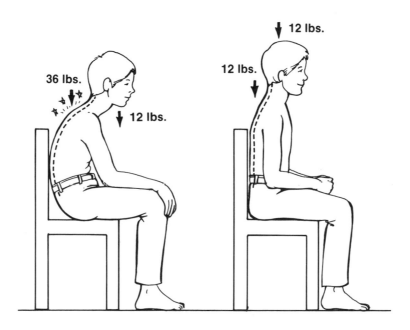

Fig. 5-10. This illustration shows how the neck acts as a lever arm, causing the development of a torque force at the base of the cervical spine. Note the slumped lumbar posture, which also must be corrected in this syndrome.

cervical and upper thoracic spine. This syndrome is characterized by generalized, non-specific pain in the neck and upper back, headaches and occasional referred pain into the upper extremities. The upper trapezius, levator scapulae and rhomboid major muscles are most often involved. A constant state of muscle guarding, spasm, ligament strain and generalized inflammation will often cause the patient to believe that the original injury has never healed even though many months or years have passed.

Treatment in this case must be directed toward: 1) restoring any loss of flexion mobility in the upper cervical spine and extension mobility in the lower cervical and upper thoracic spine; 2) strengthening of the muscles of the posterior cervical and upper thoracic area; 3) stretching the anterior shoulder and chest muscles if they have become adaptively shortened due to the postural changes and 4) making the patient aware of the correct posture that he must achieve if treatment is to be successful.

The contributing causes of forward head postural syndrome may not be as clearly defined and specific as outlined above. It is not uncommon to see several of these factors involved and it is often difficult to determine which occurred first. Therefore, treatment may need to be directed at more than one area if success is to be expected. Exercises to correct the forward head posture, stretch the anterior shoulder and chest muscles and strengthen the back, neck and shoulder girdle muscles play a key part in treatment of the forward head syndrome regardless of the underlying cause. These exercises are shown in Figs. 5-7, 5-11, 5-12, 5-13 and 5-14.

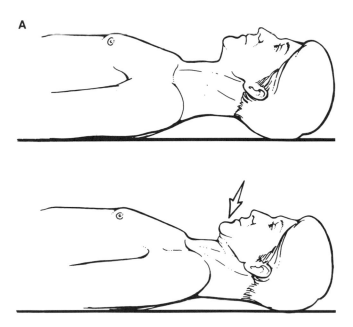

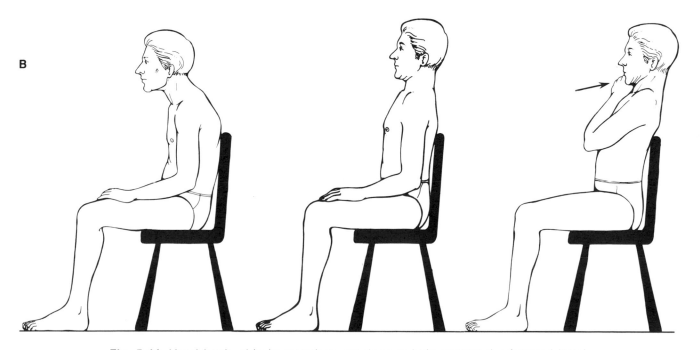

Fig. 5-11. Head back, chin in exercises are done to help correct the forward head posture. These exercises are done several times throughout the day. A) Supine B) Sitting.

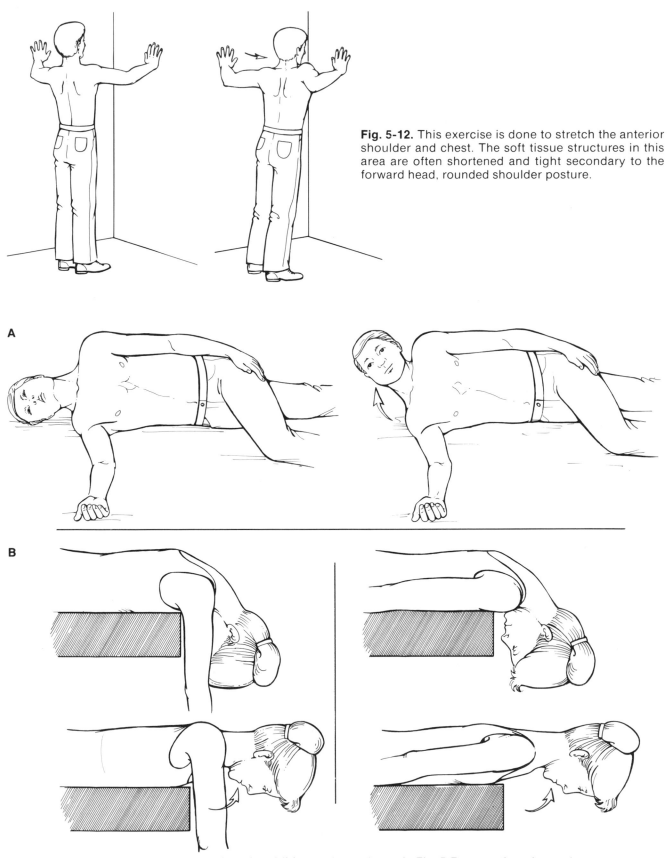

Fig. 5-12. This exercise is done to stretch the anterior shoulder and chest. The soft tissue structures in this area are often shortened and tight secondary to the forward head, rounded shoulder posture.

A

B

Fig. 5-13. These exercises, in addition to those shown in Fig. 5-7, strengthen the neck and upper back muscles. A) Sidelying exercise that is especially effective for strengthening the posterolateral neck muscles; B) Prone head back, chin in exercise to strengthen posterior neck and upper back muscles.

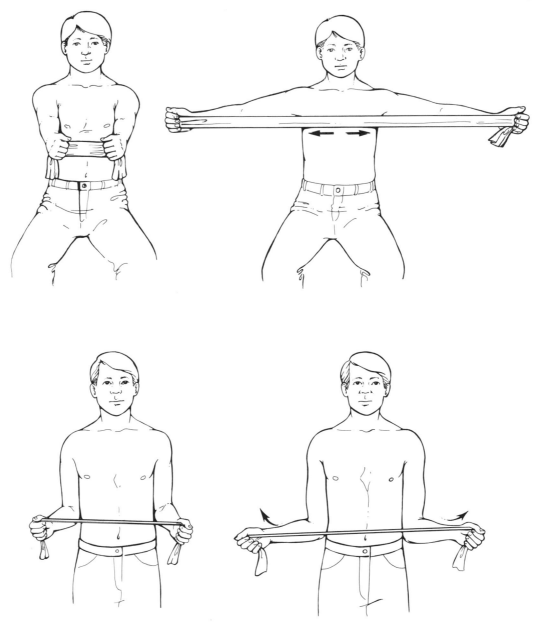

Fig. 5-14. Exercises to strengthen the posterior shoulder girdle muscles to help correct the rounded shoulders posture.

HERNIATED NUCLEUS PULPOSUS-GENERAL COMMENTS

Herniated nucleus pulposus (HNP) is classified as the disorder in which there is displacement of the nuclear material and other disc components beyond the normal confines of the annulus. Four degrees of displacement are recognized: 1) intraspongy nuclear herniation; 2) protrusion; 3) extrusion and 4) sequestration[31].

HNP-protrusion occurs gradually over a period of time. In the early stages, it is asymptomatic. As the protrusion progresses, the patient first experiences back pain, then back and leg pain, and finally, back and leg pain with signs of neurological involvement indicating impingement or irritation of the nerve root. This author chooses to classify HNP-protrusion as occurring in two stages. The first stage (mild to moderate), when the signs and symptoms are purely discogenic in nature and the second stage (moderate to severe), when the signs and symptoms also indicate involvement of the nerve root. These classifications are based on treatment concepts which often change as the condition changes. It is recommended that all other terms dealing with disc displacement such as hard disc, soft disc, disc derangement, disc prolapse, ruptured disc and slipped disc be discarded due to their lack of precision in meaning or because these terms do not describe a verifiable condition[31].

HERNIATED NUCLEUS PULPOSUS-INTRASPONGY NUCLEAR HERNIATION

Intraspongy nuclear herniation refers to displacement of the nucleus into the vertebral body through the cartilaginous endplate. It is similar to a Schmorl's node except that it is a traumatic defect rather than a developmental one[32]. Schmorl's nodes represent small invasions of the vertebral body by the nucleus protruding superiorly. According to Cyriax, they never cause any symptoms, either at their time of occurrence or later in life. In fact, Schmorl's nodes are thought to stabilize the nucleus and diminish the intra-articular centrifugal force, thus rendering posterior displacement less probable. Unfortunately, they are rarely seen where they are most needed, i.e., at the fourth and fifth lumbar levels. They occur most commonly in the lower thoracic and upper lumbar spine and are purely an adolescent phenomenon as no increased frequency is observed as age advances[33].

Traumatic intraspongy nuclear herniation is also thought to be of little clinical importance, at least there are few references in orthopaedic literature to indicate that it is of clinical significance[32].

Farfan describes a disc injury that deals with the fractured endplate of the vertebral body due to a compression injury. He maintains that these injuries can be a source of pain and that they occur in four grades:

Grade 1 = Subchondral fractures in the vertebral body.

Grade 2 = Small cracks in the endplates.

Grade 3 = A crack in which a piece of bone has shifted.

Grade 4 = A crack in which a piece of bone has shifted and disc material is forced through the crack (intraspongy nuclear herniation.)[34]

Treatment consists of rest and avoidance of compressing forces on the disc. Control of protective muscle guarding with physical therapy modalities is important because muscle guarding contributes a compressive force. Hyperextension and/or mild traction may help to restore the anatomy of a Grade 3 or 4 injury. Support with a corset or brace may also be indicated.

HERNIATED NUCLEUS PULPOSUS-PROTRUSTION (Without Spinal Nerve Root Involvement)

This classification describes the condition in which there is displacement of the nuclear material beyond the normal confines of the inner annulus, producing a discrete bulge in the outer annulus; no nuclear material escapes, however[31]. Discogenic pain arises from the outermost rings of the annulus. Most literature supports the fact that, except for the outermost rings of the annulus, the intervertebral disc itself is not a source of pain because of its lack of a sensory nerve supply [11-17,35,36]. The literature also supports disc herniation and its role in the mechanism of nerve root impingement. The agreement ends here, however, as there are divergent opinions concerning the role of the disc in spinal pain where there is no evidence of nerve root involvement [37].

In the *lumbar spine,* HNP-protrusion is most common in the L4-L5 and L5-S1 discs and is rarely seen above those levels (less than 5%.) This disorder is rarely associated with a single injury or incident. Rather, it is caused by the accumulated effects of months or even years of forward bending and lifting and/or sitting in a slumped, forward bent posture [39-42]. One usually sees a generalized loss of mobility, especially spinal extension [27,43], and an overall decline in general physical fitness [44,45]. Since mobility is necessary to maintain adequate nutrition to the disc, this loss of mobility leads to further weakening of the annular rings.

In the early stages, the patient will complain of pain, usually in the lower back, but sometimes in the posterior buttock and thigh. As a general rule, the leg pain indicates a larger protrusion than does back pain alone[27]. Usually, the patient will not hesitate when asked the question, "Which hurts more; sitting, standing, walking or lying down?" The answer will be "sitting." The patient will also often report that prolonged sitting will cause the pain to move from the lower back into the leg. He will also report difficulty in assuming an erect posture after sitting or lying down. However, after standing up and walking around, he usually obtains some relief of pain. When asked to locate the pain, the patient usually says that it is greater on one side of the lower back than the other. However, the spinal pain may be bilateral with the pain referred into the leg. This referred pain is usually unilateral and will correspond to the dermatomal pattern of the involved segment. The reason that spinal pain tends to be bilateral in these cases is that a connecting branch of the sinuvertebral nerve joins the right and left portions of that nerve[46]. It is the sinuvertebral nerve that innervates the outer annulus.

Although the patient will report sudden onset of symptoms, usually relating to forward bending or prolonged sitting, this sudden onset is believed to be "the straw that broke the camel's back." It is much more logical to assume that the onset was insidious and related, not to one incident of forward bending or sitting, but to the repetition of these activities over time (Fig. 5-15).

The patient will report an occupation or activity that relates to a long history of a flexed lumbar posture[27,38,42,47-49]. For example, truck drivers have a higher incidence of this disorder than persons in most other occupations[42]. The symptoms will gradually worsen with pain spreading from the back to the buttock and then to the posterior thigh and calf. Typically, the patient will describe having had several episodes of increasing pain and frequency of occurrence.

Fig. 5-16 shows the development of the HNP-protrusion. The first drawing is that of a normal disc; the second depicts the development of a slight posterolateral protrusion (this condition would be painless); the third drawing shows a protrusion into the posterior rings of the annulus. It is at this stage that the patient begins to experience discogenic pain and symptoms. Note also that the nerve root is not involved at this stage. Therefore, it seems reasonable to assume that the pain which the patient is experiencing is coming from the sensory innervation of the disc itself or the surrounding soft tissues.

The clinical examination will reveal a patient

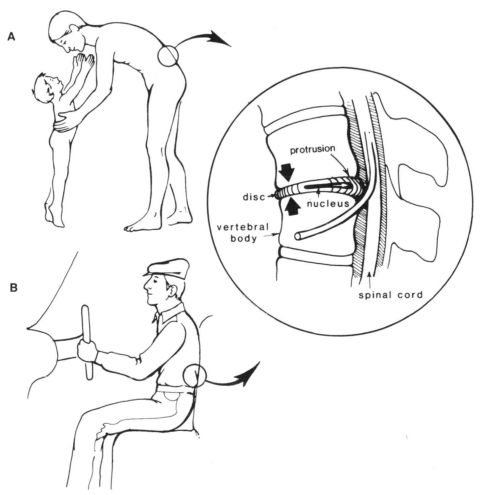

Fig. 5-15. This drawing shows what is happening in the spine with A) forward bending and B) slumped sitting (note that the bulge is not yet touching the nerve root.)

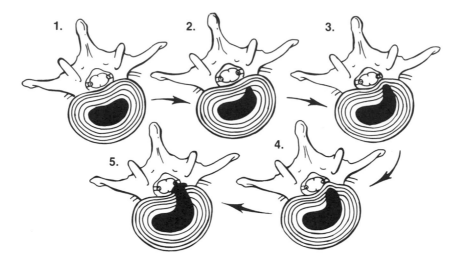

Fig. 5-16. Stages of disc herniation.

who sits in a slumped posture with the lumbar spine in flexion. He will often reach down to the chair seat with his hands to take the weight of his trunk off his lower back. The patient may have a lateral shift (lumbar scoliosis). McKenzie[27] states that 50% of the patients with this disorder have a lateral shift because of the tendency for the nuclear gel to move posterolaterally. As the gel moves posteriorly, the patient tends to shift his weight in an anterior direction, flattening the lumbar lordosis (Fig. 5-17).

He also shifts his shoulders away from the side of nuclear movement, thus producing a lateral shift (Fig. 5-18). The most important clinical features of this disorder are the flattening of the lordosis and the shift of the torso away from the painful side. Flattening of the thoracic kyphosis is also characteristic of the disorder [27, 33, 43, 50]. There will be no positive neurological signs at this stage. The involved spinal segment will be tender to palpation and routine x-rays will be negative.

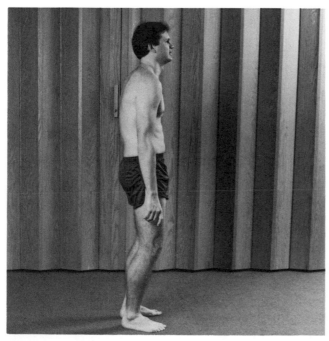

Fig. 5-17. Flattened lumbar lordosis commonly found in patients having a disc herniation with posterior or posterolateral protrusion.

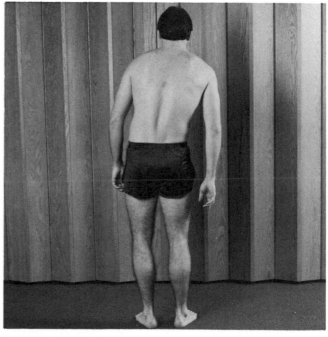

Fig. 5-18. Lateral shift commonly found in patients having a disc herniation with a posterolateral protrusion.

Some investigators imply that this HNP-protrusion indicates the early stages of disc degeneration. The exact source of pain is not well established, but there is evidence that upon intradiscal injection of hypertonic saline, it is often possible to reproduce pain similar to that which occurs naturally [14, 16, 17]. Since the recurrent sinuvertebralis nerve supplies the outermost rings of the annulus, the posterior longitudinal ligament and the duramater, it must be involved in this syndrome. The involvement of this nerve would also explain the referred pain into the extremities.

According to McKenzie, this disorder involves a situation in which the normal resting position of the articular surfaces of two adjacent vertebrae is disturbed as a result of a change in the position of the fluid nucleus between these surfaces. The alteration in the position of the nucleus may also disturb the annulus. This will cause disturbance of the normal mechanics of movement. The particular pattern will depend upon the exact area where the disturbance lies. Because the nucleus is under positive pressure at all times and slightly deforms the elastic annulus, the position of the spine in flexion or extension will add to or subtract from the pressure exerted at the posterior and posterolateral borders of the annulus. The center of the nucleus is all gel and the periphery of the annulus is all collagen fiber; one merges into the other, with the fibers becoming less dense and less frequent as one progresses into the substance of the nucleus[27] (see Chapter 4.) On extension of the spine, the intervertebral disc spaces tend to open anteriorly and close down posteriorly, thus exerting pressure on the nucleus to move it anteriorly. The converse is true with flexion (Fig. 4-1)[27, 30, 51].

McKenzie[27] theorizes that because of prolonged flexed lumbar posture and/or lifting and walking with the lumbar spine flexed, the nucleus migrates posteriorly or posterolaterally. As this condition progresses, pain sensitive structures are encountered and the patient begins to have pain in the lumbar spine (stage three of Fig. 5-16). If the condition is not corrected, it may continue to progress until the patient begins to have pain in the buttock and thigh. This may eventually progress to involve nerve root impingement.

Mechanical correction of the lateral shift will usually cause increased pain. It is important to note, however, whether the increase in pain is central in the lower back or if the increase in pain is toward the periphery. If the bulge is mild or moderate, correction of the lateral shift will cause increased pain in the central low back. Increased central pain is acceptable. If attempts at correction cause an increase in pain toward the periphery, however, they should be discontinued, at least for the present. Theoretically, if the bulge is small and the nuclear material is not displaced beyond the posterolateral edge of the vertebral body, the correction should not cause an increase in leg symptoms (Fig. 5-19).

Lumbar forward bending (flexion) is sometimes limited due to the severity of the pain and

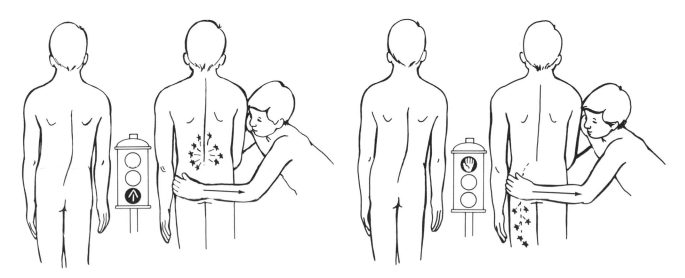

Fig. 5-19. One of these two reactions is usually seen when one attempts to correct a lumbar scoliosis when seen with HNP-protrusion. Increased central pain is acceptable; however, if attempts at correction cause an increase in peripheral pain, further attempts at correction with this method should be discontinued.

muscle guarding that may be present, but it is not uncommon for the patient to have full forward flexion mobility. When tested in the standing position, flexion will cause the pain to move peripherally. This is especially true if forward flexion is repeated several times. The pain that is produced will tend to linger for awhile after the repeated forward bending movements have been stopped. In other words, repeated forward bending causes the protrusion to enlarge, producing increased pressure on the annular wall. This enlargement does not subside immmediately, thus the tendency for the pain to linger even after the movement has stopped (Fig. 5-20).

If a lateral shift is present, it should be corrected before testing extension. Extension or backward bending after the lateral shift has been corrected will almost always be restricted and will cause increased pain. It is important to note whether the increase in pain centralizes or peripheralizes. If the bulge is mild to moderate (not displaced beyond the posterolateral edge of the vertebral body), extension may cause increased pain, but it will be central in the lower back. Let us assume for the present that extension causes increased central pain with no increase in leg symptoms (Fig. 5-21). Occasionally, extension will dramatically relieve peripheral pain.

In summary, patients with mild to moderate HNP-protrusion usually have constant pain, a reduced lumbar lordosis and limitation of lumbar extension. About 50% will have a lateral shift. If the patient is asked to perform repeated movements into flexion, the symptoms will worsen and peripheralize from the center of the spine into the leg; whereas

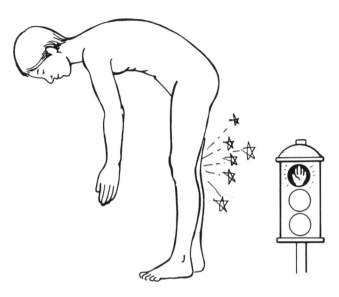

Fig. 5-20. Flexion will cause pain to move peripherally in patients who have HNP-protrusion.

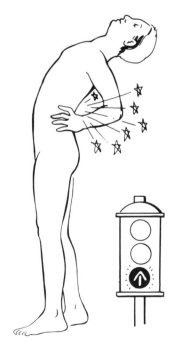 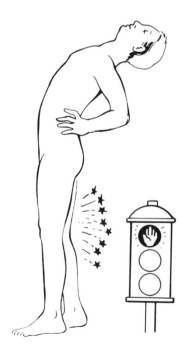

Fig. 5-21. One of these two reactions is usually seen when the patient with HNP-protrusion attempts lumbar extension. Increased central pain is acceptable; however, increased peripheral pain indicates that the condition is worsening and the movement should be discontinued.

correction of the lateral shift and extension will centralize the pain.

Treatment: McKenzie[27] advocates correction of the lateral shift and passive extension exercises to move the nucleus of the disc centrally. He also advocates constant maintenance of the correction to allow healing of the annular fibers to occur. The cardinal rule to always follow with correction of a lateral shift and the passive extension exercises which follow is: **Correction may cause increased pain in the back but must not increase the leg pain.** If the peripheral pain is increased by this corrective maneuver, it indicates that either the bulge is not being reduced by the maneuver or that the nerve root is being pulled or pushed onto the bulge by the maneuver. In either case, it is wrong to proceed. Any activity that peripheralizes the pain is probably making the condition worse, whereas something that causes pain to centralize in the lower back may not be harmful and may, in fact, be the correct thing to do. Assuming that the patient has a mild to moderate bulge, an attempt at correction should be successful.

If attempts at correcting the lateral shift in the standing position are unsuccessful, correction is attempted lying down. Sometimes elimination of the compressive force of gravity is enough to allow successful correction of the lateral shift.

Assume, then, that attempts at correcting the lateral shift are successful, in either the standing position or with the patient lying down. Fig. 5-22 shows what is believed to be happening when one is able to correct the lateral shift without increasing the peripheral signs and symptoms. One must understand that the correction is not made with one simple maneuver. Shift correction may need to be performed several times before the patient can hold the correction on his own. It then becomes the patient's responsibility over the next few days to constantly keep correcting the shift until he has successfully reduced the bulge. The methods shown in Fig. 5-23 are excellent ways for the patient to correct the shift at work or at home. All of the methods show overcorrection, which is acceptable. Assuming that the lateral shift has been successfully corrected, or that the patient did not have a lateral shift, the next step in treatment of the mild to moderate disc protrusion is passive extension exercises.

Passive extension exercises are usually started in the prone position and are progressed to the standing position as tolerated (Fig. 5-6). The first passive extension exercise simply consists of lying

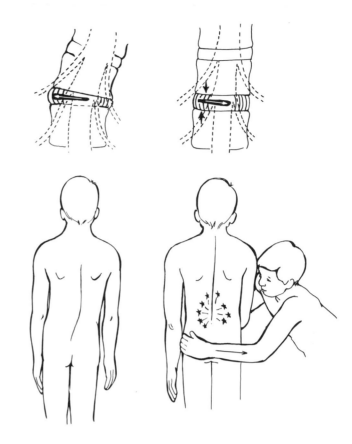

Fig. 5-22. This drawing shows what is believed to happen when one is able to correct a lateral shift without increasing peripheral signs and symptoms.

prone on a hard surface for a few minutes. This may not be necessary except for the very acute patient with a severely forward bent posture. Of course, the cardinal rule applies: if this centralizes lumbar pain, it is permissible; however, it must not increase peripheral signs. The second passive extension exercise is the "elbow prop." Here, the patient simply props himself on his elbows to allow the lower back to passively extend. A gatched treatment table is excellent for passively extending a patient in this rest position.

As the patient progresses with the passive extension exercises, he begins to do the passive press-ups. The stomach and back muscles must be completely relaxed as the patient pushes himself into an arched position. The patient is encouraged to do this exercise five to ten times, several times a day.

Often, this program will cause the patient to have dramatic relief of his leg pain and it is natural for him to become enthusiastic about doing the program because he experiences success. However, one should caution the patient not to do the exercises excessively at first because his back may

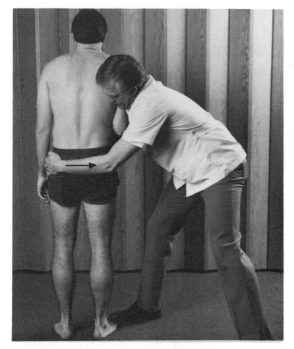
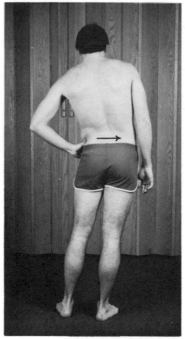
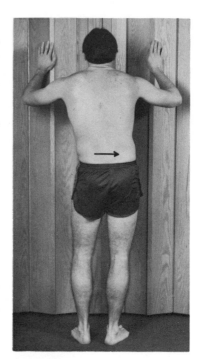

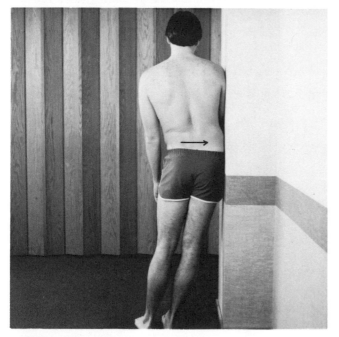
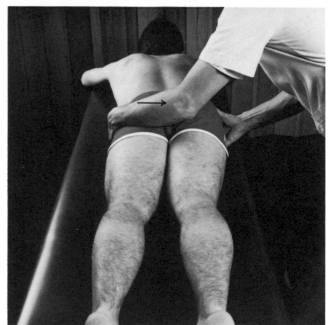

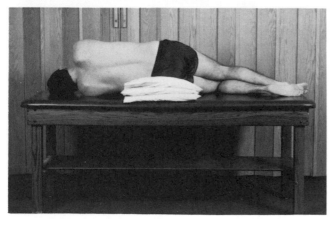

Fig. 5-23. Methods of correcting a right lateral shift.

become very sore. This, in turn, may cause increased muscle guarding and work against the patient's overall progress.

As soon as the patient has some success with the passive extension exercises in the prone position, he begins to do them in the standing position. The patient is encouraged to do this exercise four or five times, several times a day. It is very important to remember that if there is a lateral shift, it must be corrected before extension is done.

Fig. 5-24 shows what is believed to happen when the patient is able to do passive extension exercises without increasing the peripheral signs. The patient must be given clear instructions concerning the exercises and must have an understanding of what he is accomplishing with these exercises.

Fig. 5-25 shows the work of Shah[51], which demonstrates the posterior movement of the nucleus with flexion and anterior movement with extension on a cadaver specimen.

The patient must be taught to maintain the lordosis at all times in order to move the nucleus anteriorly and hold it there until healing has been effected. This means that he must use a lumbosacral corset or a lumbar roll behind his back at all times while sitting to maintain and support the lordosis and to remind him that he must not forward bend. Fig. 5-5 shows a lumbar roll that can be given to the patient. It is a foam roll approximately five inches in diameter. Small straps are attached which allow the roll to be tied to a chair or automobile seat.

Patient instructions for acute stages of herniated nucleus pulposus – protrusion consist of the following points:

1. Lordosis must be maintained at all times.

2. Bending forward will stretch and weaken the supporting structures of the back and lead to further weakening.

3. Loss of lordosis while sitting will also lead to further strain.

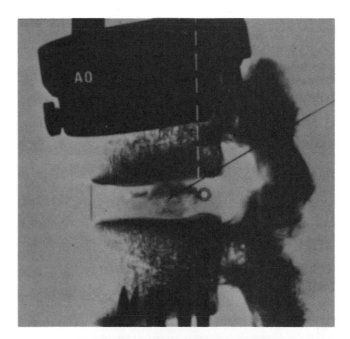

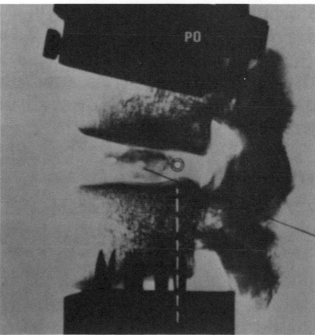

Fig. 5-25. Posterior movement of the nucleus with flexion (top) and anterior movement with extension (bottom) as demonstrated by J. Shah (reprinted with permission[51].)

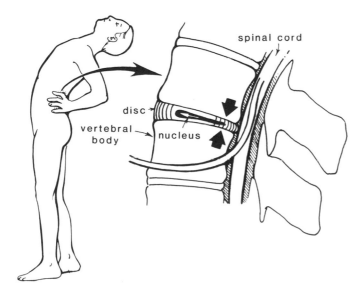

Fig. 5-24. Passive extension will reduce a small protrusion. Constant maintenance of lumbar lordosis is required to maintain this correction and allow healing to take place.

4. When in acute pain, one should sit as little as possible, and then only for short periods of time.

5. While sitting one must sit with a lordosis. This can be accomplished by placing a supportive roll in the small of the back.

6. One should try to sit on a firm, high chair if possible.

7. Avoid sitting on low, soft chairs or couches.

8. When rising from a sitting position one must maintain lordosis.

9. When in acute pain, one should drive a car as little as possible.

10. When driving a car, one should keep the seat close enough to the steering wheel to allow maintenance of the lordosis.

11. When in acute pain, one should avoid all bending and lifting.

12. If lifting cannot be avoided, one should use correct lifting techniques:
    a. The back must remain upright
    b. Stand close to the load
    c. Have firm footing and a wide stance
    d. Bend the knees and keep the back straight
    e. Have a secure grip on the load
    f. Lift by straightening the knees
    g. Lift steadily-do not jerk
    h. Pivot with the feet-do not twist

13. One should have a firm support for resting and sleeping.

14. When coughing or sneezing, stand up, bend backwards and increase the lordosis to lessen the strain[27].

The patient must absolutely avoid positions and activities that increase the intradiscal pressure or that cause a posterior force on the nucleus (flexion exercises, forward bending and slump sitting.) Exercises, mobilization or activities involving rotation must be avoided as they cause increased pressure on the disc by compressing it. Rotation also causes one-half of the oblique collagen fibers of the annular rings to become taut as the other one-half become slack. This weakens the annular structure and allows the potential for further injury.

There must be strict compliance with this program for two to ten weeks. The severity of the disorder and the initial success the patient has with the treatment program will determine the speed of recovery. There is evidence that healing of the disc can occur[12, 52-54]. The key is to reduce the bulge and then to maintain the posterior aspect of the disc in close approximation so the scar that is formed will protect from further protrusion[27, 55, 56].

Additional treatment should also be directed at pain relief and restoration of function and mobility. Modality therapy may relieve pain which, in turn, will reduce muscle guarding. Since spinal muscle guarding is a compressive force on the disc, it is important to control such guarding. Traction may also be effective in reducing the bulge[55-61]. A support or corset may be used to allow the patient more pain free activities, to aid postural correction and to reduce compressive forces on the disc[62, 63].

Patients with HNP-protrusion lose range of motion because of the bulge itself but may also become restricted because of scarring and thickening of collagen tissue in and around the disc and the facet joints (joint hypomobility.)Restoration of full mobility is a necessary component of treatment as soon as the protrusion is stable. Passive extension and flexion exercises, joint mobilization and traction are indicated if mobility is restricted. A particularly helpful technique is to passively extend the patient to the level of restriction using a gatched table and apply anterior/posterior mobilizations to the restricted segment(s). Later, active back extension exercises may be utilized to increase spinal strength and further promote correct posture (Fig. 5-7). Finally, since many of these patients have been in poor physical condition for a long period of time, a full physical fitness program should be implemented.

In the *cervical spine,* HNP-protrusion without nerve root involvement is seen less commonly or, at least, the clinical picture is less well defined. As previously discussed, many patients with cervical-upper thoracic signs and symptoms are seen with the classical forward head posture syndrome and when this postural fault is corrected, relief of symptoms is noted. Also, the progression of pain from central to peripheral (neck pain versus shoulder and arm pain) is seen as the condition worsens. At any rate, in cases where the patient reports increased shoulder/arm pain with sitting (slumped, forward head posture) and with neck flexion; and centralization of pain with neck extension (head back, chin in), one may be dealing with a mild to moderate disc protrusion(Fig. 5-26).

Treatment is directed toward: 1) returning the patient to normal posture and flexibility and 2)

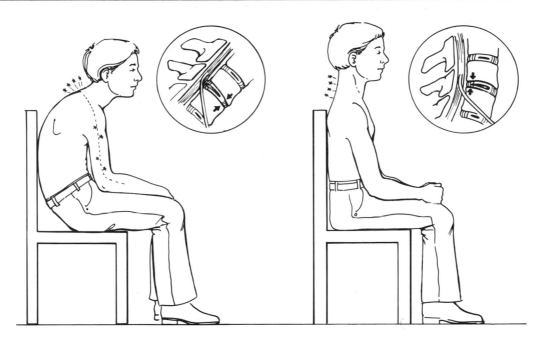

Fig. 5-26. For a patient with HNP-protrusion in the cervical spine, treatment is directed toward returning the patient to normal posture. Cervical extension exercises can help to accomplish this goal.

maintenance of correct posture to allow healing of the disc to occur. This is accomplished by starting with the head back, chin in exercises shown in Fig. 5-11 and progressing to passive cervical extension exercises (Fig. 5-27). Normal cervical lordosis must be maintained. This requires a fiber or feather pillow that can be shaped to maintain the desired amount of support while sleeping. Solid foam pillows are not recommended because some muscular tension is required to maintain the head position. Full flexibility and strength must be restored. Since slumped sitting is often associated with forward head

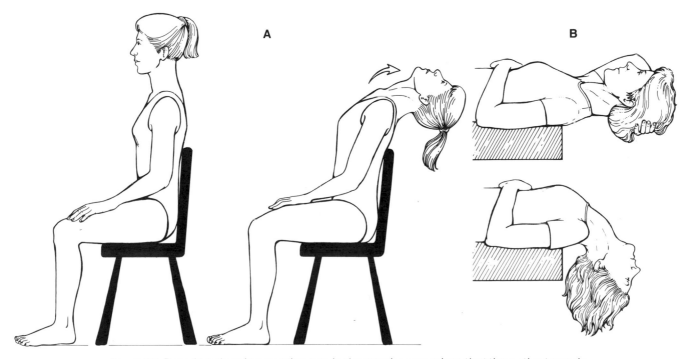

Fig. 5-27. Drawing showing passive cervical extension exercises that the patient can do to gradually restore full extension mobility to the lower cervical spine. A) Sitting and B) Supine.

posture, use of a lumbar roll and a full back and neck strengthening and flexibility exercise program is necessary (see Figs. 5-7, 5-12, 5-13 and 5-14).

NERVE ROOT SYNDROMES

Nerve root syndromes are classified as disorders caused by impingement or irritation of the spinal nerve root. They are characterized by the fact that they produce true neurological signs and symptoms.

As previously discussed, referred pain may arise from any pain-sensitive structure in the spine. It can be felt along the general distribution of the nerve roots involved. Referred pain is certainly not a true neurological finding. Nerve root pain tends to be felt as a deep, burning pain that is specific to one spinal nerve root sensory distribution, whereas referred pain is felt as a superficial aching pain that is somewhat more diffuse, tending to cover two or three dermatomes. For example, if one is experiencing referred pain because of a disc protrusion of the L5-S1 disc, the pain may be felt in the sensory distribution of both the L5 and S1 spinal nerves. This is because branches of the recurrent sinuvertebral nerve from both the L5 and S1 levels supply the L5-S1 disc. If a disc protrusion at the L5-S1 level is impinging or irritating the S1 nerve root, the nerve root pain produced is specific to the S1 sensory distribution. Of course, in the latter example, referred pain would also be present along with the spinal nerve root pain.

HERNIATED NUCLEUS PULPOSUS-PROTRUSION (WITH NERVE ROOT INVOLVEMENT)

HNP-protrusion with nerve root involvement is described as a condition in which the nucleus is bulging but is still contained within the annulus and/or posterior longitudinal ligament. The bulge is large enough to encroach into the spinal canal and/or the intervertebral foramen and is capable of impinging upon or irritating the nerve root[31].

The patient with a *lumbar* HNP-protrusion who was a candidate for mechanical correction with extension exercises and principles was presented earlier. This patient was a candidate for lateral shift correction and extension exercises because when these were attempted, there was no increase in peripheral signs. Now, however, the bulge or pro-trusion worsens and attempts to correct the lateral shift or to do extension exercises increase the signs and symptoms. If the patient otherwise has all the signs and symptoms of a disc protrusion, it is possible that the protrusion is now bulging beyond the posterior edge of the vertebral bodies and that extension or correction of the lateral shift cannot reduce the bulge. When this is the case, traction and other management techniques may be necessary before extension principles are applied. In other words, the patient has exactly the same disorder that was presented earlier, but the protrusion is simply larger (Fig. 5-28), and is probably pinching or irritating the nerve root. The patient will have all of the signs and symptoms previously discussed, with the addition of positive neurological signs such as strength loss, decreased muscle stretch reflexes, loss of sensation and a positive straight leg raise test. A radiograph may now show a narrowed disc space. Also, spinal flexion in the recumbent position may afford relief of some symptoms. This is because flexion draws the annulus taut and may bring the bulge away from the nerve root (Fig. 5-29).

Occasionally, the onset is sudden with no previous history of spinal pain, but it is more common to see disc herniation with signs of nerve root involvement as a gradually worsening condition that first appears without nerve root involvement.

Fig. 5-30 shows the bulge in relation to the nerve roots. In nearly all cases, the bulge will encroach upon the nerve root that is descending in the spinal canal to make its exit at the segmental level below the bulge. An L5-S1 bulge impinging upon the S1 nerve root is the most common example. An L4-L5 protrusion would most likely impinge directly upon or laterally upon the L5 nerve root. While it is possible that the bulge can encroach upon the nerve root that is making its exit at the same level as the bulge, this is unusual. If such is the case, the bulge usually lies medial and inferior to the nerve root. It is important to understand the relationship of the bulge to the nerve roots because this provides another explanation of why a patient may develop a lateral scoliosis. Finneson theorizes that if the bulge is lying lateral to the nerve root, the patient may shift to the opposite side in order to take the nerve root away from the bulge. Assuming that the bulge is encroaching upon the nerve root as shown in Fig. 5-30A, the patient would shift to the right. When the bulge is lying medial to the nerve root, the patient may shift toward the side of the

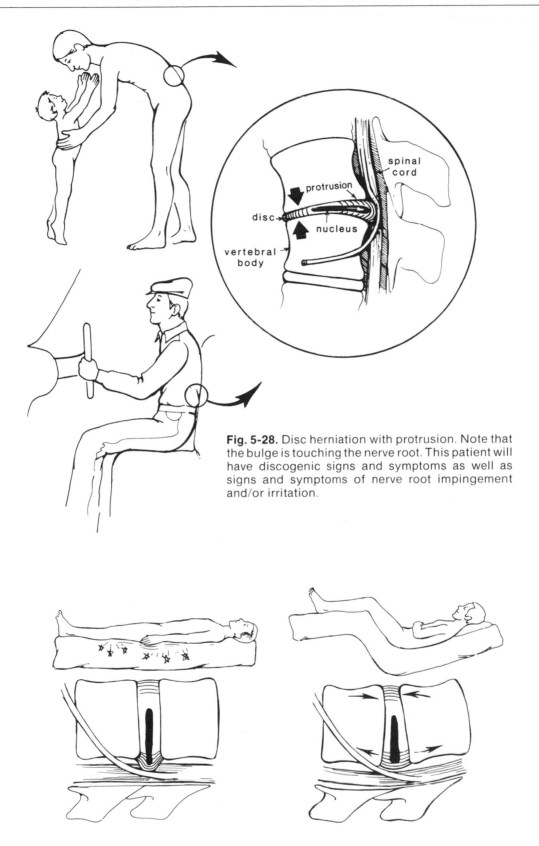

Fig. 5-28. Disc herniation with protrusion. Note that the bulge is touching the nerve root. This patient will have discogenic signs and symptoms as well as signs and symptoms of nerve root impingement and/or irritation.

Fig. 5-29. Drawing showing the effect of supine flexion on a disc protrusion that is touching the spinal nerve root. This may give the patient relief because it is drawing the bulge away from the nerve root and may be used carefully in the acute stage of treatment to relieve pain and muscle guarding. However, it is considered an ineffective, even potentially harmful, treatment in the long run because it further stretches the posterior annulus.

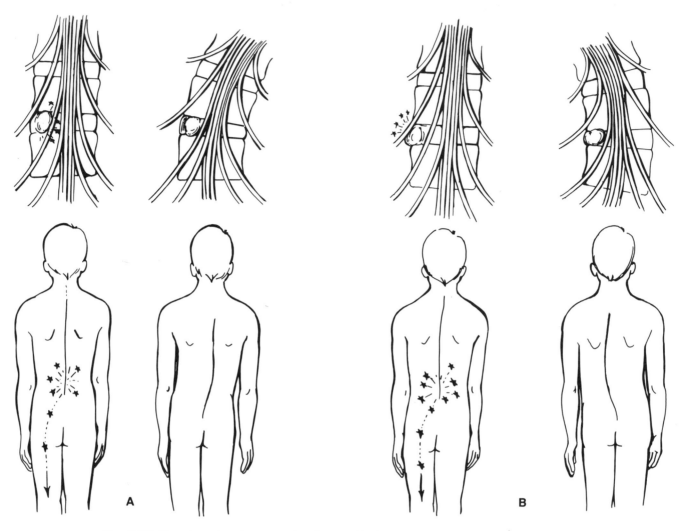

Fig. 5-30. Drawing showing a protective scoliosis sometimes seen in a patient with HNP-protrusion. If the bulge is lateral to the nerve root it is encroaching upon, the patient may experience relief by leaning away from the side of his symptoms (A). If the bulge is medial to the nerve root it is encroaching upon, the patient may experience relief by leaning toward the side of the symptoms (B).

symptoms. The example in Fig. 5-30B shows a bulge medial to the nerve root with the patient shifting to the left. Finneson calls this phenomenon "protective scoliosis". One can see that any attempt to correct the protective scoliosis will cause the nerve root to be forced back onto the bulge which would most likely increase peripheral signs and symptoms. One should also be aware that if traction is attempted with a patient in a protective scoliosis, the spine will be straightened which, again, would cause increased peripheral signs and symptoms. In such cases, traction may be beneficial in reducing the bulging disc but must be done in such a way as to preserve the protective scoliosis. In other words, unilateral or three-dimensional traction is necessary in these cases in order to apply the traction force without straightening the spine [64, 65] (see Chapter 9.)

Figs. 5-31 and 5-32 show what may happen when correction of a lateral shift or extension are attempted with a large protrusion. As these maneuvers are attempted, some of the disc material may be trapped instead of reduced. This is likely to cause the bulge to protrude further and the patient will experience increased peripheral signs and symptoms. In any case, if lateral shift correction or extension cause increased peripheralization of signs and symptoms, further attempts at doing these maneuvers should be stopped. If peripheralization occurs, treatment should include traction to reduce the bulge, which may then facilitate the use of the extension principles described earlier.

Treatment: Traditionally, at least in America, conservative treatment of HNP-protrusion has consisted of flexion positions, flexion exercises, bed

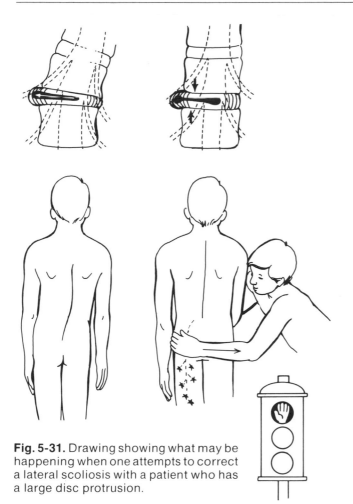

Fig. 5-31. Drawing showing what may be happening when one attempts to correct a lateral scoliosis with a patient who has a large disc protrusion.

traction and rest. Our rate of success has been poor when we recognize that there is an average of 350,000 to 450,000 back operations done in this country every year [42, 50]. These figures are eight times higher per capita than in European or Scandinavian countries [50, 66].

It is now evident that flexion positions and exercises are potentially harmful for the patient with HNP-protrusion [27, 30, 33, 51]. However, there are some reasons to believe that the recumbent flexed posture may give the very acute patient some relief. If the spine is flexed, the posterior wall of the annulus is drawn taut, which could very well take the bulge off the nerve root (Fig. 5-29). This posture may afford the patient some initial relief, but while there is separation posteriorly, there is also compression anteriorly and this could stop the disc from returning to its normal position. Nachemson[29] has shown that flexed positions increase intradiscal pressure and, from his studies, one must assume that the overall intradiscal space is also decreased. However, if the patient is in an acute state of pain with muscle guarding, this flexed, recumbent posture may be necessary in order to allow initial relief. The recumbent position also eliminates the compressing force of gravity when compared to sitting or standing postures. Also, the patient is often medicated with muscle relaxants, anti-inflammatory and pain medications while undergoing this type of treatment. All of these combined factors may give the patient considerable relief. However, the flexed

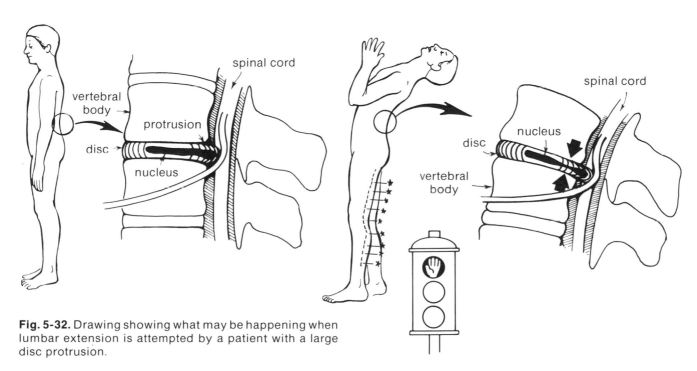

Fig. 5-32. Drawing showing what may be happening when lumbar extension is attempted by a patient with a large disc protrusion.

position is not productive in the long run and should only be used for the very acute patient. Once some pain relief is accomplished, attempts should be made to bring the patient out of the flexed posture and to restore the normal lordosis (extension principles.)

During the past 30 years while the Americans were treating the HNP-protrusion patient with rest, bed traction and flexion principles, Dr. James Cyriax and other English, European and Scandinavian physicians and physical therapists were using a different approach. In 1950, Cyriax reported that the laminectomy rate at St. Thomas Hospital in London had fallen from one in 40 patients to one in 200 patients who had been diagnosed as having a herniated disc. He advocated, in an article published in the British Medical Journal, sustained, prone pelvic traction of up to 200 pounds for ten to 20 minutes as the treatment of choice for the herniated disc. He further advocated that, after the traction had reduced the bulge, the patient be locked into an exaggerated hyperlordosis until healing of the disc was accomplished[55]. Similar references can be found in Canadian and European literature [56, 57]. Fig. 5-33 shows a disc herniation being reduced by traction[58].

Dr. James Mathews, another English physician, did studies utilizing epidurography to show that traction forces reduce the extent of a lumbar disc protrusion. Of even more importance, Mathews showed that there was a movement of the contrast medium beyond the line of the posterior longitudinal ligament into the disc space. This suggests that the traction causes a suction force on the bulging nucleus. Fig. 5-34, from Mathews' work, shows convincing evidence that a suction force is created on the nuclear material by the traction force. This work was done with a prone static traction force of 120 pounds for 20 minutes [59, 61].

In 1978, Gupta and Ramarao[57] reported clinical improvement in 11 of 14 patients with HNP who were treated with traction. Figs. 5-35 and 5-36 show disc herniations being reduced with traction. Gupta and Ramaro also show, using epidurography, evidence of the protrusion being reduced in the patients who showed clinical improvement, while they were unable to show a change in the protrusion in the patients who did not improve clinically. They also included extension exercises in the treatment protocol. Chapter 9 describes traction techniques in detail.

If a protrusion is reduced with traction, it is still unstable and the patient must not aggravate the condition for a period of time. It must be em-

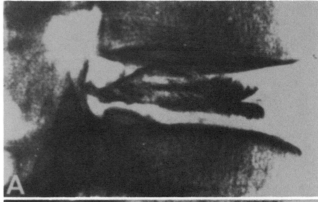
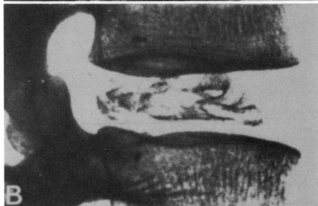
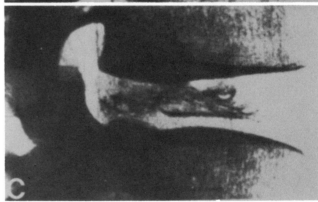

Fig. 5-33. A discogram showing a disc protrusion being reduced by traction. The top view is before traction, the middle view is during traction and the bottom view is after traction has been released (reprinted with permission from Levernieux[58].)

phasized that traction alone is usually ineffective and that a total treatment regimen must be followed or the patient will not achieve a lasting benefit. And, as with all of the previously discussed treatments and techniques, if traction increases peripheral signs and symptoms, it must not be continued.

Total management often involves passive extension exercises as soon as they can be done without increasing peripheral signs and symptoms. In other words, if the traction is successful in reducing the extent of the bulge, the patient may

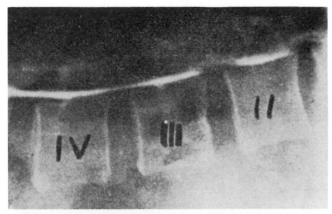

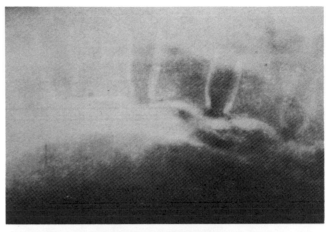

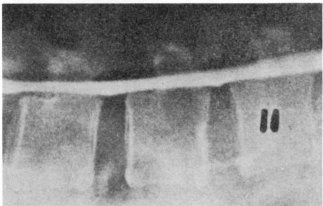

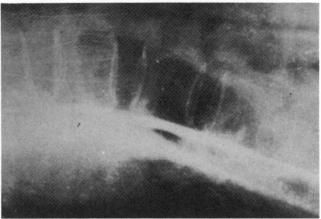

Fig. 5-35. This example is of a 35 year old woman who complained of backache with bilateral sciatica for 6 months. The clinical examination before traction revealed a bilateral positive straight leg raise test at 60° without sensory deficit. The quadriceps muscle stretch reflex was absent on the right. The photo is of lateral epidurograms showing bulging defects before traction (top) and disappearance of the defects at all levels after traction (bottom.) The clinical examination after traction revealed a bilateral positive straight leg raise test at 90° (copied with permission from Gupta and Ramarao[57].)

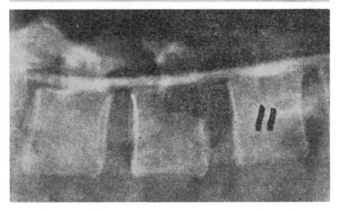

Fig. 5-34. (top) Before traction, showing bulging defects at L1-2, L2-3 and L3-4; (middle) During traction — "dimpling" of the contrast medium into the disc spaces; (bottom) Fourteen minutes after release of traction there is a partial return to the initial appearance (reprinted with permission from Mathews[59].)

then become a candidate for extension exercises and extension principles. At the very least, attempts should be made to restore the normal lordosis as the patient is able and the forward bent and slumped sitting postures should be avoided. Patients are very often slow in returning to the passive extension exercises, but they do respond well to sitting with the lumbar roll and attempting to gradually increase

their lordosis when sitting or standing. Obviously, they should avoid slumped sitting and forward bending completely at this stage.

In separate studies, Nachemson and Morris[62] and Morris, Lucas and Bresler[63] have shown that with a garment such as a lumbosacral corset, which compresses the abdomen, intradiscal pressure is diminished by approximately 25%. This significant unloading of the disc occurs in both the standing and the sitting positions. It is accomplished because the corset increases the intra-abdominal pressure and causes the abdominal cavity to become a weight bearing structure. The steel stays within the corset should be bent into a normal or hyperlordotic

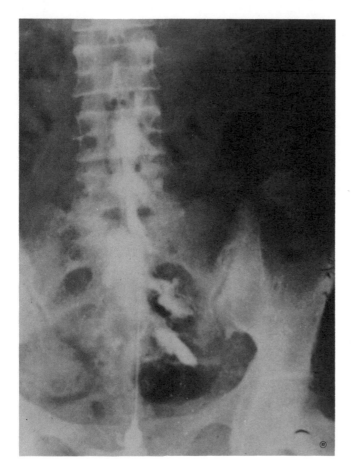 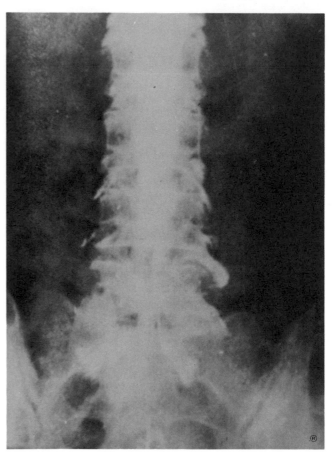

Fig. 5-36. This example is of a 40 year old woman who complained of backache with sciatica for 4 months. The clinical examination before traction revealed a positive straight leg raise test at 50° on the left. The woman had a sensory loss over the S1 distribution and an absent gastrocnemius-soleus muscle stretch reflex on the left. Posterior-anterior epidurograms show a well-defined lateral defect at the left L5 disc level before traction (left) and a normal epidurogram after traction (right.) The clinical examination after traction revealed a positive straight leg raise test at 90° bilaterally. There was no change in the sensory loss, but the gastrocnemius-soleus muscle stretch reflex was present. The woman complained of mild backache post-traction (copied with permission from Gupta and Ramarao[57].)

position and the patient should be instructed to maintain that posture at all times. The corset is especially helpful in that it reminds the patient to avoid forward bending and slumped sitting and to maintain good posture (Fig. 10-1).

Attention again must be directed toward positions and activities that cause increased intradiscal pressure. Fig. 4-3 shows that forward bending and sitting are the most hazardous positions. Also, active exercises such as straight leg raising, active back extension and, especially, sit-ups are contraindicated at this time[29]. Twisting or rotating the spine must be avoided for two reasons. First, rotation causes a narrowing of the intervertebral space and produces increased intradiscal pressure[29]. Also, as rotation of the spine occurs, there is a

relaxation of one-half of the oblique annular fibers while the other one-half are drawn taut. This puts the disc in a vulnerable position for injury.

Fig. 5-37 summarizes all of the treatment considerations for HNP-protrusion. When combined with a comprehensive educational program, these principles can be effective in treating moderate to severe protrusions. Usually, one will know within a few treatments if this program is going to be effective. There is no set length of time that is necessary to effect a complete cure, but it will usually take six to ten weeks before the patient is able to return to strenuous activities, especially those involving forward bending and/or prolonged sitting. The number of traction treatments necessary are few, as excessive treatments of traction may cause

---

Treatment:
HNP (PROTRUSION)
with nerve root impingement

Relieve compressing forces
— **Reduce muscle guarding (modalities)**
  (rest)(avoid aggravation)(medication)
— **Avoid positions that increase intradiscal**
  pressure (sitting)(forward bending)
— **Bracing**

Reduce herniation
— **Traction**

Maintain correction
— **Extension principles — Patient education**
— **Bracing — Avoid manipulation**

Fig. 5-37. Successful treatment of HNP-protrusion involves a comprehensive approach.

increased soreness in the back. For the first two or three weeks, the lumbosacral corset is used at all times when the patient is up. The patient is gradually weaned from it and may use it in the first few weeks

as he returns to work. Later, usually six to ten weeks after the initiation of treatment, the patient can be started on the back strengthening exercises shown in Fig. 5-7. The patient should start these exercises carefully and gradually build into a vigorous back strengthening program. Tight hamstring muscles can prevent the pelvis from flexing over the hip joint during forward bending, causing increased stress on the disc. If this is the case, hamstring stretching becomes a vital part of the rehabilitation program. Eventually, overall physical fitness for the improvement of flexibility, strength and endurance should become the goal of this total program. Surgical intervention (discectomy or chemonucleolysis) may be indicated if this management program fails and if there are signs of progressive neurological deficits, or loss of bowel and/or bladder function.

In the *cervical spine,* HNP-protrusion with nerve root involvement is less common than in the lumbar spine and the clinical picture is less well defined. Cervical nerve root syndromes are most common at the C5-C6 segment and involve the C6 nerve root. In most cases, cervical nerve root syndrome is caused by degenerative joint/disc

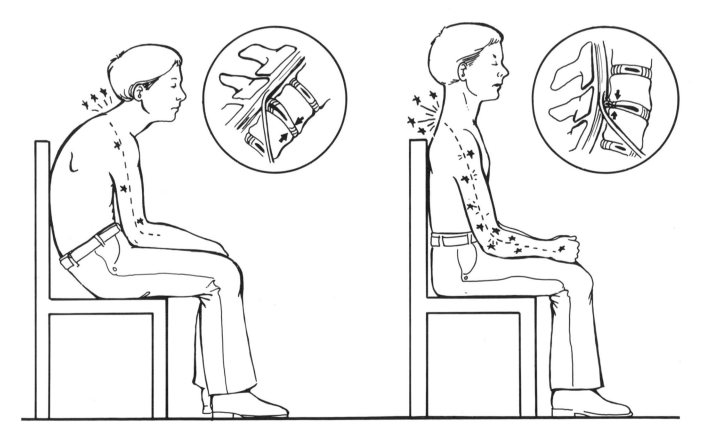

Fig. 5-38. Drawing showing what may occur if a patient with a large cervical HNP-protrusion attemps extension.

disease rather than by disc protrusion. Often, an x-ray, CAT scan or myelogram may be necessary to determine the diagnosis.

The clinical picture of cervical HNP-protrusion is one of gradual worsening with the symptoms starting centrally at the base of the neck, then spreading to the shoulder and the arm as the condition worsens. Pain is also referred to the upper thoracic spine and a trigger point may be found lateral to the T4 segment. Later, positive neurological signs appear. The slumped, forward head posture is usually seen with this disorder and attempts to do axial extension or to do backward bending of the cervical spine increase the peripheral signs and symptoms (Fig. 5-38). The x-ray may be normal or may show very slight narrowing of the disc space. This is a clue that one is dealing with HNP-protrusion rather than degenerative joint/disc disease.

Treatment goals are to reduce the protrusion with traction and maintain the correction by restoring normal posture until the disc heals. Initial attempts at restoring normal posture may be unsuccessful, but when combined with traction, may be possible. Manual traction combined with passive axial extension and/or passive backward bending exercises is often effective (see techniques in Chapters 8 and 9.) Mechanical traction may have to be done with some degree of flexion initially, but as improvement is noted, the angle of pull should be reduced in an effort to regain normal posture. Other treatment, as outlined earlier under the section on cervical HNP-protrusion without nerve root involvement, is indicated as the patient progresses.

HERNIATED NUCLEUS PULPOSUS-EXTRUSION OR SEQUESTRATION

HNP-extrusion is defined as the disorder in which the displaced nuclear material extrudes into the spinal canal through disrupted fibers of the annulus (Fig. 5-39). HNP-sequestration is defined as the condition in which the nuclear material escapes into the spinal canal as a free fragment(s) which may migrate to other locations[31]. Patients with an

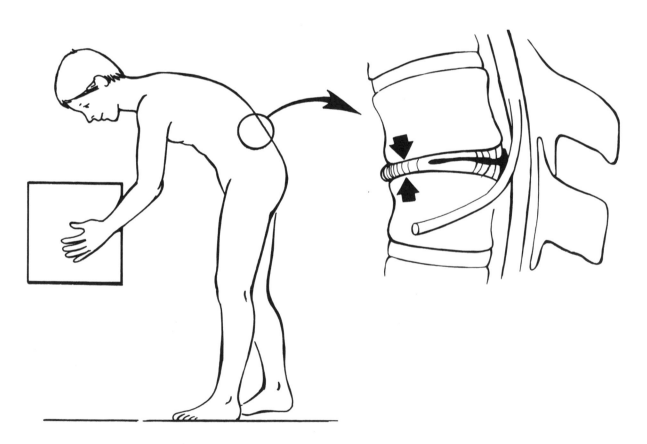

Fig. 5-39. Drawing showing HNP-extrusion. The patient with this disorder will probably have peripheral signs and symptoms which predominate over the signs and symptoms in the spine.

extrusion or sequestration will have similar histories, signs and symptoms as patients with HNP-protrusion except that the peripheral signs and symptoms will likely be predominant over the spinal signs and symptoms[67]. The patient will often have a gradually worsening history, beginning with HNP-protrusion *without* nerve root signs and symptoms, progressing to HNP-protrusion *with* nerve root signs and symptoms and, finally, to HNP-extrusion or sequestration. At this stage, there is no longer pressure on the annular wall and the pain arising from the disc bulge itself will be diminished while the signs and symptoms of nerve root irritation and/or impingement may be increased. For example, at the extrusion stage the patient's back pain may be gone and sitting may be comfortable.

Treatment: No particular form of physical therapy treatment is effective at this stage except, perhaps, electrotherapy for pain relief. Flexion exercises and the flexed recumbent position may afford relief but will not be of lasting benefit and could, theoretically, cause further extrusion of nuclear material. If extension causes increased peripheral signs and symptoms, it is contraindicated, but if extension principles can be applied without increasing the peripheral signs and symptoms, they should be implemented, but cautiously. By restoring and maintaining normal lordosis one would assume that the defect in the annulus is being closed and the disc will have a better chance to heal. A lumbosacral corset should be utilized to help reduce intradiscal loading and to remind the patient to avoid forward bending and slumped sitting. A wait-and-see attitude is justified as these disorders sometimes become "quiet" with time. However, if there are signs of possible nerve damage, surgical intervention is indicated.

Clinically, one occasionally sees what appears to be an extruded or sequestered disc (predominance of peripheral signs and symptoms) respond well to a combination of traction and extension principles. This causes one to conclude that the condition was really only a protrusion and points out the importance of a trial of physical therapy in all such cases. In other words, one cannot be certain clinically whether a condition is a disc protrusion, extrusion or sequestration and the trial of physical therapy treatments helps establish the final diagnosis.

Fig. 5-16 shows the stages of disc herniation. Stage one is normal. Stage two shows slight movement of the nuclear gel. The patient would be pain free at this stage. Stage three shows a mild to moderate protrusion. At this stage the patient may have back and leg pain but no positive neurological signs. Extension exercises and principles are usually effective treatments at this stage. Stage four shows a protrusion that is bulging and impinging against the nerve root. The patient has back pain, leg pain and positive neurological signs. Treatment includes traction, bracing, extension exercises and principles and the other measures presented in this chapter. Stage five shows disc extrusion and sequestration. In this stage, the back and leg pain diminish as the neurological signs usually increase and traction becomes ineffective.

POST-LAMINECTOMY/DISCECTOMY/CHEMONUCLEOLYSIS

Long term results from laminectomy/discectomy and chemonucleolysis are very often disappointing[37,38]. Several follow-up studies of patients who underwent laminectomies show that five years later, 50% of them were no better or worse than they were before the operation. The reason may be because little or no attention is directed toward restoring normal posture, flexibility, strength and physical fitness. Often, nothing is done to educate or motivate the patient concerning proper body mechanics or other changes of lifestyle that will be necessary if he is to have a reasonably healthy back following surgery. The surgical procedure may have removed or dissolved the disc herniation, but it has done nothing to correct the poor posture, faulty body mechanics, stressful living and working habits, loss of flexibility and poor physical fitness which are the **real** causes of the problem. Therefore, a full rehabilitation program should be implemented for all patients who have had surgery. This program should start with restoration and maintenance of normal posture (extension principles) and eventually involve a full flexibility, strengthening and fitness program.

Sometimes patients who have previously had back surgery begin to have signs and symptoms indicating that another disc disorder is developing. In such cases, treatment protocol need not be altered because of the fact that the patient has had surgery. In other words, if extension principles and/or traction are indicated because of the signs and symptoms, they should be given. The only exception is the patient who has had a recent (within one year) spinal fusion or a complete laminectomy. In these cascs, the surgeon should be consulted concerning specific treatment before proceeding[68].

DEGENERATIVE JOINT/DISC DISEASE (LATERAL STENOSIS)

Degenerative joint/disc disease may occur with or without neurological complications. It is classified here as a disorder in which true neurological signs are present. The term which describes this disorder is lateral spinal stenosis. The advent of the CAT scan seems to be attracting renewed attention to this disorder.

The reason nerve root impingement may occur with this disorder is threefold: First, it may be due to a decrease in size of the intervertebral foramen because of disc space narrowing; second, it may be due to osteophytic and bony changes in and around the foramen; and third, it may be due to hypertrophy, thickening and bulging of the ligamentum flavum and other soft tissues in and around the intervertebral foramen (Fig. 5-40 and 5-41). There may or may not be a disc herniation present. Because of the compression of the facet joint which occurs with narrowing of the disc space, joint hypomobility will usually be seen along with this disorder. Other signs and symptoms of degenerative joint/disc disease were discussed earlier. Degenerative joint/disc disease is most common in older persons and is most commonly seen in the cervical spine. As previously stated, this disorder accounts for most nerve root syndromes in the cervical spine.

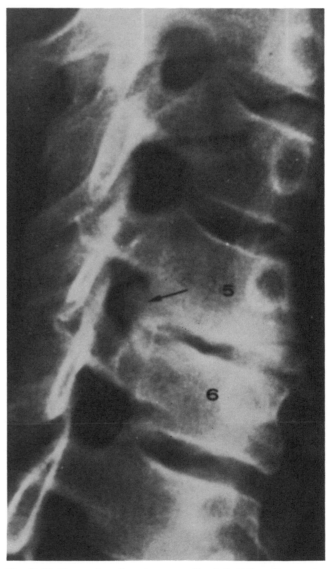

Fig. 5-41. X-ray showing degenerative joint/disc disease in the cervical spine. This disorder accounts for most nerve root syndromes seen in the cervical spine (reprinted with permission from Peterson and Kieffer[69].)

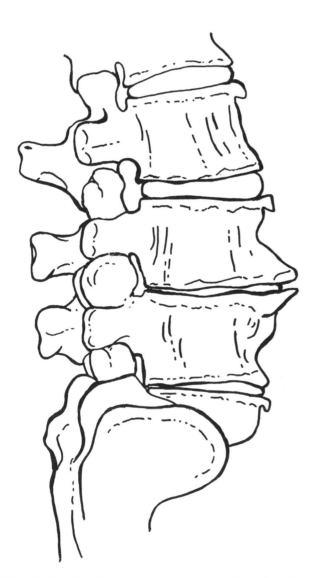

Fig. 5-40. Drawing showing degenerative joint/disc disease (lateral stenosis) in the lumbar spine.

Treatment described earlier for degenerative joint/disc disease consisted of mobilization, manual or mechanical traction, flexibility and strengthening exercises and modalities. All of these methods of treatment may be applicable in this case also. Caution should be used with joint mobilization because it may increase nerve root irritation. Traction is probably safer than mobilization at this stage.

Since many of these patients are restricted in both spinal flexion and extension (forward and backward bending), exercises to increase mobility in both directions are indicated, provided they do not aggravate the degenerative joint/disc disease or any nerve root irritation. Many practitioners have avoided extension exercises with these patients because they believed that extension would close the foramen, further irritating the nerve. While it is true that extension does close the foramen in a normal, healthy spine, it is questionable whether the foramen closes at a spinal segment where there is already narrowing of the disc space and the facet joints are already in their maximum close packed position (full extension.) If the facet joints are indeed in maximum extension, then further extension recruitment will take place about an axis at the joints themselves and only *widening* can occur at the intervertebral foramen and disc spaces (Fig. 5-42). Therefore, both flexion and extension exercises should be attempted with this disorder and those which give relief of signs and symptoms should be utilized. Clinical experience shows that the response to these exercises can only be determined by assessment of the patient's reaction to them individually (see previous discussion of flexion versus extension exercises for patients with degenerative joint/disc disease without neurological involvement.)

NERVE ROOT SWELLING AND INFLAMMATION (NEURITIS)

Nerve root swelling and inflammation may be severe enough to cause impingement or irritation

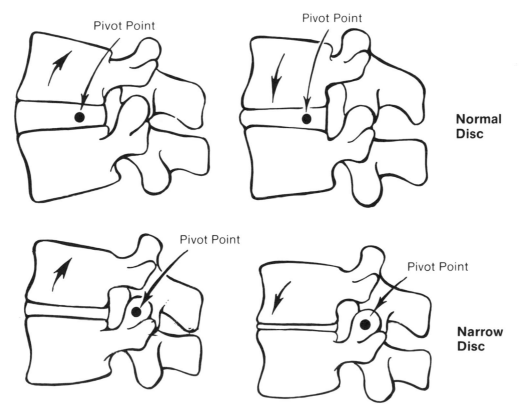

Fig. 5-42. Drawing showing that spinal flexion and extension occur about an axis slightly posterior to the nucleus in a spinal segment with a normal disc, but that the same movements may occur about an axis within the facet joint when a narrow disc is present. This implicates that flexion widens and extension narrows the intervertebral foramen with a normal disc, but that the reverse may be true in the presence of a narrow disc space.

within the intervertebral foramen; this will produce true positive neurological signs.

Nerve root swelling and inflammation can have an insidious onset of unknown etiology or can accompany joint and muscle inflammation. This condition is usually seen within a few days following severe injury as an inflammatory response to the injury.

Treatment should be similar to that used for other inflammatory disorders. Measures to maintain normal posture and promote healing and a gradual return to full strength and mobility as healing occurs are the important aspects of treatment. Although traction is sometimes prescribed for this disorder when it accompanies an acute cervical strain (whiplash), it should be avoided because the extent of any ligamentous damage cannot be determined at this stage and traction may overstretch already damaged ligaments.

NERVE ROOT ADHESIONS

Occasionally, the spinal nerve root becomes entrapped by scar tissue. Probably the most common occurrence of this disorder is seen following spinal surgery. As a preventive measure, many surgeons are now mobilizing the spinal nerve root following surgery by advocating a program of passive straight leg raising, starting the day following surgery and continuing until appreciable healing is accomplished. Nerve root adhesions may also form following an episode of disc herniation. As the body attempts to heal the bulge or defect in the annulus, collagen tissue is laid down. If the nerve root is lying in proximity, it may become entrapped by the scar tissue. Thus, historically, the patient with nerve root adhesion is likely to have had spinal surgery or, at least, a history of disc herniation. He is likely to still have at least some of the signs and symptoms of the previous disability or he may have had a period of complete recovery with subsequent insidious onset of spinal pain and/or referred pain with or without positive neurological signs. The outstanding diagnostic characteristic of this syndrome is the **marked absence of lumbar flexion in standing** versus little or no restriction of lumbar flexion when tested sitting or supine, bringing the knees to the chest. The straight leg raising test will also show the restriction. In other words, when the lumbar spine alone is flexed, no restriction is present, but when the spinal nerve is pulled through the intervertebral foramen, such as in forward bending while standing or straight leg raising, the restriction will be shown. Other classical disc protrusion signs and symptoms, such as increased pain with sitting, will not be present.

Treatment for this disorder consists of mobilizing the nerve root adhesion by passive straight leg raise stretching. Unilateral lumbar traction is also especially beneficial for this disorder. Prevention of this disorder, by passive straight leg raising exercises soon after surgery and other rehabilitation measures described earlier for the post-laminectomy/discectomy patient, is of the greatest importance.

MISCELLANEOUS DISORDERS

CONGENITAL ABNORMALITIES

One often sees patients with various disorders such as lumbarized sacral vertebrae, sacralized lumbar vertebrae, assymmetry of the facet joints or other congenital anomalies. The clinical signs and symptoms that these patients have are quite varied and do not seem to present a clear clinical picture that can be consistently related to a definable pathological disorder. In other words, except for the radiological evidence, it is difficult to determine the real significance of many of these congenital anomalies. It is this author's belief that, except as these anomalies contribute to joint hypermobility or hypomobility or, perhaps, to degenerative joint/disc disease, they are insignificant and are often unrelated to the patient's real problem. In fact, there is a certain danger in diagnosing one's condition by the radiological findings when there is no direct cause and effect relationship established during a complete evaluation and assessment. When a patient is told he has a congenital anomaly or "birth defect" in his back, will he be as likely to carry out the self-help program that he has been given? Perhaps everyone would be better off not knowing that these probably insignificant abnormalities exist in the first place. Certainly, caution should be used when applying this cause and effect relationship to cases such as degenerative joint/disc disease (lateral stenosis) and spondylolisthesis. One should always be on guard against the temptation to use one or two isolated findings as the basis for a diagnosis.

TRAUMATIC FRACTURES

It is this author's belief that x-rays need not be taken of every patient who complains of spinal pain.

However, when trauma is involved, a radiological exam is absolutely necessary to determine whether or not a fracture is present.

Treatment: Management of spinal fractures is not within the scope of practice for a physical therapist. When a spinal fracture has healed, however, it is important to evaluate strength, mobility and posture and rehabilitate the patient as needed.

COMPRESSION FRACTURES- OSTEOPOROSIS

Although osteoporosis is associated with dorsal and lumbar spinal pain, it is not likely to be a cause of symptoms by itself. The pain associated with osteoporosis is probably caused by the presence of fractured bone (compression fracture) and the resulting pressure on nerve roots or upon sensory fibers in the periosteum. Osteoporosis has many known causes; the majority are classified as post-menopausal and senile. Genetic abnormalities, nutritional dysfunctions, endocrine disorders, corticosteroids, pregnancy, prolonged immobilization, inactivity and weightlessness are all known causes of osteoporosis[46].

Diagnosis of compression fracture is by x-ray. The patient will often have sharp pain that may be referred with or without signs of nerve root compression. In the acute state the pain will be especially sharp with movement. Flexion of the spine is usually painful, is harmful and should be avoided. A single thoracic compression fracture will be characterized by the presence of a prominent spinous process and a wide interspinous space below the prominent spinous process. Multiple thoracic compression fractures are characterized by progressive increase of kyphosis, which can eventually lead to severe disability.

Treatment: In most cases, only the anterior portion of the vertebral body fractures, creating a wedge. If the posterior aspect of the body has fractured, management must be directed by an orthopaedic surgeon on an individual basis. Therefore, the assumption here is that one is dealing with an anterior compression fracture only, and that the posterior edge of the vertebral body is structurally intact.

Education of the patient concerning positions and activities that are beneficial or potentially harmful is absolutely necessary. Active and passive extension exercises are indicated as soon as the patient's pain has decreased to the point that he can tolerate them (see Figs. 5-6 and 5-7). All positions and activities involving spinal flexion must be avoided. Modalities such as moist heat and electrical stimulation may relieve some of the pain.

SPONDYLOLISTHESIS

Spondylolysis is a defect involving the pars interarticularis of the neural arch of the vertebra. When the defect in the neural arch is bilateral, separation of the anterior and posterior elements at the site of these defects may occur. This displacement is called spondylolisthesis. The most common site for occurrence is L5 on S1.

Diagnosis is by x-ray, but clinically, a "step-off" of the spinous processes may sometimes be appreciated. The patient will often have hyperlordosis and complain that prolonged standing increases pain, sitting relieves it and various types of vigorous physical activities aggravate the condition. The original onset of symptoms can often be traced back to athletic or other vigorous physical activities. There is almost certainly a congenital weakness associated with this disorder, and it is thought that the defect actually occurs as a stress fracture. Many people have spondylolisthesis and are symptom-free. It is important to remember that once a diagnosis of this nature is made, the diagnosis may seem to "follow" the patient. There may, however, be another cause for the patient's complaint. For example, there is an increased incidence of herniated disc at the level above the spondylolisthesis in patients who have this disorder, yet it often goes undiagnosed because it is assumed that the patient's complaint is related to the spondylolisthesis[69].

If a spondylosisthesis is the true cause of a patient's symptoms, it will probably be because the segment is unstable and aggravation is due to the excessive movement and stress at the segment when physical activities are attempted. If, on the other hand, a spondylolisthesis is stable, it will probably not be the source of the patient's complaint. Frequently, in the presence of an unstable spondylolisthesis, the patient will describe a slipping sensation or movement occurring in the back when assuming a certain position or doing certain activities. As previously mentioned, a step-off can often be felt when palpating the spinous processes. If the spondylolisthesis is unstable the step-off can usually be felt when the patient is standing and side lying, but it will disappear when the patient lies prone with pillows under the lumbar spine.

Treatment: The presence of this disorder makes the patient more vulnerable to joint sprains and muscular strains, and such a patient may need to avoid heavy labor and vigorous physical activities. General postural improvement is necessary, especially abdominal muscle strengthening and other flexion exercises. It is often necessary to fit the patient with a lumbosacral support or brace to be used when performing any activities that may aggravate the condition. In such cases, a chairback spinal brace may be effective in immobilizing the involved segments or at least may serve as a reminder to the patient that vigorous activity should be limited.

In a hyperlordotic state, or in the case of obesity and weak abdominals, the vertical shear forces between the two elements which are slipping apart is greatly magnified. Reduction of the hyperlordosis can reduce the shear forces. These patients can often be effectively managed in a brace designed to reduce the lumbar lordosis and/or with flexion exercises with an emphasis on abdominal strengthening.

Children in their preteen ages indulging in sports requiring excessive lumbar lordosis (i.e., gymnastics) and teenagers indulging in contact sports are more frequently found to have spondylolysis. The assumption is made that the break in the pars interarticularis represents a stress fracture. If a bone scan demonstrates an increase in metabolic activity over the pars interarticularis, this assumption is justified. Such patients can be treated with the use of a brace that reduces the lumbar lordosis in an attempt to heal the stress fracture. There are not suffucient data to confirm that such healing takes place, although pain can readily be eliminated. In patients whose scans are not "hot", the assumption is made that nonunion has resulted. If pain is a problem in these cases, a lumbar brace often provides relief[46]. During acute episodes, rest and modality treatments are indicated. If the displacement is great enough there may be signs of neurological impingement of the cauda equina. In such cases, Cyriax advocates traction[70]. Surgical fusion may be necessary in severe cases.

SPINAL STENOSIS

In the past two decades, encroachment upon the *cervical* spinal cord resulting from a stenotic cervical spinal canal has been generally accepted as a recognizable clinical entity. This disorder is characterized by neurological symptoms that may initially lead to diagnosis of multiple sclerosis or other neurological diseases[71]. Mixed hyper- and hypoactive reflexes are sometimes observed in the upper extremities, depending upon the level of encroachment. Hyperactive reflexes may be observed in the lower extremities. There may be paresthesia, pain and motor weakness in the extremities. Symptoms are aggravated by extension of the neck. There are a number of ways encroachment can occur. Annular protrusions of the cervical disc, osteophytes, folding or bulging of the ligamentum flavum, subperiosteal thickening over the vertebral body and the laminal arch and congenital smallness of the spinal canal are all factors. Smith states that a combination of these factors is frequently involved[71].

Lumbar spinal stenosis is also known as Neurogenic Intermittent Claudication of the Cauda Equina. This disorder has received increased emphasis in the past few years. Spinal stenosis occurs much the same way in the lumbar spine as it does in the cervical spine in that it is usually associated with degenerative joint disease and a combination of factors that act together to diminish the size of the spinal canal (Fig. 5-43).

The chief symptoms are pain in the lower back and one or both legs, numbness and tingling in the feet and legs, decreased muscle stretch reflexes and motor weakness in the legs. Often these symptoms are present only after walking and are relieved by rest and/or flexing the lumbar spine. Spinal extension produces an overall decrease in the volume of the lumbar spinal canal and increased nerve root bulk. Bulging of the ligamentum flavum is also most pronounced in spinal extension. Based on this

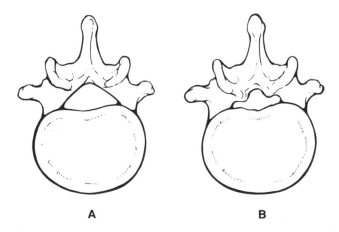

A   **B**

Fig. 5-43. Drawing showing A) a normal spinal canal and B) a reduced size spinal canal. This reduced size is usually caused by a combination of degenerative changes and congenital smallness.

information it is easy to see why the symptoms are most pronounced when the patient is standing or lying flat with the lumbar spine extended. Blau and Logue state that the ultimate mechanism that produces the symptoms is vascular insufficiency of the cauda equina nerve roots[72].

Treatment centers around educating the patient to avoid aggravating or irritating the disorder. A soft collar or lumbar support is often helpful. Physical therapy modalities may provide temporary relief of pain. Measures to increase mobility and flexibility (exercises and/or traction) are sometimes helpful. A decompression laminectomy is indicated in severe cases.

SACROILIAC DISORDERS

Sacroiliac disorders are often present with lumbar spine and/or hip joint problems. This makes the evaluation process more difficult, but is another aspect of spinal pain/dysfunction which the therapist must consider. The sacroiliac is difficult to assess properly, the mechanics of which go beyond the scope of this text. However, some basic concepts are presented for the sake of completeness.

Movement at the sacroiliac may be thought of as actually occurring at two joints, depending on whether the spine is weight bearing or non-weight bearing:

1. Iliosacral — These movements are those of the ilia (innominate) moving on the sacrum and usually involve an anterior or posterior rotation, with a posterior rotation being the most common. In essence, one-half of the pelvis moves in relation to the other half. These movements may range from 3-18mm[30] and may be assessed fairly easily by the clinician or on x-ray through changes in the anterior-posterior diameter of the brim.

2. Sacroiliac — These movements are those of the sacrum within the ilia and may occur on one or more of the several axes of motion which have been identified. Normally, the sacrum should simply flex and extend (nutate and counternutate) during forward and backward bending and respiration.

In a person with a dynamic spine (curvatures pronounced), the sacrum tends to lie in a more horizontal position within the ilia and is quite mobile. Conversely, in a person with a static spine (curvatures de-

creased), the sacrum lies in a more vertical position and is less mobile. Dysfunctional movements usually take the form of torsions about oblique axes, rotations about a vertical axis, tilts about an anterior-posterior axis and flexion-extension about transverse axes. Torsions and flexion lesions are the most common.

Of the two functional joints, iliosacral and sacroiliac, iliosacral dysfunctions are more common and more easily treated. Therefore, the remaining discussion will address this type of lesion only; however, since it is really one aspect of the entire sacroiliac joint, it will be called such for simplicity.

Since the sacroiliac joint is a synovial joint, it can be injured in the same manner as any other synovial joint. In other words, any of the following disorders can develop at the sacroiliac joint: 1) sprain; 2) inflammation; 3) hypomobility; 4) hypermobility; 5) degenerative joint disease or 5) subluxation.

Quite often when there is a lesion in the sacroiliac joint, the patient reports pain and tenderness in the region medial to the posterior-superior iliac spine. The patient may report falling backward onto the ischial tuberosity (posterior rotation of the ilium on the sacrum) or tripping, stumbling forward or twisting (anterior rotation of the ilium on the sacrum.) Perhaps the most common mechanism of injury is the forward bend with the knees locked in lifting. This produces a posterior rotation lesion. A sprain/inflammation may be the result of this type of injury or the joint may become subluxed. As healing of the sprain occurs, hypomobility may develop. Sacroiliac hypermobility is common in pregnant or post-pregnant women. This disorder is easily aggravated and many of these patients report a general soreness across the sacroiliac joints. Hypermobility frequently allows the joint to become subluxed or "stuck" in either anterior or posterior rotation.

When a subluxation is present, there may be a noticeable change of alignment at the pubic symphysis (Fig. 5-44). The structural exam will frequently show uneven iliac crests and posterior-superior iliac spines with level anterior-superior iliac spines and trochanters. Special evaluation techniques are helpful in determining if the problem is in the sacroiliac joint. These include the spring test, the long-sitting leg length versus supine leg length test

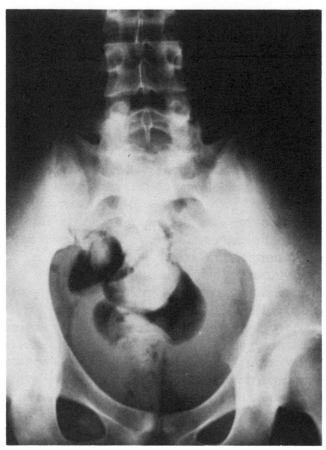

Fig. 5-44. X-ray showing change of alignment of the public symphysis that sometimes occurs with sacroiliac subluxation.

and sacroiliac mobility tests (see Chapter 3.)

Treatment should include mobilization if the joint is hypomobile. Modality therapy may be helpful to relieve pain and/or promote healing. Strapping or support is often helpful if the joint is hypermobile or with an acute sprain (see Chapter 10.) If subluxation has occurred secondary to joint hypermobility, manipulation will be necessary to reduce the subluxation (see Chapter 8.) Stabilization with a sacroiliac support will then be necessary to allow the joint to heal and regain normal structural integrity. This may take many weeks or even months to accomplish.

ANKYLOSING SPONDYLITIS

Ankylosing spondylitis is characterized by progressive joint sclerosis and ligamentous ossification which first appears in the sacroiliac joints and later spreads into the lumbar and thoracic spine and rib cage. In severe cases the cervical spine and hip joints may also become involved. Onset typically occurs between 20 and 35 years of age and first appears as a vague lower back pain and stiffness which is usually worse upon waking and eased by exercise. The symptoms are intermittent with episodes lasting for weeks or months at a time. The onset of each acute episode seems to be insidious, unrelated to exertion or activities. Complete ankylosis of the involved joints may eventually occur. This eases pain, but may lead to disability depending upon the position the joints are in when they become fixed. The younger the patient is at onset, the worse the prognosis; men usually do worse than women[33].

Clinically, one sees a flattening of the lumbar lordosis and increased rounding of the thoracic and cervical spine. Since the two upper cervical joints are affected later, hyperextension may be seen here in contrast to the tendency otherwise for a spinal flexion deformity to develop. In severe cases, if the hip joints also become fixed in flexion, the patient may become seriously disabled. Certain laboratory tests (elevated sedimentation rates) may be helpful in diagnosis. X-ray diagnosis may be possible only after several years, with the earliest abnormalities being seen in the sacroiliac joint [33, 46].

Treatment: Patient education is of great importance. If the patient is young at the onset of the disease, it is important to direct him toward a career that does not involve heavy work. It is best to tell the patient that the spine will eventually stiffen in a way that does not interfere with sedentary work, and that the pain is controllable.

Certainly, positioning and exercises to resist the gradual development of the flexed spine (and hip joints, in severe cases) play an extremely important part. The patient must sleep on a firm mattress and should avoid lying curled up on his side or using more than one pillow when lying supine. Some prone lying is necessary and both the passive and active extension exercises outlined in Figs. 5-6 and 5-7 should be emphasized. Use of the lumbar roll (Fig. 5-5) when sitting and avoidance of prolonged sitting and flexion postures is recommended. Manual mobilization to maintain spinal extension is also indicated and can often be taught to family members. Use of a lumbar support, medication and physical therapy modalities may be helpful during acute episodes[33].

COCCYX

Injury to the sacro-coccygeal joint may occur as a sprain, subluxation or fracture. As healing occurs, the joint gradually becomes sclerosed and passive movement becomes restricted[73]. The classic patient will be one who has been to many doctors and has had very little help. The patient will have a history of a fall directly on the coccyx or a childbirth injury. The x-ray may show a healed fracture. The patient will be unable to sit on both buttocks at the same time. External and internal examination will reveal tenderness to palpation of the coccyx and mobility of the coccyx may be very limited or absent.

The normal coccyx flexes while sitting and extends when standing; when the coccyx is injured, it may heal in the more extended position and become hypomobile, or it may become subluxed and heal in extension (i.e., childbirth.) If this happens, the soft tissue directly over the end of the coccyx develops a painful pressure point when the patient sits.

The coccyx can also be dislocated or fractured and heal in a flexed position or become fragmented or unstable in a flexed position. This disorder can be diagnosed by palpating the position of the coccyx and testing the passive mobility of the sacro-coccygeal joint, or it may be diagnosed by radiological exam.

Treatment: Surgical removal of the coccyx may be indicated if it is hypermobile (unstable) or dislocated in a flexed position. The physical therapist can expect good results with ultrasound and passive mobilization along with other conservative management, such as a coccyx pillow, if the joint is hypomobile/subluxed and positioned in extension (see Chapter 8.)

LEG LENGTH DISCREPANCIES

Leg length discrepancies are classified as either being true (actual bony assymmetry due to fracture, growth abnormalities, coxa vara/valga, etc . . .) or functional (positional due to a pronated foot, genu valgus, tight adductor muscles, sacroiliac lesions, etc . . .) One must determine the cause of the leg length discrepancy before deciding if the disorder can be treated.

A lumbar scoliosis (convexity toward the short leg) will develop secondary to an uneven leg length (Fig. 5-45A). This will cause unequal biomechanical stresses on the structures of the spine and can, over a long period of time, contribute to the development of adaptive muscle shortening, ligamentous and capsular hypomobility, degenerative joint disease

and, at least theoretically, to disc protrusion. The adaptive muscle shortening and joint hypomobility will develop on the concave (long leg) side. Degenerative joint disease develops in the facets on the concave side and osteoarthritic (traction) spurring has been observed on the convex side. If a disc protrusion develops, it will most likely be toward the convex (short leg) side.

When assessing active mobility of the lumbar spine in the presence of uneven leg length, one must correct the leg length discrepancy by placing a lift under the foot of the short leg before any observation is made.

Treatment involves correcting the cause (i.e., sacroiliac subluxation) or compensating for it with the use of a shoe lift. If the problem has been long-standing and adaptive muscle shortening and joint hypomobility are present, *one must be absolutely certain that full mobility, strength and normal posture are restored. Correcting uneven leg length in the presence of joint hypomobility will not correct the lumbar scoliosis and, in fact, will increase the compensatory or secondary thoracic curve (Fig. 5-45).* Therefore, treatment such as ultrasound, unilateral lumbar traction, positional traction, joint mobilization and home exercises are a necessity in these cases to restore full mobility.

Although full correction of any consistently measurable leg length discrepancy is the final goal, it may be advisable to make corrections gradually as mobility, strength and normal posture are being regained. Sometimes small corrections are made with a heel lift only. While this does correct standing leg length, it does not correct the discrepancy at toe-off during gait. Therefore, correction with the use of a heel lift only is often not adequate treatment.

SYSTEMIC DISEASE AND REFERRED PAIN FROM THE VISCERA

Venereal disease, gout, lupus erythematosis, rheumatoid arthritis and urological infections are among the systemic diseases that can cause spinal pain. Metastatic lesions can be a source of pain and pain can also be referred from visceral structures.

Increased pain with rest and during the night, pain that is not associated with movement or body position, pain of insidious onset, pain covering large, non-specific areas and pain migrating from one joint to another are all signs of systemic or visceral origins and should alert the physical therapist that he may not be dealing with a musculoskeletal disorder. Changes in the general health of the patient such as weight gain or loss, fever or previous carcinoma are indications of systemic diseases. In addition, any patient who does not respond in a timely fashion to a reasonable trial of physical therapy treatment should be suspected of having a systemic disease or a visceral problem. Although the diagnosis of these disorders is the responsibility of the physician, the physical therapist should be aware of signs and symptoms unique to these disorders and in the absence of any musculo-skeletal findings, the patient should be referred to the physician for further evaluation and assessment.

SUMMARY

It has been the purpose of this chapter to show that many factors contribute significantly to spinal pathology and that each disorder has its own unique pathology and should also have its own unique treatment plan. An attempt has also been made to

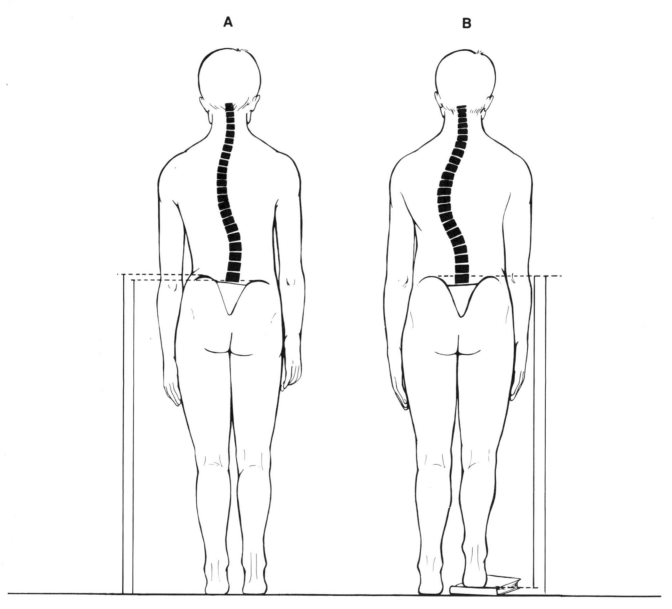

Fig. 5-45. A leg length discrepancy is shown on the left. If the condition has been present for a long period of time, joint hypomobility and adaptive muscle shortening may have developed on the concave side of the lumbar scoliosis. If this is the case, correction of the discrepancy with a shoe lift will not change the lumbar scoliosis and may actually cause the secondary curve in the thoracic spine to worsen. Full mobility (flexibility) must be restored to the spine if the shoe lift is to be an effective treatment.

show that although each disorder is unique, many are related, in that one disorder may eventually progress to another, more serious disorder if left untreated (Fig. 5-46). It also must be stressed that clinically, the patient often presents more than one of these disorders at the same time.

There is no substitute for a complete and thorough evaluation and assessment of the patient before planning an effective treatment program. Likewise, there is no substitute for complete and thorough knowledge of spinal pathology before making a meaningful evaluation and assessment.

Interrelationship of Certain Spinal Disorders

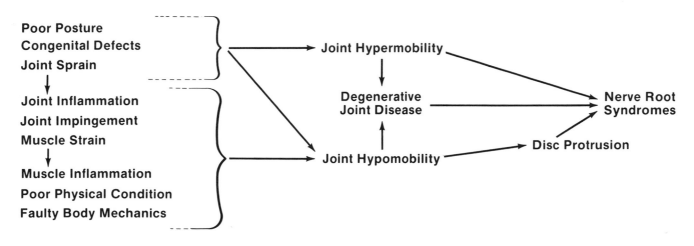

Fig. 5-46. Drawing showing the interrelationship of certain spinal disorders.

CLASSIFICATION OF MUSCULOSKELETAL SPINAL PATHOLOGY

(Chart reads across to next page.)

CONDITION	HISTORY	STRUCTURAL EXAM	MOBILITY EXAM
MUSCLE			
Muscle Spasm Muscle Guarding	Is present with all painful spinal conditions. May need to be treated before primary condition can be evaluated and treated. Is not considered a primary condition itself.	Musculature stands out. Protective scoliosis or torticollis.	Generalized restricted movement.
Acute Muscle Strain Contusion	Onset traumatic (heavy lift or blow) or aggravation from repeated activity. Movement aggravates. Rest relieves but stiffens.	Normal.	Restricted & painful active movement. Painful resisted movement. Passive mobility tests normal. Tortuous recovery.
Muscle inflammation (Myositis)	Onset insidious often following strain. Pain & stiffness with rest as well as movement.	Normal.	As above.
JOINT			
Facet Joint Impingement (Blockage) (Subluxation) (Fixation) (Locking)	Sudden unguarded movement. Very little trauma. Rest relieves, movement hurts.	Normal unless protective scoliosis, torticollis or other postural change.	Specific loss of active & passive mobility. Cervical = side bending and rotation pain/ restriction will be in same direction. Lumbar-Thoracic = side bending and rotation pain/ restriction will be in opposite directions.
Acute Joint Sprain	Sudden onset. Mild to severe trauma. Rest relieves, movement hurts.	As above.	Localized loss of active & passive mobility with pain.
Joint Inflammation	Insidious onset. Often follows joint sprain. Migrating pain. Pain & stiffness with rest as well as movement.	Normal.	Localized loss of active & passive mobility with pain.
Chronic Postural Strain/Sprain	Gradual onset over several years. Rest relieves. Pain comes on after standing or sitting several hours. (End of day)	Sway Back Flat Back. Slump Sitting. Forward Head.	General hypermobility. (Sway Back) Loss of extension mobility (Flat Back & Forward Head)
Joint Hypomobility (Dysfunction)	Sprain, strain or fracture that has healed, or some other immobilization. Pain associated with movement. Associated with chronic working postures. Industrial worker, male.	Flat back postures.	Localized loss of active & passive mobility.
Joint Hypermobility (Instability)	Long standing postural problem. Severe trauma. Overuse of manipulation. Hypomobility nearby. Describes joint "movement". Athlete. Female.	Hyperlordosis	Excessive movement at certain levels.
*Degenerative Joint/Disc Disease (Osteoarthritis) (Spondylosis)	Long standing pain & stiffness. Old spinal injury. Pain with movement. Frequent episodes of impingement, sprain and/or inflammation.	Normal.	Loss of active & passive mobility at one or more levels. Is sometimes hypermobile instead of hypomobile.
*Disc Herniation — Protrusion	Forward bending. Slump sitting. Sitting increases pain. Difficulty standing up. Walking relieves.	Decreased lordosis. Slump sitting. Lateral shift.	Decrease of extension mobility. Extension centralizes pain. Flexion peripheralizes pain.

Chart compiled by H. Duane Saunders.

*Without neurological complications.

CLASSIFICATION OF MUSCULOSKELETAL SPINAL PATHOLOGY (Continued)

NEUROLOGICAL EXAM	PALPATION EXAM	OTHER SIGNS & SYMPTOMS	SUGGESTED TREATMENT
Normal.	Muscles tense. Muscles may be tender to palpate if condition has been present for a few days or more. Pain spreads and spans several spinal levels. Stance Shift Test (+).	X-ray (-). Lab (-).	Look for primary cause of pain. Moist heat, short wave diathermy, electrical stimulation, ice, cold packs, and/or massage.
Normal.	Muscle palpation painful. Joint palpation painless. Spans several segments. Unilateral pain. May radiate distally.	X-ray (-). Lab (-).	Acute ⁻ support, rest, ice. Subacute = gentle movement, heat & massage. See that full mobility, strength and posture are restored as healing takes place.
Normal.	As above, except often bilateral. Temperature and color changes? Painful area spreads.	X-ray (-). Lab (-).	Rx same as acute muscle strain/contusion.
Normal.	Tender to palpate one joint. Unilateral pain. May radiate distally. Positional changes (pinch test).	X-ray (-), except mobility x-ray. Lab (-).	Modalities to relieve pain and guarding. Treat with mobilization.
Normal.	Tender to palpate joint(s). May radiate distally.	As above.	Acute = support, rest, ice. Subacute = mild mobilization, heat, ultrasound, massage. Restore mobility, strength and posture as healing takes place.
Normal.	As above.	X-ray (-). Lab (-).	Acute = rest & modalities. Subacute = ultrasound, gentle mobilization. Restore mobility, strength and posture as healing takes place.
Normal.	Bilateral spinal pain often referred bilateral. Pain covers large area. Cannot pinpoint pain.	X-ray (-). Lab (-).	Postural exercises. General conditioning exercises. Modalities for symptomatic relief. Brace or support extreme cases.
Normal.	As above. Thick, dry skin and subcutaneous tissue. Thickened supraspinous ligament.	As above.	Ultrasound. Mobilization. Traction.
Normal.	Tender to palpate joint(s). Unilateral or bilateral pain. May radiate distally. Generalized pain.	X-ray diagnosis? Patient changes position frequently.	Muscular strengthening & posture training. Brace or support. Modalities for symptomatic relief. Look for hypomobility nearby.
Normal.	As above. Thickened supraspinous ligament.	X-ray diagnosis. Often symptom free.	Treat hypo or hypermobility as appropriate. Brace or support as last resort.
Normal.	Tender to palpate joint(s). Bilateral spinal pain referred unilaterally.	X-ray (-). Lab (-).	Modalities to control muscle guarding. Correct lateral shift. Extension exercises & principles. Traction. Support to allow activities. Patient education to avoid further injury and recurrence. Lumbar pillow.

CLASSIFICATION OF MUSCULOSKELETAL SPINAL PATHOLOGY (Continued)

(Chart reads across to next page.)

CONDITION	HISTORY	STRUCTURAL EXAM	MOBILITY EXAM
NERVE ROOT			
*Disc Herniation — Protrusion	Forward bending. Slump sitting. Sitting increases pain. Difficulty standing up.	Decreased lordosis. Slump sits. Lateral shift.	Decrease of extension mobility. Extension/shift correction may peripheralize pain.
Disc Herniation — (Extrusion or Sequestration)	Previously had disc herniation (protrusion) signs & symptoms. Sitting now ok. Standing may be worse.	Normal.	Extension may peripheralize pain.
*Degenerative Joint/Disc Disease	Long standing pain & stiffness. Old spinal injury. Pain with movement. Frequent episodes of impingement, sprain and/or inflammation.	Normal.	Loss of active & passive mobility at one or more levels. Is sometimes hypermobile. Usually hypomobile.
Nerve Root Adhesion	Surgery. Disc herniation. Sitting (-).	Normal.	Loss of standing lumbar flexion, but sitting or supine lumbar flexion normal.
Nerve Root Swelling (Neuritis)	Insidious onset. Present with joint or muscle trauma, and/or inflammation.	Normal.	Vague limitation of active & passive mobility.
MISCELLANEOUS			
Fractures	Trauma. Sharp pain with movement. Aching pain at rest.	Normal.	Guarded, vaguely limited.
Osteoporosis (Compression Fracture)	Variety of metabolic problems. Onset of pain following compression, cough, forward bend, or lifting. Sharp pain with movement.	Increased Kyphosis?	Generalized limited movement. General weakness.
Spondylolisthesis	Stress fracture. Congenital defect. Frequent episodes of strains & sprains. Heavy physical labor/athletics Describes joint "movement".	Hyperlordosis?	May be hypermobile or stable.
Spinal Stenosis (Cervical) (Lumbar)	Long history of problem. Degenerative joint disease. Lumbar symptoms come on only after exercise in the standing position. Flexion relieves. Extension aggravates.	Normal.	Generalized restricted mobility.
Sacroiliac	Fall on ischial tuberosity or tripping, twisting injury. Other injury or aggravation. Pregnancy. Anterior hip pain.	Uneven sacral base.	Mobility tests may be hypomobile or hypermobile. Sacroiliac spring tests (+).
Coccyx	Old history of injury or fall on coccyx. Childbirth injury. Cannot sit on both buttocks at the same time.	Normal.	Internal examination reveals hypomobility in extension, or hypermobility and subluxation in flexion.

Chart compiled by H. Duane Saunders.

*With neurological complications.

CLASSIFICATION OF MUSCULOSKELETAL SPINAL PATHOLOGY (Continued)

NEUROLOGICAL EXAM	PALPATION EXAM	OTHER SIGNS & SYMPTOMS	SUGGESTED TREATMENT
True neurological signs (+)	Bilateral spinal pain often referred unilaterally. Tender to palpate joint(s). Spinal pain greater than peripheral pain.	Joint space narrow. Traction relieves. Myelogram (+). Lab (-). CT Scan (+).	Heat, ultrasound to relieve symptoms & reduce guarding. Heavy traction. Extension exercises & principles. Careful return to activities. Brace or support. Patient education.
True neurological signs (+)	Same as disc herniation — protrusion, except peripheral pain and symptoms worse than spinal pain.	As above.	Probably none successful, but trial of heavy traction is necessary because this condition cannot be differentiated from other nerve root syndromes. TENS for pain. "Wait and see" attitude if neurological signs are not getting worse.
True neurological signs (+)	Tender to palpate joint(s). Thickened supraspinous ligament. Bilateral spinal pain may radiate unilaterally.	X-ray shows degeneration, narrow joint space, osteophytes. Myelogram (+). Lab (-).	Ultrasound. Heavy traction to relieve nerve root impingement and to mobilize joints. Brace or support severe cases.
True neurological signs (+), especially SLR	Normal.	X-ray (-). Myelogram (-). Lab (-).	Ultrasound. Unilateral traction. Straight leg stretch.
May have true neurological signs (+)	Generalized tenderness. Other muscle & joint signs.	X-ray (-). Lab (-).	Rest. Modalities. promote healing. Avoid aggressive treatment (traction) if history of severe trauma.
True (+) neurological signs possible	Pinpoint tenderness.	X-ray diagnosis.	Restore mobility, strength and posture after fracture has healed.
True (+) neurological signs possible	Joint tenderness. Wide space between spinous processes.	X-ray diagnosis of compression fracture. Lab to find cause? Predominance of older women.	Avoid forward bending. Hyperextension exercises. Hyperextension brace. Heat & massage for symptomatic relief. Patient education.
True (+) neurological signs possible	Joint tenderness. Palpate "step off."	X-ray diagnosis. Predominance of males. Lab (-). Some are symptom free.	Postural improvement. Strengthen abdominals. Modalities for pain relief. Brace or support severe cases. Look for other problem.
True (+) neurological signs possible Hyperactive reflexes below a cervical stenosis.	Normal.	X-ray diagnosis? DJD on X-ray. Myelogram diagnosis.	Patient education. Support with brace. Decompression surgery.
Neurological exam (-)	Tenderness over sacroiliac. Pain may be referred distally.	Long-sitting vs. supine leg-length test (+). X-ray findings? X-ray may show DJD.	Ultrasound if hypomobile. Mobilize if hypomobile or subluxed. Rest & support if acute or inflamed. Support if hypermobile.
Neurological exam (-)	Tenderness to external palpation.	Patient sits on donut cushion.	Ultrasound if hypomobile. Mobilization if hypomobile. Avoid aggravation. Surgical removal.

CLASSIFICATION OF MUSCULOSKELETAL SPINAL PATHOLOGY (Continued)

(Chart reads across to next page.)

CONDITION	HISTORY	STRUCTURAL EXAM	MOBILITY EXAM
MISCELLANEOUS (Continued)			
Ankylosing Spondylitis	Insidious onset of LB & SI pain. Morning stiffness. Improves with exercise. Young adult males. Gradually worsening — spreading.	Stands with flat lumbar spine and increased kyphosis.	Very stiff in back & SI joints. Eventually may involve all of spine and even hips.
Leg Length Discrepancies.	Old Leg Injury	Uneven sacral base. Lumbar Scoliosis.	Lumbar spine hypomobile in sidebending toward and rotation away from short leg.
Systematic Disease Pain referred from the viscera	No history of injury. Gradual onset. Pain unrelated to movement. Migrating pain. Night pain. No other musculoskeletal findings. No improvement with physical therapy.	Normal.	Normal.

Chart compiled by H. Duane Saunders.

*Without neurological complications.

CLASSIFICATION OF MUSCULOSKELETAL SPINAL PATHOLOGY *(Continued)*

NEUROLOGICAL EXAM	PALPATION EXAM	OTHER SIGNS & SYMPTOMS	SUGGESTED TREATMENT
Neurological Exam (-)	Pain over SI joints and low back. Bilateral. Vague — non specific.	Lab diagnosis. X-ray diagnosis later. May become seriously disabled in flexed posture.	Patient education. Exercises to resist the development of a flexed posture. Posture training and aides. Modalities and mobilization for acute episodes.
Neurological exam (-)	Normal.	Standing X-ray. Shows uneven sacral base and lumbar scoliosis.	Shoe lift. Mobilize hypomobility.
True (+) neurological signs possible	No pinpoint tenderness. Non-specific area of pain.	Lab diagnosis. Fever. Other related illness.	Consult physician.

References:

1. Tabary, J, et al: Experimental Rapid Sarcomere Loss in Concomittant Hypoextensibility. Muscle Nerve 4:198-203, 1981.

2. Tabary, J, et al: Physiological and Structure Changes in the Cat's Soleus Muscle Due to Immobilization by Plaster Casts. Joul Physiol 224:231-244, 1972.

3. Cummings, G: Proceedings, Ninth Annual Dogwood Conference, Atlanta, GA, 1984.

4. Mennell, J: Differential Diagnosis of Visceral From Somatic Back Pain. Joul of Occ Med 8:477-480, Sept 1966.

5. Mooney, V and Robertson, J: The Facet Syndrome. Clinical Orthopaedics and Related Research 115:149-156, March/April 1976.

6. Kos, J and Wolf, J: Intervertebral Menisci and Their Possible Role in Intervertebral Blockage. Bul of the Orth Sec Amer Phy Ther Assn, Winter 1976.

7. Kraft, G and Levinthal, D: Facet Synovial Impingement. Surg Gynecol and Obstet 93:439-443, 1951.

8. Maitland, G: Palpation Examination of the Posterior Cervical Spine: The Ideal, Average and Abnormal. Aust J Physiother 28:3-12, 1982.

9. Sprague, R: The Acute Cervical Joint Lock. Physical Therapy 63:1439-1444, Sept 1983.

10. Cailliet, R: Low Back Pain Syndrome. 2nd ed, FA Davis, Philadelphia, 1970.

11. Jayson, M and Barks, J: Structural Changes in the Intervertebral Disc. Annuls Rheum Dis 32:10-15, 1973.

12. Hirsch, D and Schajowicz, F: Studies of Structural Changes in the Lumbar Intervertebral Discs. JBJS 36B:304-322, 1954.

13. Harris, R and McNab, I: Structural Changes in the Lumbar Intervertebral Discs. JBJS 36B:302-322, 1954.

14. Hirsch, C; Ingelmark, B and Miller, M: The Anatomical Basis for Low Back Pain. Studies on the Presence of Sensory Nerve Endings in Ligamentous, Capsular and Intervertebral Disc Structures in the Human Lumbar Spine. Acta Ortho Scand 33:1-17, 1963.

15. Jackson, N; Winkelman, R and Bickel, W: Nerve Endings in the Lumbar Spinal Column. JBJS 48A:1272-1281, 1966.

16. Roofe, P: Innervation of Annulus Fibrosis and Posterior Longitudinal Ligament: Fourth and Fifth Lumbar Level. Arch Neurol Psych 44:100-103, 1940.

17. Lindblom, K: Technique and Results of Diagnostic Disc Puncture and Injection (Discography) in the Lumbar Region. Acta Ortho Scand 20:315-326. 1951.

18. Travell, J and Rinzler, S: The Myofascial Genesis of Pain. Postgraduate Med 11:425, 1952.

19. Burkart, S: Personal Communications. Physical Therapy Department, University of West Virginia, Morgantown, WV.

20. Paris, S: Course Notes. The Spine. Atlanta Back Clinic, Atlanta, GA.

21. Griffin, J: Physiological Effects of Ultrasonic Energy As It Is Used Clinically. Phys Ther 46:18-21, 1966.

22. Amato, V, et al: The Normal Vascular Supply of the Vertebral Column in the Growing Rabbit. JBJS 41B:782-795, 1959.

23. Broden, H: Paths of Nutrition in Articular Cartilage and Intervertebral Disc. Acta Orthop Scand 124:171-183, 1954-55.

24. Brown, J: Tsaltas II Studies on the Permeability of the Intervertebral Disc During Skeletal Maturation. Spine 1:240-244, 1976.

25. Holm, S and Nachemson, A: Variations in the Nutrition of the Canine Intervertebral Disc, Induced by Motion. Spine 8:866-873, 1983.

26. Kramer, J: Pressure Dependent Fluid Shifts in the Intervertebral Disc. Ortho Clinics of N Amer 8:211-216, Jan 1977.

27. McKenzie, R: The Lumbar Spine. Spinal Publications, Waikanae, New Zealand, 1981.

28. Nachemson, A: Low Back Pain, Its Etiology and Treatment. Clinical Medicine 18-24, 1971.

29. Nachemson, A: The Lumbar Spine, An Orthopaedic Challenge. Spine 1:50-71, 1976.

30. Kapandji, I: The Physiology of the Joints. Spine, Vol 3, 2nd ed, Churchill-Livingstone, London-New York, 1974.

31. A Glossary on Spinal Terminology. American Academy of Orthopaedic Surgeons, Chicago.

32. Brown, K: Personal Communication. Orthopaedic Surgeon, Miami, FL, 1983.

33. Cyriax, J: Textbook of Orthopaedic Medicine; Diagnosis of Soft Tissue Lesions. Vol 1, 8th ed, Bailliere-Tindall, London, 1982.

34. Farfan, H: Proceedings International Federation of Orthopaedic Manipulative Therapists. B. Kend ed, Vail, CO, 1977.

35. Wyke, B: The Neurological Basis of Thoracic Spinal Pain. Rheumatology and Physical Medicine, 10:356-367, 1970.

36. Nachemson, A: Low Back Pain, Its Etiology and Treatment. Clinical Medicine, 18-24, 1971.

37. Quinet, R; Hadler, H: Diagnosis and Treatment of Backache. Sem in Arth and Rheu 8:261-287, 1979.

38. Spangfort, E: The Lumbar Disc Herniation. ACTA Orthop Scand (Suppl 142):5-95, 1972.

39. Chaffin, D: Manual Materials Handling. Joul of Environmental Pathology and Toxicology 2:31-66.

40. DePalma, A and Rothman: The Intervertebral Disc. Saunders, Philadelphia, 1970.

41. Park, W: Radiological Investigation of the Intervertebral Disc. The Lumbar Spine and Back Pain, ed Jayson, Grune and Stratton, 1976.

42. Nordby, E: Epidemiology and Diagnosis in Low Back Injury. Occupational Health and Safety 50: 38-42, Jan 1981.

43. Waitz, E: The Lateral Bending Sign. Spine 6:388-397, 1981.

44. Kramos, P: New Rules to Fight Back Injuries. Health and Safety 44:42-44, 1975.

45. Cady, L, et al: Strength and Fitness and Subsquent Back Injuries in Firefighters. Joul of Occ Med 21:269-272, 1979.

46. Finneson, G: Low Back Pain. Lippincott, Philadelphia, 1973.

47. Davis, P: Reducing the Risk of Industrial Bad Backs. Occupational Health and Safety 45-47 May/June, 1979.

48. White, A and Gordon, S: Synopsis: Workshop on Idiopathic Low Back Pain. Spine 7:141-149, 1982.

49. Snook, S: The Design of Manual Handling Tasks. Ergonomics 12:963-985, 1978.

50. Spagfort, E: Personal Communication. Orthopaedic Surgeon, Huydinge, Sweden, 1982.

51. Shah, J: Structure, Morphology and Mechanics of the Lumbar Spine. The Lumbar Spine and Low Back Pain, Jayson, M, ed. , Pitman Medical, London, 1980.

52. Farfan, H: Mechanical Disorders of the Low Back. Lea and Febiger, Philadelphia, 1973.

53. Lipson, S and Juir, H: Proteoglycoms in Experimental Intervertebral Disc Degeneration. Spine 6:194-210, 1981.

54. Harris, R and McNab, I: Structural Changes in the Lumbar Intervertebral Discs. JBJS 37B:304-322, 1954.

55. Cyriax, J: Treatment of Lumbar Disk Lesions. Brit Med Joul 2:1434-1438, 1950.

References: (Continued)

56. Parson, W and Cummings, J: Mechanical Traction in the Lumbar Disc Syndrome. Can Med Assoc Joul 77:7-11, 1957.
57. Gupta, R and Ramarao, S: Epidurography in Reduction of Lumbar Disc Prolapse by Traction. Arch Phy Med and Rehabil 59:322-327, 1978.
58. Levernieux, J: Traction Vertebrate. Expansion Scientifique, 1960.
59. Mathews, J: Dynamic Discography; A Study of Lumbar Traction. Ann Phy Med. 9:275-279, 1968.
60. Hood, L and Chrisman, D: Intermittent Pelvic Traction in the Treatment of the Ruptured Intervertebral Disc. Phys Ther 48:21-30, 1968.
61. Mathews, J: The Effects of Spinal Traction. Physiotherapy 58:64-66, 1972.
62. Nachemson, A and Morris, J: In Vivo Measurements of Intradiscal Pressure. JBJS 46A:327-351, April 1964.
63. Morris, J; Lucas, M and Bresler, M: Role of the Trunk in Stability of the Spine. JBJS 43A:327-351, April 1961.
64. Saunders, H: Unilateral Lumbar Traction. Phys Ther 61:221-225, Feb 1981.
65. Saunders, H: The Use of Spinal Traction in the Treatment of Neck and Back Conditions. Clinical Orthopaedics and Related Research, 179:31-38, October, 1983.
66. White, A and Bordon, S: Idiopathic Low Back Pain. Spine 7:141-149, 1982.
67. Mennell, J: Differential Diagnosis of Visceral From Somatic Back Pain. Joul of Occ Med 8:477-480, Sept 1966.
68. Brown, C: Personal Communication. Orthopaedic Surgeon. Great Bend, KS, 1978.
69. Peterson, H and Kieffer, S: Introduction to Neuroradiology. Harper and Row, Philadelphia, 1972.
70. Cyriax, J: Textbook of Orthopaedic Medicine; Treatment by Manipulation, Massage and Injection. Vol 2, 10th ed, Bailliere-Tindall, London, 1980.
71. Smith, B: Cervical Spondylosis and Its Neurological Complications. Thomas, Springfield, 1968.
72. Blau, J and Logue, V: The Natural History of Intermittent Claudication of the Cauda Equina. Brain 101:211-222, 1978.
73. Turck S: Orthopaedics. 2nd ed, Lippincott, Philadelphia, 1967.

CHAPTER 6

PATHOLOGY AND TREATMENT CONCEPTS — EXTREMITIES

Musculoskeletal disorders of the extremities may be classified as either contractile (muscle and tendon) or noncontractile (joint, ligament, bursa, nerve, bone and capsule) in origin. Spinal cord and nerve root disorders may cause symptoms such as weakness, numbness and pain in the extremities. Pain can also be referred into the extremities from any of the pain-sensitive structures in the spine[1-4].

Extremity pain may also be caused by visceral or systemic pathology. Although medical diagnosis of visceral and systemic pathology is not within the scope of the physical therapist's musculoskeletal evaluation and assessment, one must be aware that disorders such as venereal disease, gout and rheumatoid arthritis can cause joint and muscle pain. Angina and myocardial infarctions may radiate pain to the left shoulder, arm and neck. Shoulder symptoms may also be related to irritation of the diaphragm, gall bladder or spleen, which share the same spinal nerve root innervation. Numerous other examples could be given. The physical therapist must be concerned with recognition of certain characteristics of visceral and systemic pathology such as involvement in more than one joint, migrating pain, night pain and, above all, symptoms that are unrelated to and unaltered by movement and position. If the patient's complaint does not present any concrete musculoskeletal findings, one should be concerned. One should also become concerned when a patient does not respond in a timely fashion to physical therapy treatment. These are clues to the physical therapist that he may be dealing with something other than a musculoskeletal disorder and physician consultation should be made before further treatment is considered.

MUSCLE DISORDERS

Muscle disorders occur within the contractile unit. The contractile unit consists of the muscle belly, the musculotendinous junction, the tendon and its bony attachment.

ADAPTIVE MUSCLE CHANGES

Muscles rapidly adapt to length changes due to joint hypomobility, joint hypermobility, structural changes or abnormal posture. This is a non-pathological response, but it must be treated[5,6].

Treatment that emphasizes normal physiological function (active exercise) is more effective than passive stretching or other passive exercises in treating adaptive muscle length changes[7]. Primary treatment, of course, must be directed toward the cause of the adaptive changes.

MUSCLE GUARDING AND INTRINSIC MUSCLE SPASM

Muscle guarding nearly always accompanies pain, regardless of the underlying cause. Muscle guarding may develop wherever pain is felt, even if it is referred from elsewhere in the body. Prolonged muscle guarding leads to a circulatory stasis and the retention of metabolites. The muscle then may become inflamed (myositis) and a localized tenderness develops in the muscle. This intrinsic muscle spasm adds additional pain and discomfort (Fig. 5-1).

Without a thorough examination, it is easy to incriminate muscle guarding and the resulting intrinsic muscle spasm as the primary cause of the patient's problem. It is unwise to make this assumption as an underlying cause must exist to produce the muscle guarding in the first place. It is, however, often necessary to treat muscle guarding and intrinsic muscle spasm even though it may not be the primary musculoskeletal disorder.

Treatment may consist of various combinations of rest, medication, heat or cold, support, massage, electrotherapy, hydrotherapy and stretching exercises.

STRAIN (STRESS, PULL, RUPTURE)

Strain may be defined as damage of some part of the contractile unit caused by overuse (chronic strain) or overstress (acute strain.) O'Donoghue grades strains as mild (first degree), moderate (second degree) and severe (third degree)[8]. A mild strain (I) may involve a small amount of mechanical injury to the tissue (bleeding and swelling), irritation and inflammation, but no structural damage occurs. In a moderate strain (II), some portions of the contractile unit are damaged (torn) and some degree of functional loss is present, but the entire unit is intact. In a severe strain (III), there is loss of function of the muscle, tendon or its attachment due to a complete tear. The strain will occur at the weakest link of the muscle-tendon unit. Under stress the muscle may tear, the musculotendinous junction may give way or the damage may be to the tendon or to its bony attachment. The patient will also often report that he felt a tearing or pulling sensation or, less commonly, a "snap".

Resisted (isometric) muscle tests will cause pain with mild and moderate strain, whereas a complete rupture will show loss of function and may be painless. Passive stretching of the muscle may also cause localized pain in the case of mild and moderate strains. The involved structure(s) will be tender to palpation. A rupture is often easy to palpate or may be visible as a lump or a depression in the otherwise normal surface anatomy. Rest from movement gives relief of pain. The patient will often complain that rest also stiffens the involved structure(s) and that movement initially hurts but does help loosen up the stiffness.

Acute strain, in distinction to chronic strain, is the result of a single violent force applied to the contractile unit resulting in the disruption of some of the fibers of the unit. There may be rupture of a few muscle or tendon fibers, or of the entire muscle or tendon. The tendon may be partially avulsed from the bone or completely torn away.

Treatment of mild and moderate strain consists of rest and protection from further injury. Initially, ice and compression may be indicated, followed by local heat, massage, electrotherapy and gradual resumption of activities. Full restoration of mobility and strength should be achieved before the patient is dismissed. Severe strains involving rupture of the muscle, tendon or its insertion may require surgical repair.

Chronic strain from overfunction causes fatigue of the muscle. This, in turn, may result in muscle spasm, myositis and ischemia. Overfunction may also irritate the musculotendinous junction or tendon, resulting in tendinitis or tenosynovitis. Crepitus may be felt over the involved structure. Although these may seem to be different conditions, they are basically the same and require the same treatment regime.

Treatment of chronic strain consists of rest, local heat and protection against further strain, followed by gradual return to activities. Cyriax advocates massage when there is muscular involvement and transverse friction massage for tenosynovitis[9, 10]. During transverse friction massage, the inner aspect of the sheath is moved repeatedly to and fro across the external aspect of the tendon. With chronic strain, prevention is of more importance than cure. Gradual build-up of activities so that the musculotendinous unit is able to withstand a progressively heavier workload is the key.

CONTUSION (BRUISE)

Contusion may be defined as a direct blow against the muscle. This results in capillary rupture and bleeding, followed by edema and an inflammatory reaction.

Treatment consists of limitation of bleeding by application of cold, a pressure bandage and immobilization and protection from further injury. When the bruise begins to show signs of resolution, measures to promote healing may be started. Local heat, electrotherapy, rest, protection and pain free movement are vital at this stage. Finally, the therapist should be certain that full function (strength and mobility) is restored before the patient is discharged.

INFLAMMATION (MYOSITIS, TENDINITIS, TENOSYNOVITIS)

Inflammation of the contractile group (myositis, tendinitis, tenosynovitis) occurs on rare occasions as a result of sleeping or sitting in a draft or as the aftermath of influenza or other systemic diseases. More commonly, inflammation is seen as a natural reaction following strain or contusion, or accompanying intrinsic muscle spasm.

Many of the same characteristics of muscle strain and contusion, such as pain with resisted muscle tests and passive stretching and localized tenderness to palpation, will also be present with muscle inflammation. Nodules and crepitus may be felt over the involved structures and the muscle fibers may be thick and cordlike. Temperature and color changes may also be present. Pain and stiffening with rest and loosening up with activity is characteristic of muscular inflammation. Occasionally, calcific deposits will be seen in the tendon (calcific tendinitis.) The presence of calcium in such a situation denotes an attempt by nature to heal and does not alter the treatment.

Treatment of rest, local heat or cold, electrotherapy, massage (myositis) and transverse friction massage (tendinitis and tenosynovitis) are recommended. Ultrasound with hydrocortisone ointment (phonophoresis) may be effective, especially with calcific tendinitis[11]. Ion transfer treatment (Phoresor® with Decadron® and Xylocaine®) is also an effective treatment if the lesion is superficial[12]. Steroid injections are sometimes effective. All use of steroids should be conservative as studies have shown that repeated steroid injections cause weakening of the tendon and erosion of bone[10, 13].

MYOSITIS OSSIFICANS

Myositis ossificans is an occasional complication of trauma (strain or contusion) and hematoma involving the muscle. The disorder may appear as a simple exostosis having a broad base with a sharp extension into the muscle and may seem to be an involvement of the periosteum rather than the muscle. In this case, the mass is true bone and is firmly attached to the parent bone. In another type there is actually a plaque of bone lying within the muscle. Myositis ossificans may result either from repeated slight injuries or from a single, more severe traumatic event. It may occur in various regions of the body but is most frequent in the thigh, in the upper arm and about the elbow joint. Myositis ossificans will often be evident by palpation before x-rays will show the calcified mass[8]. Diagnosis is not difficult once the ossification has matured. However, it is much more important to recognize the early stages of the condition and prevent the ossification from occurring. If a strain or contusion of the arm or thigh does not resolve promptly, one should be on guard against myositis ossificans. This is why rehabilitation of strains and contusions should take place within the limits of pain; in addition, return to normal activities should not depend upon any predetermined time, but upon the resolution of symptoms.

Treatment: Early treatment of myositis ossificans is preventive; i.e., proper care of strains and contusions. As the impending condition is recognized, the muscle should be put to rest. Local heat is permissible. Active motion in the form of mild stretching is permitted only if it is painless.

O'Donoghue states that ultrasound, massage, passive stretching and any more vigorous activity than outlined above is contraindicated[8]. However, this author has had considerable success treating myositis ossificans with ultrasound and knows of many athletic trainers and sports physical therapists who have as well. Perhaps the intensity of treatment and stage of progression determine the appropriateness of ultrasound. Certainly caution should be used if the disorder is progressing to the mature stage and perhaps it is at this stage that ultrasound is indeed contraindicated. Subsequent rehabilitation should be carried out well within the limits of pain, at least for the first several months.

It is imperative that the physical therapist recognize the clinical picture of myositis ossificans because he will often be the only medical practitioner having day-to-day contact with the patient as the potentially crippling disorder develops.

CONTRACTURE

Considerable attention is paid to contractures and tightness of muscles, tendons and fascia. Tight hamstrings, hip flexors and heel cords are frequently encountered in physical therapy practice. Zohn and Mennell advocate the use of the term "myostatic spasm" to describe the muscular tightness that is often seen around joints following immobilization or after a patient has been at bed rest for any prolonged period of time[14]. This brings the concept of intrinsic muscle spasm due to the retention of metabolites and circulatory stasis, described earlier, and true muscle contracture more into focus. True contractures, in which there is increased laying down of collagen fiber and/or scarring within the muscle, do occur, but usually as a complication of surgery, severe trauma, or as a complication of neuromuscular diseases.

Myostatic spasms (tight muscles) are reversible with proper physical therapy, whereas true contractures are extremely difficult to overcome. Often they are not pain-producing but require treatment because of severe limitation of function. Occasionally, progressive contractures involving tendons and/or fascia, such as Dupuytren's contracture of the palmar fascia, are seen. Often the etiology is unknown in these disorders (see earlier discussion of adaptive muscle shortening.)

Treatment consists of stretching exercises and return to functional activities. In more severe cases massage, modality treatment and more vigorous stretching may be necessary. Ultrasound applied during passive stretch is often effective treatment for true muscular contractures.

FIBROSITIS (FIBROMYOSITIS)

Fibrositis is a term that is used synonymously with fibromyositis and myofibrositis. This condition is usually defined as acute or chronic inflammation of the fibrous tissue in the muscle which gives rise to pain and stiffness. Sometimes painful nodules and/or crepitus are felt, hence the impression that fibrositic nodules or deposits are present. Studies by Awad have shown histological changes indicating the presence of a disorder primarily involving the connective tissue of muscle. He demonstrated the presence of a metachromatic mucoid substance in massive amounts in these nodular areas. In addition, he found some mast cells and platelet clots[15]. However, the specific pathological entity of a fibrositic nodule has not been consistently demonstrated. For this reason, many authorities refuse to recognize the condition of fibrositis as a true pathological disorder[13]. It is reasonable, therefore, to assume that the nodules and crepitus often attributed to fibrositis are sometimes simply manifestations of myositis and tendinitis (see earlier discussion.)

Treatment — Regardless of the exact pathological entity, treatment for conditions of this nature should include modalities to relieve pain, promote healing, improve circulation and restore function. Local heat or cold, electrotherapy, massage and stretching exercises are especially effective.

ATROPHY

Muscle atrophy may be perceived by inspection. It can also be checked quite accurately in most situations by manual muscle testing and, in some cases, by circumferential measurements. However, *to use only circumferential measurement as a method to determine muscle weakness can be misleading.* When a muscle is strengthened it will lose some of its fat content and may appear leaner, yet when tested will show strength equivalent to or above the uninvolved side. Muscle atrophy can occur secondary to disuse or from a neurological deficit. For this reason, it is not sufficient just to recognize muscle atrophy and weakness, but it is also necessary to determine the reason why it is present.

Treatment should focus on alleviating the cause of the weakness, strengthening exercises and return to functional activities.

JOINT DISORDERS

For classification purposes, the following structures are considered part of the joint: 1) subchondral bone; 2) hyaline cartilage; 3) menisci; 4) synovial lining; 5) capsule; 6) ligament and 7) bursae. They are referred to as the non-contractile or "inert" structures.

Although there are certain exceptions, joint (noncontractile) disorders are characterized by the fact that both active and passive movements are painful and/or limited in the same direction and the pain appears as the limit of range is approached. Except in very acute cases, resisted muscle tests are not painful (see discussion in Chapter 3.) The patient will often be able to describe the exact mechanism of injury, thus leading the examiner to the exact area of injury. The palpation exam is very important in determining joint involvement, as many of the structures can easily be palpated in the extremity joints.

SPRAIN

A sprain may be defined as an injury to the joint capsule and/or the supporting ligaments resulting from overstress which causes some degree of damage to the fibers or their attachments. The function of the joint capsule is to hold the bone ends together while allowing free movement at the joints. Ligaments reinforce the capsule at points of special stress. A ligament is designed to prevent abnormal motion of a joint while permitting normal functional motion. The collagen fibers of ligaments are arranged in a parallel fashion, thus allowing very little, if any, elasticity. Therefore, if a ligament is overstressed to any appreciable degree, permanent laxity may develop. The collagen fibers of the joint capsule are arranged in an irregular fashion. This arrangement allows a certain degree of "play" even though the individual collagen fibers are nonelastic (Fig. 5-8).

Sprains may be classified as mild, moderate or severe (I, II, III.) In a mild sprain, some of the fibers have been torn with a small amount of hemorrhage present. The ligament is not weakened. A moderate sprain is one in which some portion of the ligament and/or capsule is torn and some degree of functional loss is present. In severe sprain, there is loss of function of the ligament and/or capsule due to a complete tear[8,13].

Treatment: As a *mild* sprain heals, stiffness is inherent. Therefore, treatment is aimed at prevention of joint hypomobility and disuse atrophy. Movement and activities are allowed within pain free limits. Modality treatments, especially high-voltage electrical stimulation, are helpful to promote healing. Ice, compression bandaging and elevation are indicated to prevent or reduce edema. Gradual and progressive return to normal function is encouraged as healing is accomplished.

A *moderate* sprain must be treated with considerably more precaution to guard against further injury. The capsule and/or ligament(s) are already in a weakened state and must be protected from further injury. Even after the "healed" joint is pain free, it is still vulnerable to re-injury. However, if a moderate sprain is left alone entirely to heal, joint restriction and disuse atrophy may develop. Therefore, pain free range of motion and joint mobilization must be integrated into the treatment regime, along with modalities for symptomatic relief, to reduce edema and to promote healing. The greatest challenge in the treatment of sprain is in the moderate type. The fact that it takes six, eight or ten weeks for a ligament to heal after surgery is readily accepted by both doctor and patient. O'Donoghue believes it is a mistake if the same amount of time is not allowed for a moderate sprain to heal[8]. It is not uncommon for a moderate sprain to be relatively pain free with normal mobility within two to three weeks following injury, but the injured tissue is still in a weakened state. If the patient returns to vigorous physical activity at this time he may suffer a second, often more serious, sprain. It is under these exact circumstances that many severe sprains occur in athletics.

Sometimes, the *severe* sprain must be surgically repaired or joint laxity (hypermobility) will likely be present when all healing has taken place. The trend, however, seems to be toward nonsurgical management of many severe sprains. Splinting, supporting or cast bracing the joint in a position to allow optimal healing is often the treatment of choice. Gradual return to functional activities and restoration of full strength and mobility is the final phase of treatment.

DISLOCATION

Dislocation is defined as an actual displacement of the opposing surfaces making up a joint. This, of necessity, presumes loss of function of some of the ligamentous and capsular structures of the joint. Subluxation is a partial dislocation. Either of these conditions may spontaneously reduce or the bones may lock in the dislocated position. It is also possible to have a chronically dislocating joint without acute ligamentous damage. In this case, one may assume that the ligament(s) and/or capsule has been stretched or torn previously.

Treatment: In an acute dislocation one visualizes a complete tear of the ligament(s) and surgical repair must be considered. Otherwise, since acute dislocation is simply the end result of a severe sprain, it can be treated as such. In the case of chronic dislocation it is assumed that the joint is hypermobile or unstable and it is treated as such.

INFLAMMATION (CAPSULITIS, SYNOVITIS, ARTHRITIS)

Joint inflammation, like muscle inflammation, usually follows as a natural reaction to injury. It is rarely seen without a history of aggravation or injury. The involved joint may show signs of swelling, redness and warmth. As with all joint disorders, movement will hurt, but it is also characteristic for inflammatory disorders to be painful and stiff with rest. Joints which have undergone degenerative changes are more vulnerable to developing inflammation following overuse or overstress.

Treatment consists of rest, pain free movement and activities, modalities to promote healing and restoration of strength and mobility as healing progresses.

BURSITIS

A bursa is a sac or saclike cavity filled with viscid fluid and situated at places in the tissues at which friction would otherwise develop. "Adventitious" bursa occur at sites of friction caused by such abnormalities as pathological bony prominences and protruding metallic inserts. The bursa is highly vascularized and has a rich sympathetic nerve supply. Bursitis is inflammation of a bursa. It rarely occurs as a primary disorder. Bursitis usually occurs secondary to strains, sprains or contusions and is often present in cases of tendinitis and myositis. Calcific deposits (calcific bursitis) are occasionally seen as a further complication of bursitis. Palpation is often the key to diagnosis. Active and passive range of motion and resisted muscle tests will allow the examiner to determine if joint and/or muscle inflammation is also present. Bursitis may herald the onset of systemic disease, particularly a collagen disease such as rheumatoid arthritis or gout. Naturally, unless there is a bursa anatomically in a place from which pain appears to be emanating, the pain cannot be coming from bursitis (Fig. 6-1). There are no primary bursae located in the back unless they are adventitious. Traumatic bursitis is usually limited to olecranon, ischial, calcaneal, metatarsophalangeal or intermetatarsal bursae[14].

Treatment consists of rest, protection from further aggravation, modalities to promote healing and restoration of functional activities (strength and mobility) as healing progresses. Ultrasound with hydrocortisone ointment (phonophoresis[11]) or ion transfer (Phoresor® with Decadron® and Zylocaine®[12]) are effective treatments.

HYPOMOBILITY (DYSFUNCTION)

Joint hypomobility or dysfunction occurs in two ways: joint impingement and joint contracture.

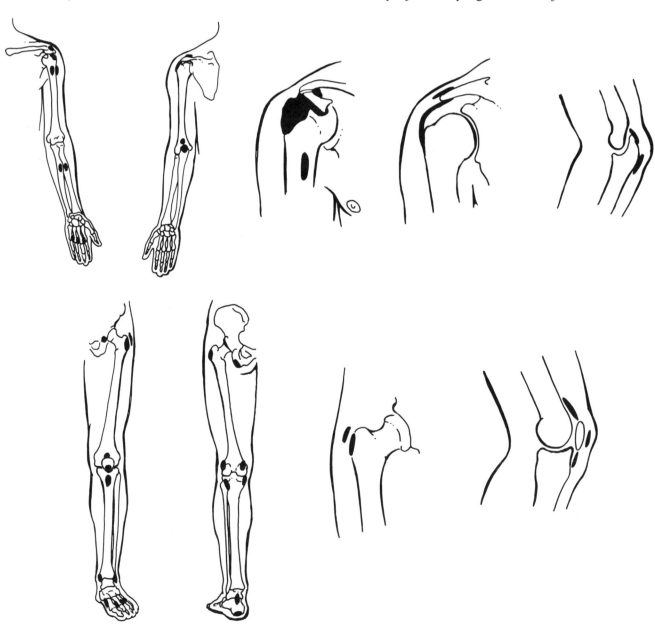

Fig. 6-1. Drawings showing location of bursae in the body (adopted from Zohn and Mennell[13].)

Impingement

Although joint impingement or locking occurs occasionally in the spine, it happens rarely in the extremity joints. The mechanism of injury is usually a sudden unguarded movement with little or no trauma. The joint seems to lock or be blocked in one particular direction, but may be free to move in other directions (articular pattern.) The cause of the blockage is usually a roughened cartilage or menisci, a loose body or osteophyte or a nipping of the synovial lining. Joint impingement is most frequently seen in joints that are hypermobile (unstable) or that show signs of degenerative joint disease.

Treatment: Joint manipulation is occasionally indicated as treatment, although the patient will often know how to "treat" the disorder himself. Patient education in avoiding the circumstances that cause the locking is often effective. Surgery may be indicated if a torn meniscus or other joint obstruction is the cause of the impingement.

Contracture (Adhesive Capsulitis)

Joint contracture is a disorder that generally involves the entire capsule, although certain parts of the capsule (movements) may be more contracted than others due to specific areas of injury and/or the position of the joint at rest. Joint contracture is usually the end result of prolonged immobilization following an injury such as a sprain or fracture or surgery.

Joint contracture develops when the individual collagen fibers adhere to each other during immobilization. This prevents the play that is normally present between these fibers as the joint moves. This disorder is further complicated when additional collagen is laid down in response to injury (scarring) and when adhesions are formed. The end result is a thickened, tight, constricted capsule.

Ligaments do not become contracted nearly as quickly as the capsule does because the individual collagen fibers are laid down in a parallel arrangement within the ligament and there is normally very little play within the fibers of the ligament. Ligaments do hypertrophy and become thick and stiff and do contribute to joint contracture in cases involving long periods of immobilization[16].

Active and passive movements will be restricted in a capsular pattern, and resisted muscle tests will be painless[9,16]. Muscle atrophy and weakness may be present. The joint capsule will often be tender to palpation. The patient's chief complaint will often be that of stiffness and restriction of movement rather than pain. Although initially joint contracture will not show up on x-ray, prolonged joint hypomobility may lead to joint degeneration which will be evident with x-rays.

Treatment consists of mobilization using articulating and stretching techniques. Heat, and especially ultrasound, is useful preceding mobilization. Ultrasound energy produces a deep heating effect precisely at the joint structures (muscle-bone interface) and therefore is the most effective form of heat. It also acts to break down molecular binding that causes the criss-crossed collagen fibers in the joint capsule to adhere to one another[17]. Range of motion, hold-relax stretching exercises and active (functional) exercises are also indicated due to the adaptive muscle shortening that is also often present following prolonged periods of immobilization. Joint contracture can be prevented in most cases by proper physical therapy management of acute sprains, strains and inflammations and utilization, when possible, of fracture management techniques that allow some joint movement early.

HYPERMOBILITY

Joint hypermobility involves laxity of the joint capsule and/or ligament(s) and is commonly associated with congenital defects or severe trauma. Patients with joint hypermobility often complain of pain following vigorous activity. They often cannot maintain any joint position for more than a few minutes without pain. The patient will often describe a "slipping" or "popping" in the joint with certain movements. This slipping or popping can be repeated over and over again. Occasional, inconsistent popping of a joint is usually meaningless. Chronic dislocation may be a complaint in severe cases (see discussion of joint play and ligament stress tests in Chapter 3 and description of specific tests in Chapter 8.) Joint hypermobility may lead to early joint degeneration because of the increased wear and tear and abnormal biomechanical stresses to which the joint is subjected.

Treatment: Joint hypermobility should be treated with muscle strengthening or, in extreme cases, support such as bracing or splinting or surgery. Strengthening of the rotator cuff muscles is especially effective if the glenohumeral joint is unstable.

DEGENERATIVE JOINT DISEASE (OSTEOARTHRITIS)

Degenerative joint disease is characterized by degenerative loss of articular cartilage, subchondral bony sclerosis, cartilage and bone proliferation at the joint margins with subsequent osteophyte formation and capsular thickening with synovial inflammation.

In severe, advanced stages of this disorder, pain is present with all movement, especially activities that cause approximation of the joint surfaces such as lifting a heavy weight (upper extremity) or weight bearing (lower extremity.) This is because the protective articular cartilage is worn away and bone is moving on bone. In other stages the degenerative joint disease itself is usually symptom free. *The pain associated with mild to moderate degenerative joint disease is more likely to be because of joint contracture than degenerative joint disease itself.* One can easily distinguish between the two by determining whether joint approximation or joint movement increases the patient's pain. Patients with degenerative joint disease are more vulnerable to joint sprain and inflammation because often only a slight amount of overstress or overuse is enough to aggravate the symptoms.

There are many theories as to the cause of degenerative joint disease. Although there is evidence of genetic, metabolic and endocrine factors all related to degenerative joint disease, *three principle causes* are commonly seen:

1) Joints which are **hypomobile** are susceptible to degenerative joint disease. The hyaline cartilage is avascular and receives its nutritional supply via the synovial fluid. Normal movement is vital to this exchange. Laboratory experiments have shown that a joint which is immobilized will soon begin to show signs of degenerative joint disease[18].

2) Joint **hypermobility** or instability will lead to degenerative joint disease because of abnormal biomechanical stresses. Clinical experience shows that joints which are unstable or hypermobile due to old injury, repeated overstress or congenital defects will often develop degenerative joint disease. Examples include the "football knee", dancing and gymnastics injuries and spondylolisthesis.

3) **Traumatic** or "wear and tear" factors often play an important role in development of degenerative joint disease. A joint that is subjected to abnormal biomechanical stresses or repeated injuries will often show signs of joint degeneration.

Treatment: Since mild to moderate degenerative joint disease is usually symptom free in and of itself, treatment is directed toward correcting and/or supporting abnormal biomechanical stresses, mobilizing hypomobility and managing the joint sprains and/or inflammations which are often the true cause of the patient's complaint. An example of abnormal biomechanical stress is uneven leg length. The patient is likely to stand more on the short leg, thus increasing the weight bearing stress on that leg. He is also apt to develop genu recurvatum of the short leg due to an abnormal hyperextension factor at toe-off[19]. The spine will develop a compensatory scoliosis with increased weight bearing and decreased facet joint mobility on the concave side. Any of these factors could cause early degenerative joint disease in the involved joint(s). Such a condition can easily be corrected with a shoe lift (see previous discussion.) Numerous other examples of abnormal biomechanical stresses can be cited, such as pes planus, pronated foot, genu valgus, genu varus and depression of the metatarsal arch. Joint hypermobility or instability can also cause abnormal stress.

If joint hypomobility is present with degenerative joint disease, mobilization should be attempted. If successful, restoration of normal joint mobility may interrupt the degenerative process. In severe degenerative joint disease, any attempt to increase the mobility or activity may result in increased pain and/or inflammation. In such cases, correction of abnormal biomechanical stresses may still be feasible, as well as support with braces, foot orthoses, splints and use of other assistive and labor saving devices.

OSTEOCHONDRITIS DESSICANS

Osteochondritis dessicans consists of the separation of a fragment of articular cartilage from the underlying matrix. It occurs most frequently at the knee and elbow. Some believe that the disorder results from spontaneous ischemic necrosis due to circulatory insufficiency, while others believe it is due to repeated trauma. The latter seems most probable[20].

Treatment varies from no treatment, except for protection from further trauma, to surgical excision. The physical therapist's interest in this condition concerns the awareness of such a disorder and it again points out the need for x-ray examination in cases involving trauma, repeated or unusual stresses or conditions that do not respond in a timely fashion to physical therapy management.

NERVE DISORDERS

Although positive neurological signs and symptoms are often found in the extremities, they are usually due to pathology in the brain or spinal cord (upper motor neuron) or to spinal nerve root impingement. The former is not within the scope of a text dealing with musculoskeletal disorders and the latter is discussed in the chapter on spinal disorders. Only the neurological disorders directly associated with pathology in the extremities are dealt with here.

NERVE INJURY

Contusion

The peripheral nerves most often contused are the axillary nerve at the shoulder, the radial nerve in the radial groove of the humerus, the ulnar nerve at the elbow and the peroneal nerve behind the fibular head.

The injury is usually from a direct blow on the nerve, causing pain and numbness. The condition may be entirely transient or there may be persistent aching along the distribution of the nerve because of swelling and congestion within the nerve and nerve sheath. In isolated cases, there may be paralysis of the muscles supplied by the nerve[8].

Treatment should include measures to protect from overuse and further contusion. Cold compresses initially, followed by local heat or hydrotherapy on the second or third day, are indicated to promote healing. Recovery is almost always complete and fairly rapid[8]. Muscle strengthening and re-education may be necessary in cases of prolonged paralysis.

Nerve Stretch

Another type of nerve injury is caused by overstretch. Examples include overstretching of the common peroneal nerve after rupture of the lateral collateral ligaments of the knee, or of the median nerve following elbow dislocation. The symptoms will vary with the severity of the injury. If there is a complete avulsion there will be immediate and complete loss of function; if the nerve is stretched but not torn, there will be hemorrhage and shock to the fibers and perhaps subsequent scarring around the nerve, in which case function will return more slowly and less completely[8].

Treatment: In most cases gradual recovery will take place. Physical therapy measures are important to maintain joint function and prevent deformity during a time of complete paralysis and to regain muscle strength as the nerve function returns. Surgical exploration and repair is sometimes necessary, but should be approached conservatively[8].

PERIPHERAL NERVE ENTRAPMENT

Peripheral nerve entrapment can cause pain, numbness and muscle atrophy in the structures supplied by the entrapped nerve. Kopell and Thompson is an excellent reference concerning the diagnosis, classification and treatment of these disorders[21]. Peripheral nerve entrapment symptoms follow the specific nerve distribution as opposed to a dermatome pattern which is characteristic of spinal nerve root syndrome (Fig. 6-2). The patient with peripheral nerve entrapment will often have normal muscle stretch reflexes. Night pain may be the primary symptom.

Thoracic Outlet Syndrome

The thoracic outlet syndromes have one common denominator. Their signs and symptoms are attributed to compression of the neurovascular bundle in the region of the cervical-thoracic dorsal outlet. The neurovascular bundle is a grouping of the brachial plexus nerve fibers and the subclavian artery and vein (Fig. 6-3). As a general rule, thoracic outlet syndromes involve the C8-T1 nerve roots, whereas cervical nerve root syndromes are most common at the C5, 6, and 7 levels.

Scalenus-Anticus/Cervical Rib Syndrome

The subclavian artery and brachial plexus pass over the first rib through a normally occurring space between the scalenus anticus and scalenus medius muscles. Occasionally, due to an accessory cervical rib or its fibrous extension, or congenital or acquired abnormalities of the scalene muscles, the neurovascular bundle is entrapped, causing neurological and circulatory changes in the upper extremity. Adson's test is a maneuver to determine if one of these conditions is present. The patient is instructed to take and hold a deep breath, extend his neck fully, and turn his chin toward the side being examined. At the same time, the examiner is taking

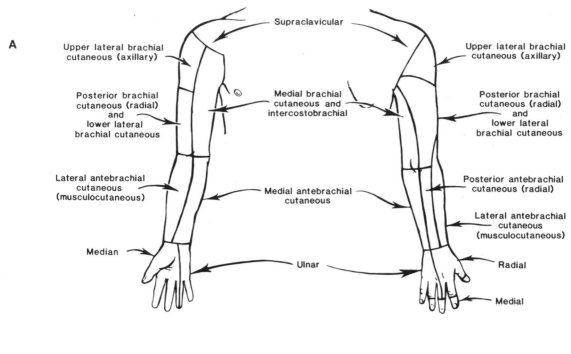

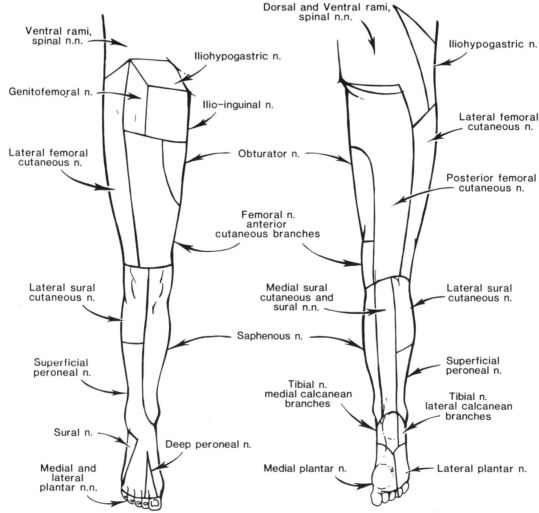

Fig. 6-2. Cutaneous sensory nerve distribution: A) Upper extremity; B) Lower extremity (adopted from Merck Manual[22].)

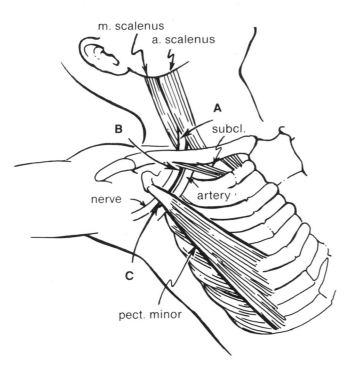

Fig. 6-3. Drawing showing the three thoracic outlet syndromes: A) Scalenus-anticus/cervical rib syndrome; B) Costoclavicular syndrome and C) Hyperabduction syndrome.

the patient's radial pulse. If the pulse disappears and the pain and other symptoms are reproduced in the arm, the test is positive. A diminished pulse alone is not a true positive finding. In some subjects, a greater effect upon the neurovascular bundle is exerted by turning the head to the opposite side. Therefore, both positions should be tested (Fig. 3-76).

Treatment includes local heat, massage, ultrasound, traction and stretching of the scalenus muscles. Active strengthening exercises of the upper trapezius and levator scapulae muscles should be emphasized to bring the carriage of the shoulder girdle upward and backward.

Costoclavicular Syndrome

The subclavian artery and brachial plexus can also be entrapped as they pass between the clavicle and the first rib. The test to determine this syndrome requires the patient to take and hold a deep breath as he retracts and depresses his shoulders. Again the examiner determines if the radial pulse disappears and if there is reproduction of the symptoms in the arm (Fig. 3-77).

Treatment includes exercises and posture training to elevate the shoulder girdle. Mobilization

of the clavicle may be indicated if hypomobility is present at the sternoclavicular joint(s).

Hyperabduction Syndrome

The subclavian vessels and brachial plexus can also be entrapped beneath the tendon of the pectoralis minor muscle and under the coracoid process. The arm is held in a hyperabducted position while the examiner feels if the radial pulse disappears and if there is reproduction of the symptoms in the arm (Fig. 3-78). The patient suffering from this syndrome will often complain that the symptoms come on while he is sleeping on his back or stomach with his arm overhead.

Treatment should emphasize patient education to correct the habit or occupational posture that causes the symptoms. Stretching of the pectoral muscles is also often helpful.

Carpal Tunnel Syndrome

Carpal tunnel syndrome occurs from compression of the median nerve at the wrist. The compression occurs between the carpal bones and the transverse carpal ligament. Symptoms are confined exclusively to the median nerve distribution of the hand (Fig. 6-4). The symptoms are paresthesia, pain, numbness, clumsiness and trophic changes in the fingers and hand. Symptoms often wake the patient during the night[23]. A valuable test is to reproduce the symptoms by holding the wrist firmly in flexion for a minute (Phalen's test.) This test should also be done with the wrist in extension. Nerve conduction velocity testing confirms the diagnosis.

Treatment is either conservative, by immobilization of the wrist in a neutral position, or is accomplished by surgical release of the transverse carpal ligament (flexor retinaculum.) Cailliet reports permanent cure in some patients using the conservative approach for a period of two weeks[23]. Treatment with ultrasound is sometimes effective.

Piriformis Syndrome

Piriformis syndrome is a frequently mentioned, yet rarely encountered syndrome that allegedly entraps the sciatic nerve against the ischium as it passes in front of the piriformis muscle. In approximately 15% of the population, the sciatic nerve actually pierces the muscle belly of the piriformis and may become entrapped if the muscle spasms. Many osteopaths believe that the piriformis syn-

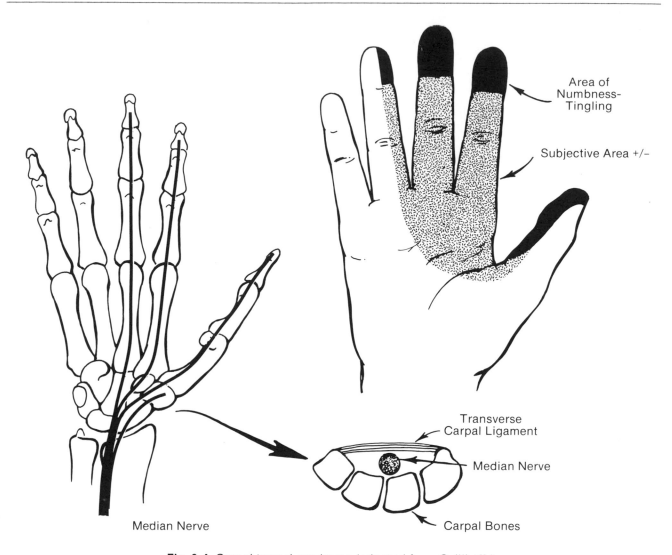

Fig. 6-4. Carpal tunnel syndrome (adopted from Cailliet[23].)

drome is secondary to sacral torsions which can stretch the piriformis. The region of entrapment is located just superior to a point midway between the ischial tuberosity and the greater trochanter (Fig. 6-5).

Resisted (isometric) muscle testing of external rotation of the hip should cause pain if the piriformis muscle is involved, as it is an external rotator of the femur. Another diagnostic feature of this syndrome is reproduction of sciatic pain upon straight leg raising (which causes the hip to be internally rotated) but relief upon externally rotating the leg while still in the straight leg raised position.

Treatment includes local heat, ultrasound and massage to the piriformis muscle, along with passive stretching exercises (internal hip rotation) and, possibly, manipulation of the sacroiliac joint.

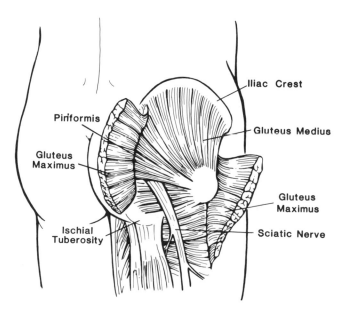

Fig. 6-5. Piriformis syndrome involves entrapment of the sciatic nerve by the piriformis muscle.

Common Peroneal Syndrome

The common peroneal nerve is exposed to direct injury or to sustained pressure at the point where it winds around the lateral aspect of the neck of the fibula (Fig. 6-6). Scar tissue resulting from fracture of the fibular head, surgery (Baker's cyst), sprain of the superior tibio-fibular joint or from direct nerve injury can encroach upon the nerve. Since the nerve supplies the tibialis anterior, extensor hallucis and peroneal muscles, drop foot may result and the outer foot and calf may become anesthetic.

Treatment: Mobilization of the fibular head is often helpful in releasing the scar tissue binding the nerve. In severe cases, surgical release may be necessary.

BONE DISORDERS

FRACTURE

Any case involving trauma should be x-rayed to determine if a fracture is present. Although diagnosis of fracture is done primarily with x-ray, certain signs and symptoms should cause one to suspect fracture. Pain in locations unusual for sprain or strain, such as superior to the malleoli with an ankle injury, should be suspect. Deep aching pain at rest is another symptom of fracture. Such obvious signs as grinding or grating sensations with movement should be immediately recognized as fracture symptoms. Since fractures are occasionally missed with x-rays one should be aware of these signs and symptoms and seek further radiological examination if the patient's symptoms persist beyond a normal expected treatment time.

Treatment involves medical managment of the fracture. The physical therapist is concerned with preservation and/or restoration of full mobility and strength as healing progresses.

STRESS FRACTURE

A particularly puzzling disorder is the stress, or fatigue, fracture. The term "march fracture" was coined to describe the fracture of the metatarsal shaft that is caused, not by acute injury, but by repeated stress. Stress fractures are usually seen in people who have experienced a rather rapid increase in their level of physical activity. Included are military recruits, athletes starting quickly into a new activity, runners who have increased their mileage rapidly or anyone who has gone from a sitting occupation to one that requires standing and walking (waiters/waitresses.) This disorder is particularly deceptive since there is no history of traumatic injury. Early x-rays are negative, yet the symptoms still persist. Only by the appearance of the new bone formation that develops at the site of the insult is the diagnosis confirmed by x-ray. These circumstances often occur without an actual fracture line ever appearing across the bone. A useful diagnostic procedure is a bone scan, which will be "hot" within 24 hours of onset of the symptoms.

While this disorder is common in the foot, it can appear almost anywhere, especially in the lower extremities and pelvis. Careful examination that reveals pain and tenderness over the bone occurring without specific trauma but under unusual stresses adds to the diagnostic picture. The use of a tuning fork over a suspected fracture site will produce pain. Fracture pain is felt as a deep aching that often persists even at rest.

Treatment: Once the diagnosis is confirmed, the treatment is protection against further stress until the lesion is solidly healed, followed by gradual resumption of activities.

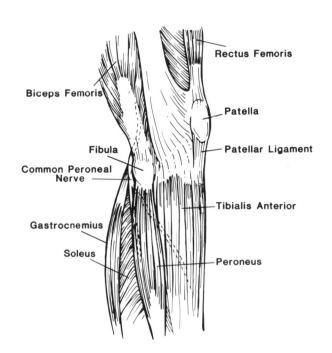

Rectus Femoris

Biceps Femoris

Patella

Fibula

Patellar Ligament

Common Peroneal Nerve

Gastrocnemius

Tibialis Anterior

Soleus

Peroneus

Fig. 6-6. The common peroneal nerve may become entrapped by scar tissue at a point where it winds around the lateral aspect of the neck of the fibula.

SPECIFIC DISORDERS

SUPRASPINATUS TENDINITIS/ SUBDELTOID BURSITIS

Subdeltoid or subacromial bursitis occurs most frequently secondary to degenerative lesions of the rotator cuff and thus is not a primary phenomenon. Other precipitating factors may be: 1) immobilization; 2) working on a tedious task in a slumped position; 3) sudden movements in an abnormal direction and 4) normal movements in a moment of fear, tension or anxiety.

Most subdeltoid bursitis can be traced to fatigue and/or weakness of the rotator cuff musculature during activity. The fatigue and/or weakness of these muscles decreases the efficiency of the rotator cuff mechanism in seating the humeral head in the lower portion of the glenoid fossa during active abduction and flexion. The greater tuberosity tends to "run into" the acromion and presses against the suprahumeral tissues when these movements are attempted (Fig. 6-7). Thus, subdeltoid bursitis is often superceded by supraspinatus strain or tendinitis. Repeated irritation of the supraspinatus tendon causes it to swell and cause compression between the humeral head and the overhanging acromial process and corocoacromial ligament and arch.

The tendon may rupture and material is extruded outwardly and downwardly into the lower portion of the subdeltoid bursa. Pain is more severe and more constant, regardless of movement, and may be felt lower in the arm at the mid-humerus where the deltoid inserts onto the humerus. Constant deep pain is caused by the constant tension in these tissues held within the confines of the narrow container. Movement is prohibited by mechanical obstruction, by pain and by protective muscle spasm.

Tenderness to palpation is felt at the insertion of the supraspinatus tendon which is felt just anterolateral to the acromion with the glenohumeral joint in full internal rotation and hyperextension.

Bursitis will have a swift onset. Pain is the initial symptom and varies in intensity. Pain is usually localized in the shoulder region and is initially at the anterolateral aspect of the glenohumeral joint. Limitation in passive movement occurs rather quickly and is of a non-capsular pattern with internal and external rotation free, but with flexion and abduction restricted. The non-capsular pattern with free rotation is diagnostic for this disorder. Flexion and abduction force the greater tuberosity against the acromion and suprahumeral tissues, thus causing pain. Shoulder "shrugging" replaces smooth, effortless scapulohumeral motion. The clinician may also detect an empty end feel with passive movement. A painful arc in the mid-range of motion is also diagnostic for subdeltoid bursitis. This painful arc of abduction also may involve the

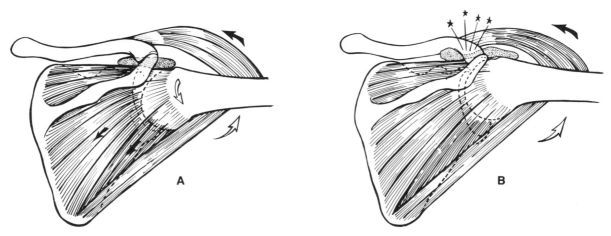

Fig. 6-7. A) Force couple action that occurs with shoulder abduction or flexion. As the deltoid muscle lifts the humerus, the rotator cuff muscles act to pull the head of the humerus inferiorly in the glenoid fossa. This action allows sufficient space for the supraspinatus tendon, subdeltoid bursa and greater tubercle to move under the acromion as full flexion or abduction is achieved. B) If the rotator cuff muscles are weak or are otherwise unable to function properly, the humeral head remains in the superior portion of the glenoid fossa causing impingement of the soft tissues between the humeral head and acromion.

tender area of the supraspinatus tendon as it is in intimate contact with the undersurface of the acromion. Calcific deposits are sometimes observed within the bursae and/or tendon. This does not necessarily change the treatment considerations.

Treatment: Ice is an effective modality. Ultrasound with hydrocortisone ointment used as the coupling agent (phonophoresis) may also be beneficial[11]. Protection from further injury and aggravation is necessary to allow healing to occur. Transverse friction massage across the insertion of the supraspinatus tendon is especially effective[9, 10]. A home exercise program to prevent capsular involvement (joint contracture) is also required. Codman's and rotation exercises in the pain free range of motion to maintain the joint capsule mobility should be used. Gentle joint mobilization is also used to prevent joint contracture, but it must not aggravate the condition. *Since weakness of the rotator cuff muscles (external and internal rotators) is almost always one of the underlying causes of supraspinatus tendinitis/subdeltoid bursitis, strengthening of these muscles is the ultimate cure.* Usually, these exercises can be started early in the treatment program because internal and external rotation are relatively painless. An effective exercise program is shown in Fig. 6-8. Ideally, when supraspinatus tendinitis is involved, the internal and external rotation exercises shown in Fig. 6-8 should be done with the shoulder in some abduction (30° to 40°) to avoid "wringing" of the supraspinatus tendon. These exercises should be started mildly and progressed as tolerated. A little pain with the exercise is acceptable as long as it does not linger afterward. Short arcs of range of motion may be necessary if pain is experienced at the end of range.

The use of steroid injections for treatment of tendinitis should be used sparingly, as repeated injections have been shown to cause weakening of the myotendinous structures [10, 13], and at best are only treating the inflammation rather than the cause (weakness of the glenohumeral rotator muscles.) Typically, patients treated with steroid injections experience short-term relief but gradual worsening of the disorder occurs with long-term use.

TEAR OF THE ROTATOR CUFF

Rupture of the supraspinatus tendon is a common and important cause of shoulder disability. In severe cases, the tear may be extensive and may involve the entire rotator cuff of the shoulder.

The mechanism of injury is varied. It may involve a fall or direct blow onto the point of the shoulder or a sudden powerful elevation of the arm, but spontaneous tears are common in patients over 50 years of age, especially those patients who have had repeated steroid injections[10, 16].

The diagnosis of tear of the rotator cuff is arrived at with the loss of the stabilization function of the rotator cuff; thus, the patient cannot maintain abduction passively attained (drop arm test[24]). This test is not exclusive for tears of the rotator cuff, however, as any acute, painful condition of the shoulder may have this reaction. Zohn and Mennell describe another test for rotator cuff tear when at the extreme of painless abduction. The arm is taken gently through external and then internal rotation by the examiner. If the patient experiences a sharp pain, and there is a click at the same point in both external and internal rotation at the point of pain, the diagnosis of a tear of the rotator cuff is established[14]. The patient will often describe a slipping or "popping" sensation when certain motions are repeated (usually rotation movements with the arm abducted.) When diagnosis is in doubt, arthrography may help.

Treatment: Complete, or extensive tears probably should be repaired surgically, but for the most part surgical repair is not necessary[14]. For acute tears, physical therapy that promotes healing and allows pain free movement to prevent contracture and muscle atrophy is indicated. One must allow a considerable length of time for healing (6-10 weeks) and must protect the joint from further injury during this time. Gradual return to activity under the guidance of a physical therapist is an absolute necessity if maximal results are to be obtained. If the disorder is chronic, strengthening of the rotator cuff muscles is often surprisingly effective.

FROZEN SHOULDER (ADHESIVE CAPSULITIS)

Frozen shoulder or adhesive capsulitis is a common disorder which develops when the individual collagen fibers adhere to each other or as the result of formation of adhesions (scar tissue) (Fig. 6-9). This disorder is more common in women than in men and is sometimes idiopathic in nature, although one often sees it develop secondary to

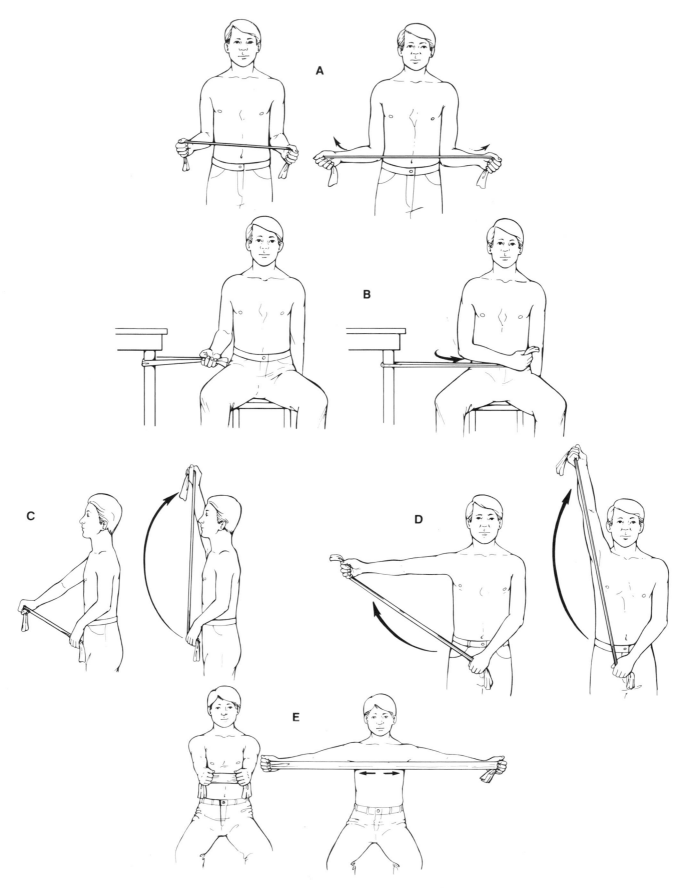

Fig. 6-8. Exercises to strengthen the shoulder muscles: A) external rotation; B) internal rotation; C) flexion; D) abduction; E) horizontal abduction.

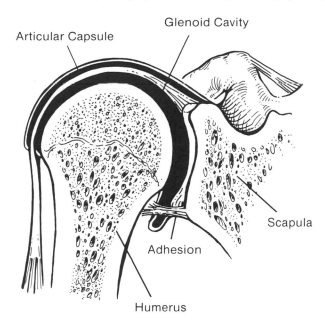

Articular Capsule

Glenoid Cavity

Scapula

Adhesion

Humerus

Fig. 6-9. Adhesions which form at the anterior-inferior aspect of the glenohumeral joint capsule are sometimes the cause of frozen shoulder.

periods of immobilization or inactivity, inflammation (tendinitis-bursitis) and postural changes (increased thoracic kyphosis[14].)

The patient with frozen shoulder will usually complain of loss of function, such as an inability to comb his hair, rather than pain. If pain is a predominant complaint it may be at night when the patient attempts to lie on the involved side. Many times the loss of mobility will be quite severe before the patient notices that he has a problem.

Range of motion will be restricted in a capsular pattern with external rotation and abduction being restricted the most. Pain with passive movement will be felt only after the joint is moved into the restriction and a capsular end feel will be present (see Chapter 3.) It can be assumed that some adaptive muscle shortening will also be present.

Treatment: Since most of the joint contracture/adhesion forms in the anterior-inferior portion of the capsule, treatment to mobilize that portion of the joint capsule is of primary concern. Physical therapy modalities, especially ultrasound, are effective when given in preparation to mobilization and stretching. The ultrasound should be given with the arm supported in an abducted and externally rotated (stretched) position and directed toward the anterior-inferior portion of the capsule. Stretching (range of motion) exercises are ineffective in the early stages of treatment because the stretching is

opposed by acute muscle guarding. Joint mobilization techniques such as those described in Chapter 8 are most effective in the initial stages of treatment. Codman's exercises with cuff weights attached to the wrist for passive distraction of the glenohumeral joint are especially effective. As treatment progresses, it may be necessary to become quite vigorous with the joint mobilization treatment. Active and passive range of motion and stretching exercises such as the wand exercises shown in Fig. 6-10 are gradually included in the treatment program. The patient should initially concentrate more on external rotation and flexion than on abduction with the range of motion exercises that he is doing himself because abduction may cause pinching of the subacromial tissue. This is not the case, of course, if the therapist is passively depressing the humeral head while doing stretching and manual joint mobilization techniques. Ice packing with the arm supported and the shoulder joint in a maximum externally rotated and abducted position is very effective following vigorous joint mobilization and stretching. (Fig. 6-11).

Since adaptive muscle shortening and muscle weakness are almost always present with this disorder, strengthening exercises are started as soon as possible. Since active movement through full available range of motion is often painful, short arc exercises using an elastic band for resistance are usually most effective (Fig. 6-8). In other words, the emphasis here is strengthening and physiological activity of the muscles which can be done in the pain free range of motion. The joint mobilization and stretching exercises, on the other hand, are done to increase capsular mobility and must be carried to a point where there is a stretch on the joint capsule. The latter may of necessity be painful.

If the patient has rounded shoulders and an increased kyphosis, special emphasis should be directed toward strengthening external rotation and horizontal abduction and stretching the anterior shoulder/chest (Fig. 6-12).

Some sources claim that adhesive capsulitis is a self-limiting disorder and resolves spontaneously in about twelve month's time[10]. This has been disputed by other sources[16] and is not consistent with this author's experience. Improvement tends to be characterized by spurts and plateaus and satisfactory results sometimes take as long as three to four months.

An alternative to physical therapy treatment is surgical manipulation under anesthesia. Clinical

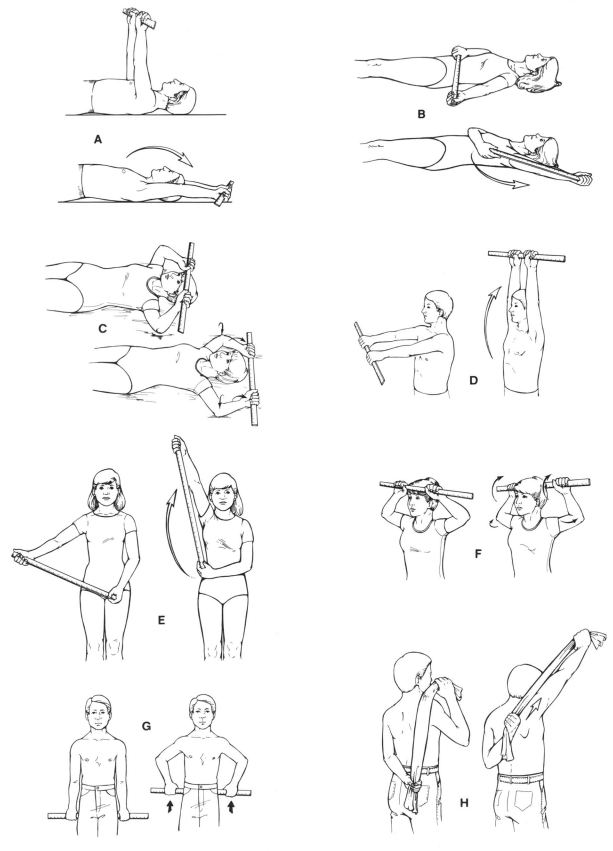

Fig. 6-10. Wand exercises to increase range of motion in the shoulder: A) supine flexion; B) supine abduction; C) supine external rotation; D) standing flexion; E) standing abduction; F) standing external rotation; G) standing internal rotation and H) standing internal rotation with towel.

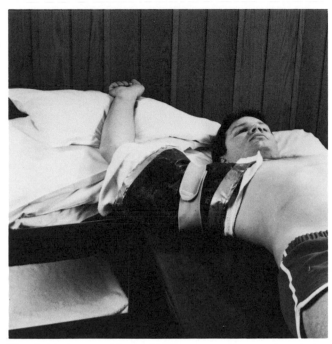

Fig. 6-11. Ice packing with the arm supported and the shoulder in a maximally externally rotated and abducted position is very effective following vigorous joint mobilization and stretching.

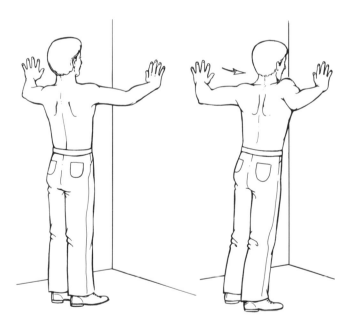

Fig. 6-12. Exercise to stretch soft tissue structures of the anterior shoulder/chest.

experience shows that some patients seem to do quite well with surgical manipulation while others actually seem to develop greater pain and disability following this procedure. Theoretically, this wide variation in clinical results may be explained by the original cause of the restriction. If, on one hand, the restriction is caused by a distinct adhesion(s) that has formed at the inferior or anterior-inferior aspect of the joint and is binding together the capsular fold, vigorous manipulation or range of motion may tear the adhesion(s) and considerable improvement may be noted almost immediately. This is characterized by a distinct "pop" or "snap" during the maneuver. Some pain and swelling (bleeding) may be present but it is usually not so severe that the increased range of motion that has been gained cannot be maintained with physical therapy management. On the other hand, if the restriction is caused by thickening and tightening of the capsule itself (binding and proliferation of individual collagen fibers), one will not experience a distinct "pop" or "snap", but will feel a gradual, rather non-specific tearing sensation while the joint is taken through the range of motion[25]. It has been this author's experience that these patients return from the recovery room with considerable pain, increased swelling and often have increased disability as a result of such treatment.

Since one cannot be certain if it is an adhesion(s) or general tightness of the capsule that is causing the restriction, a trial of physical therapy management should always be given before surgical manipulation is considered. The therapist should always begin treatment mildly and with caution, but should not be afraid to progress to vigorous mobilization and stretching in some cases. If a "pop" or a "snap" is experienced during the stretching or mobilization treatment, it is almost always a good sign and is followed by improved range of motion.

SHOULDER-HAND SYNDROME

The shoulder-hand syndrome is a painful shoulder disability associated with sympathetic upset, swelling and pain in the entire extremity. It is often associated with and may become the end result of glenohumeral joint contracture (frozen shoulder.) The disorder may follow any painful shoulder lesion. It may be a sequel to myocardial infarction, pleurisy, painful intrathoracic lesions, cerebrovascular accidents, trauma, cervical nerve root syndrome or any of the cervical joint and muscle disorders. It may arise from any circumstance that causes the patient to keep the arm immobile such as Colle's fracture. The clinical picture is one of both joint and muscle pain, stiffness, edema, poor circulation and eventually muscle atrophy and joint contracture.

Treatment should be aggressive with emphasis toward the patient being involved in the treatment program. Active and passive range of motion, joint mobilization and massage are important treatment considerations. The elastic band resistance exercises shown in Fig. 6-8 are especially effective. Heat or cold may give relief. Intermittent positive pressure cuff treatment may also be helpful.

TENNIS ELBOW

It is generally unwise to use a diagnostic term such as tennis elbow. Zohn and Mennell point out that there are several different conditions that are often lumped together under the term "tennis elbow"[14]. However, lateral humeral epicondylitis is most commonly referred to as true tennis elbow. Specifically, the disorder involves strain and inflammation of the common extensor tendon at its insertion on the lateral epicondyle, somewhere in the common tendon or at the musculotendinous junction. The disorder may develop a painful adherent scar in the tendon and x-rays may show calcification adjacent to the lateral epicondyle in the tendon. Pain over and just distal to the lateral epicondyle may be severe and radiate to the outer side of the forearm. It is aggravated by extension of the wrist, supination of the forearm against resistance and squeezing or gripping with the hand. Weakness of the wrist extensors may develop.

Treatment: In mild cases, avoiding the pain-producing movements will result in gradual improvement. Local heat or ice, massage, ultrasound with hydrocortisone cream and Phoresor® with Decadron® and Zylocaine® are effective treatments[11,12]. A two-inch strap worn tightly around the forearm just distal to the elbow has the effect of transferring the origin of the affected muscles distally and is often effective in preventing further aggravation. Transverse friction massage is also quite effective. Pain free movement is encouraged, followed by full rehabilitation (strengthening.) Activities will usually be more aggravating with the elbow extended, therefore all exercises should be started with the elbow in flexion.

DUPUYTREN'S CONTRACTURE

Dupuytren's contracture is a contracture of the palmar fascia due to progressive fibrous proliferation resulting in flexion deformities and loss of function of the fingers. The ring finger is involved most often. Diagnosis is by visual inspection and palpation.

Treatment: Ultrasound, applied during passive stretching, and splinting have been shown to be beneficial. Advanced contractures may require surgery. Whirlpool, stretching, splinting and ultrasound may be helpful post-operatively.

DEGENERATIVE ARTHRITIS OF THE HIP

Osteoarthritis pain is usually associated with either capsular/ligamentous tightness (moderate stage) or wearing away of the joint surfaces (severe stage.) The development of degenerative arthritis in the hip shows a good example of this progression. Initially, the patient may complain of pain at night, especially when side lying on the unaffected side with the painful hip joint internally rotated and adducted. Other problem-causing positions include prolonged sitting and any position that causes the joint to internally rotate, abduct or adduct. It is not until the later stages of this disorder that the patient complains of pain with weight bearing (joint surface pain) (Fig. 6-13). Restriction of range of motion will

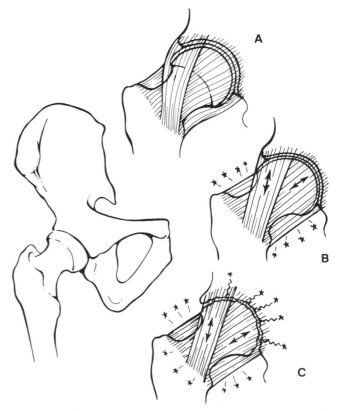

Fig. 6-13. Degenerative arthritis of the hip: A) normal; B) moderate (pain source = ligament and capsule tightness); C) severe (pain source = ligament and capsule tightness and joint surfaces.)

be greatest in internal rotation and abduction (capsular pattern) and pain will be noted at the end of range.

Treatment: Unfortunately, many patients with moderate degenerative arthritis of the hip are told that they are not ready for surgery and that at this stage there is nothing that can be done except rest and medication. This is certainly not the case, since ultrasound and vigorous mobilization and stretching, followed by strengthening exercises, can be very effective at this stage. In fact, restoration of full mobility to an arthritic hip may interrupt the progression of the degenerative joint disease by restoring the normal nutritional supply to the joint. Severe degenerative arthritis (bone-on-bone) may require surgery.

MENISCUS INJURIES OF THE KNEE

Meniscus injuries of the knee are common. The history is one of twisting on a semi-flexed knee (internal tibial rotation = medial meniscus injury, external tibial rotation = lateral meniscus injury), or hyperextension of the knee. Injury usually occurs during weight bearing. The patient experiences immediate deep pain associated with giving way of the joint. Occasionally, immediate locking of the joint is experienced so that the last 20° to 30° of extension is lost. Effusion nearly always accompanies a medial tear, but is not always present with a lateral tear. The patient will note pinpoint pain along the joint line. If the acute effusion and pain have subsided, the patient may complain of intermittent buckling of the joint and an occasional or persistent "clicking" of the joint. If full flexion is possible, a consistent click may be elicited on combined external rotation of the tibia on the femur, valgus stress and extension (tear of the posterior portion of the medial meniscus) or on combined internal rotation, varus stress and extension (tear of the posterior portion of the lateral meniscus.) This is known as McMurray's test. Apley's compression test is another procedure designed to aid in the diagnosis of a torn meniscus. With the patient lying prone with the leg flexed to 90°, the therapist applies pressure on the heel to compress the medial and lateral menisci between the tibia and femur. Then, the tibia is rotated internally and externally. Pain on the medial side indicates a medial meniscus tear and pain laterally suggests a lateral meniscus tear[24]. Weight bearing flexion and extension is often impossible[16].

Treatment: Once it has been determined that a meniscus tear exists, it is important to determine if the tear is confined to the periphery or if it involves the body of the meniscus. When a tear of the body of the meniscus is diagnosed, treatment is usually surgical and if left untreated may lead to early degenerative changes. Tears or sprains localized to the periphery (coronary ligament) do heal and surgery is usually not required. If an acute tear of the meniscus is suspected on examination, a physician should be consulted. Often arthroscopy or arthrography will assist the physician in determining the course of management[8,16]. If surgery is not indicated, the physical therapist will assume a primary role in management. Treatment is aimed at prevention of joint stiffness and disuse atrophy. Movement and activities are allowed within pain free limits. Modality treatments, especially high-voltage electrical stimulation, are helpful to promote healing. Ice, compression and elevation are indicated if effusion is present. Gradual and progressive return to normal function is encouraged as healing is accomplished.

OSGOOD-SCHLATTER'S DISEASE

Osgood-Schlatter's disease occurs predominantly in active boys between 10 and 15 years of age. A visible swelling and direct tenderness over the tibial tuberosity are the major findings and they worsen with exercise. X-rays show irregular ossification of the tibial tubercle[8].

Treatment by immobilization in extension is advisable for a period of at least five weeks. Weight bearing is usually permitted. Subsequent treatment should focus on prevention of recurrence by gradual reconditioning and avoidance of rapid increase of aggravating activities such as running[8].

CHONDROMALACIA PATELLAE

Chondromalacia patellae is a degenerative process that involves the cartilage of the articular surface of the patella. The degenerative changes may follow acute, severe trauma or repeated minor trauma. It occurs most often in young females. Patients with chondromalacia patellae often have an old history of injury to the knee followed by a later onset of catching, instability, locking, weakness and swelling in the knee. Descending stairs is often particularly difficult for patients with this disorder. The clinical examination reveals patellar tenderness, crepitus under the patella and swelling. Frequently, the tenderness will be on the lateral facet of the patella and is associated with genu valgus and a pronated foot (Fig. 6-14A). This results in the patella rubbing laterally at the knee. Walker and Schreck found a high percentage of patients with chondromalacia patellae to have leg length inequalities with the shorter leg on the involved side. These patients were also found to hyperextend the involved knee during the stance and push-off phase of the gait pattern. When a heel lift was used to correct the leg length inequality and the patient was taught to walk without knee hyperextension, the symptoms of chondromalacia were relieved[19].

Treatment: Mild cases should be treated with rest and modalities (ice, electrical stimulation and ultrasound) and protection from further injury. Since muscle weakness will almost certainly have occurred, isometric or pain free arc quadriceps and hamstring exercises are indicated. One must always assess leg length and correct it if necessary. Since many cases involve genu valgus and a pronated foot, appropriate correction with a foot orthosis (medial lift) is imperative (Fig. 6-14B). These cases may also respond to specific strengthening of the vastus medialis. High frequency electrical stimulation with short "on" time (10-15 seconds) and long "off" time (45-50 seconds) is an effective adjunct to muscle strengthening and is particularly effective in this case because it can be applied specifically to the vastus medialis muscle[26].

PLICA SYNDROME

A plica is a distinct permanent fold of the synovium of the knee that is present in 20% to 60% of the population. Three distinct plica have been described. First, the suprapatellar plica is that portion that courses from the lateral patellar tendon to the medial wall of the knee joint. The medial patellar plica is that portion that runs along the medial wall of the knee joint to the infrapatellar fat pad. Lastly, the infrapatellar plica is that portion running parallel to the anterior cruciate ligament. The plica is stretched in a bowstring fashion across

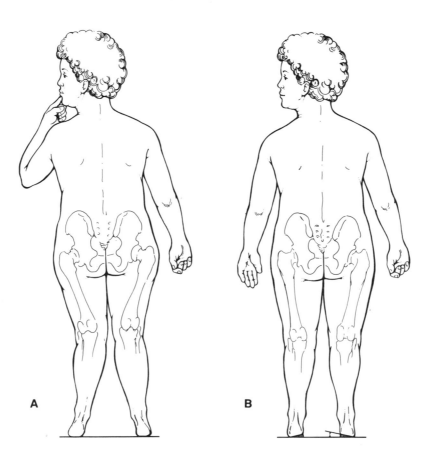

Fig. 6-14. A) This posture is often seen (especially in adolescent females) with lateral patellar pain. B) Correction with foot orthoses (medial lift) is often effective.

the medial femoral condyle underneath the patella. Normally the plica is a soft, pliant and highly elastic tissue, and is able to pass back and forth over the femoral condyles during flexion and extension of the knee joint[27].

Injury to the plica may occur as a contusion or a strain from a single, traumatic event or from repeated high levels of activity. Inflammation, edema and thickening may result. Continued trauma will lead to a tough, inelastic fibrotic band.

The patient will report a history of trauma followed by swelling and a dull, aching pain along the medial patella. Sitting for any length of time with the knee flexed will be especially uncomfortable. Pain is generally increased with activities requiring flexion of the knee and quadriceps activity (squatting, stair climbing.) Tenderness and swelling may be palpated just medial to the superior border of the patella.

Treatment: Conservative treatment can be successful, especially in the acute phase. Modalities and medications to reduce inflammation, quadriceps strengthening and hamstring stretching are effective. Quadriceps strengthening must not be aggravating and is probably most effective when done isometrically or in short arcs avoiding very much flexion. Surgery may be indicated if the

patient's symptoms do not subside in a six to eight week course of conservative treatment. Post-surgical management must be directed at restoring full function, yet at the same time avoiding irritation of the synovium for a time[27].

CHRONIC FOOT STRAIN

If excessive stress is repeatedly placed on the foot, chronic foot strain may develop. Ultimately, degenerative arthritic changes will take place and become an added source of pain. The breakdown process follows a sequence. Ligaments exposed to strain elongate and undergo inflammatory changes which results in pain. If the condition persists, the ligaments degenerate, lose their supporting function and permit eventual degenerative joint disease to develop[28].

Five common foot disorders arise from chronic foot strain: 1) metatarsalgia; 2) Morton's neuroma; 3) clawed toes; 4) plantar fasciitis and 5) pronated foot (Fig. 6-15).

Metatarsalgia

Metatarsalgia is pain and tenderness of the three middle metatarsal heads due to depression of

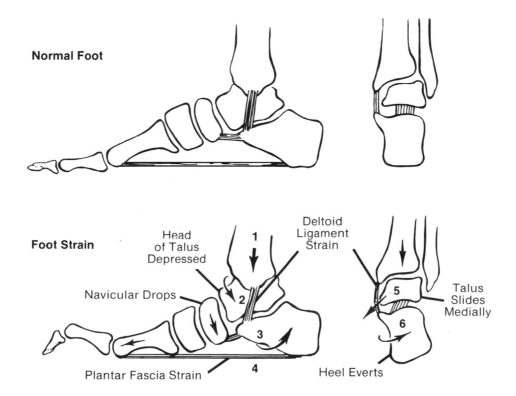

Fig. 6-15. Drawing showing the chronic foot strain process (adopted from Cailliet[28].)

the metatarsal arch which is usually caused by chronic foot strain or degenerative changes in the foot. Tender callouses may be present under the ball of the foot and are indications of excess weight bearing on the heads of the metatarsals. The patient will also describe the condition as "walking with a pebble in the shoe". Pain is usually greatest while weight bearing and is present regardless of whether the patient is wearing shoes or not. In severe cases, patients will walk with weight bearing only on the heels and will develop a "hips flexed, knees straight" gait with short, choppy steps.

Treatment: Metatarsalgia is treated by elevating the middle portion of the metatarsal arch which restores the normal weight bearing distribution. This is best accomplished by using a foot orthosis in the patient's shoe with a metatarsal support. The metatarsal support should lift under the shafts of the 2nd, 3rd and 4th metatarsals and should not press against the metatarsal heads. This treatment may also be effective for Morton's neuroma in which case the support should be smaller and lift only the fourth (third) metatarsal shaft. Surgery may be indicated if conservative management is ineffective.

Morton's Neuroma

Morton's neuroma is described as a fibrous swelling of the fourth digital nerve, resulting from irritation caused by rubbing or nipping between the metatarsal bones. It occasionally occurs between the third and fourth metatarsals[28]. It is another disorder that may cause pain in the area of the metatarsal heads, but can be distinguished from metatarsalgia because it is usually pain free if the patient is not wearing shoes and is characterized by occasional episodes of sharp, severe pain rather than the more constant pain with weight bearing caused by metatarsalgia. In other words, it is compression of the metatarsal heads in the medial-lateral plane that causes irritation of the nerve in Morton's neuroma, whereas it is weight bearing on the plantar surface of the metatarsal heads that is the cause of pain with metatarsalgia.

Treatment: See discussion of treatment of metatarsalgia above.

Clawed Toes

Clawed toes are also associated with a flattened metatarsal arch. As the arch flattens, the metartar-sophalangeal joints are pushed into extension. At the same time, the interphalangeal joints flex. The problem associated with clawed toes is the development of a callous on the top of the toe as it rubs against the roof of the shoe and a callous on the tip of the toe as it rubs against the sole of the shoe.

Treatment: This problem can also be alleviated by restoring the normal metatarsal arch. In severe case, it is sometimes necessary to provide the patient with extra-depth shoes in order to provide room for the clawed toes.

Plantar Fasciitis

Plantar fasciitis is the most frequent cause of pain felt under the heel. It occurs with or without a calcaneal spur. It is most common in a pronated foot which has a flattened longitudinal arch. As the patient with a flattened longitudinal arch walks, there is a constant pulling of the plantar fascia at its insertion on the calcaneus. Over a period of time, ossification and calcification result because of the constant traction of the plantar fascia on the periosteum. Examination reveals a point of deep tenderness at the anteromedial aspect of the calcaneus. X-rays may reveal nothing or a typical spur coming forward from the calcaneus. The spur is secondary to the primary problem of plantar fasciitis.

Treatment: Although traditional treatment is often only directed toward alleviating the pressure of weight bearing on the anteromedial aspect of the calcaneus and relieving the pain and inflammation, treatment of the primary problem (the flattened longitudinal arch) should take precedence. Therefore, a foot orthosis to restore the longitudinal arch is of primary importance. The heel of this orthosis should be contoured to the heel in order that the weight be distributed evenly. A hole or depression can be made in the orthosis at the point on the anteromedial aspect of the calcaneus in order to alleviate the weight bearing entirely at that point. It is rare that surgical removal of the spur is necessary. A high incidence of recurrence after surgery is claimed by many, due to the fact that such treatment is directed toward a symptom rather than toward the primary cause[28]. Although physical therapy modalities such as whirlpool and ultrasound seem to provide temporary relief, it is only symptomatic relief that is achieved. This, again, is because the treatment has been directed toward the symptoms rather than the primary cause.

Pronated Foot (Valgus Heel)

Pronated foot is actually a valgus position of the calcaneus on the talus. It is commonly seen in conjunction with fallen longitudinal and metatarsal arches and is a contributing factor to chronic foot strain. Assessment for pronated foot is made by viewing the patient standing from the rear. The heel should be in a central position directly under the calf of the leg and the Achilles tendon should go straight down into the calcaneus (Fig. 6-16).

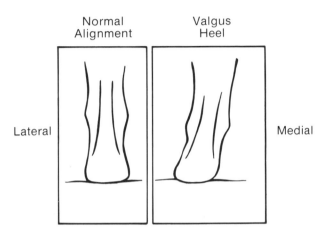

Normal
Alignment

Valgus
Heel

Lateral

Medial

Fig. 6-16. Valgus heel. The left foot is shown in this illustration.

A pronated foot can cause pain on both the medial and the lateral aspects of the foot. Medial pain can arise because of the additional strain upon the deltoid ligament and lateral pain can arise when synovium is pinched between the bony structures.

Treatment: Pronated foot should be corrected by placing a medial wedge in the patient's shoe. One should remember that flattened longitudinal and metatarsal arches may also be present with this condition and all of the necessary corrections should be built into a foot orthosis.

Treatment of all of the above disorders associated with chronic foot strain should include muscle strengthening exercises for the foot.

OTHER FOOT AND ANKLE DISORDERS

It is beyond the scope of this text to deal with other specific biomechanical and alignment problems that can develop at the foot and ankle, other than make the reader aware that they do exist. It is true that many foot and ankle problems can be effectively treated with rather simple mechanical corrections; on the other hand, a complete understanding of foot and ankle biomechanics and orthotics is necessary to evaluate and treat certain other cases, especially those involving alignment of the forefoot with the talus and calcaneus.

References:

1. Mooney, V and Robertson, J: The Facet Syndrome. Clinical Orthopaedics and Related Research 115:149-156, March/April 1976.
2. Cloward, R: The Clinical Significance of the Sinu-Vertebral Nerve of the Cervical Spine in Relation to the Cervical Disk Syndrome. Joul of Neuro and Psych 12:321-326, 1960.
3. Jayson, M and Barks, J: Structural Changes in the Intervertebral Disc. Annals Rheum Dis 32:10-15, 1973.
4. Wyke, B: The Neurological Basis of Thoracic Spinal Pain. Rheumatology and Physical Medicine 10:356-367, 1970.
5. Tabary, J, et al: Experimental Rapid Sarcomere Loss in Concomitant Hypoextensibility. Muscle Nerve 4:198-203, 1981.
6. Tabary, J, et al: Physiological and Structural Changes in the Cat's Soleus Muscle Due to Immobilization by Plaster Cast. Joul Physiol 224:231-244, 1972.
7. Cummings, G: Proceedings, 9th Annual Dogwood Conference, Atlanta, GA 1984.
8. O'Donoghue, D: Treatment of Injuries to Athletes. Saunders, Philadelphia, 1962.
9. Cyriax, J: Textbook of Orthopaedic Medicine; Diagnosis of Soft Tissue Lesions. Vol 1, 8th ed. Bailliere-Tindall, London 1982.
10. Cyriax, J: Textbook of Orthopaedic Medicine; Treatment by Manipulation, Massage and Injection. Vol 2, 10th ed. Bailliere-Tindall, London 1980.
11. Griffin, J, et al: Patients Treated with Ultrasound Driven Hydrocortisone and With Ultrasound Alone. Physical Therapy 47:594-601, 1967.
12. Bertolucci, L: Introduction of Anti-Inflammatory Drugs by Iontophoresis: Double Blind Study. Joul of Ortho and Sports Phys Ther 4:103-108, 1982.
13. Noyes, F: Advances in the Understanding of Knee Ligament Injury, Repair and Rehabilitation. Medicine and Science in Sports and Exercise 16:427-443, 1984.
14. Zohn, D and Mennell, J: Musculoskeletal Pain. Little-Brown, Boston, 1976.
15. Awad, E: Interstitial Myofibrositis: Hypothesis of the Neck. Arch of Phy Med and Rehab 54:449-453, 1973.
16. Kessler, R and Hertling, D: Management of Common Musculoskeletal Disorders. Harper and Row, Philadelphia 1983.
17. Griffin, J: Physiological Effects of Ultrasonic Energy As It is Used Clinically. Phys Ther 46:18-23, 1966.
18. Paris, S: Course Notes. The Spine. Atlanta Back Clinic, Atlanta GA 1975.

References: (Continued)

19. Walker, H and Schreck, R: Relationship of Hyperextended Gait Pattern to Chondromalacia Patellae. Phys Ther 55:259-262, 1975.
20. Turck, S: Orthopaedics. 2nd ed, Lippincott, Philadelphia 1967.
21. Kopell, H and Thompson, W: Peripheral Entrapment Neuropathies. Krieger, Huntington, NY, 1975.
22. The Merck Manual. Merck, Sharp and Dohme, Rahway NJ, 1977.
23. Cailliet, R: Neck and Arm Pain. FA Davis, Philadelphia, 1964.
24. Hoppenfeld, S: Physical Examination of the Spine and Extremities. Appleton, Century and Crofts, New York, 1976.
25. Brown, C: Personal Communication, Orthopaedic Surgeon, Great Bend, KS 1978.
26. Johnson, D; Thurston, P and Ashcroft, P: The Russian Technique of Faradism in the Treatment of Chondromalacia Patellae. Physiotherapy, Canada 29:266-268, 1977.
27. Blackburn, T; Eiland, W and Bandy, W: An Introduction to the Plica. Joul of Ortho and Sports Phys Ther 3:171-177, 1982.
28. Cailliet, R: Foot and Ankle Pain. FA Davis, Philadelphia, 1964.

CHAPTER 7

TEMPOROMANDIBULAR JOINT

Steven L. Kraus, P.T.

INTRODUCTION

Recognition and treatment of temporo-mandibular joint (TMJ) afflictions by man have been recorded as early as 3000 BC[1]. The earliest known surgical text, *The Edwin Smith Papyrus,* includes one case, a "dislocation of the mandible", which describes the method of reduction that is still used today[2]. In 1842, Cooper is said to have reported snapping in the TMJ. Another 19th century surgeon, Annandale, repositioned the articular disc and sutured it to the outer side of the joint[3]. Lanz, in 1909, introduced disc removal as a treatment choice[4].

Symptoms attributed to the TMJ first appeared with Costen's original article in 1934[5]. Costen, an otolaryngologist, described such symptoms as hearing loss, burning sensations in the tongue and throat, tinnitus and many others. These symptoms were presumably related to overclosure of the mandible (distalization of the condyle.) This overclosure was considered the etiological reason for the above symptoms for 15 years. Sicher and Zimmerman later demonstrated that there was no anatomical basis for Costen's proposal that distal pressure of the condyle on post-articular nerves or arteries caused such symptoms[6,7].

Today, seemingly based upon empirical observations, a host of symptoms are being attributed to a TMJ affliction. Suggested symptoms range from obvious ones such as pre-auricular pain to seemingly unrelated symptoms such as stiff neck, leg aches, numb or tingling arms and hands, profuse nervous perspiration and indigestion to mention only a few[8,9].

With so many symptoms supposedly related to a TMJ affliction, a variety of terms has been used in the literature in an attempt to describe disturbances of the TMJ. To the novice reader, these varied terms may be confusing and may detract from the actual topic under question. A plethora of terms has been introduced into the literature to describe the genesis of a TMJ affliction. Some of these terms are as follows:

1. Costen Syndrome
2. Mandibular Pain-Dysfunction Syndrome
3. Oto-Dental Syndrome
4. Occluso-Mandibular Disturbances
5. Arthrosis Temporomandibularis
6. Myoarthropathy of the TMJ
7. Temporomandibular Joint Arthrosis
8. Dysfunctional TMJ Arthritis
9. Pain Dysfunction Syndrome
10. Myofascial Pain-Dysfunction Syndrome
11. Temporomandibular Joint Pain-Dysfunction Syndrome
12. Dysgnathogenic Distress Syndrome
13. Craniomandibular Syndrome
14. Craniomandibular-Cervical Syndrome

Due to the variety of symptoms and terms associated with describing a TMJ affliction, it should not come as a surprise that the etiological factors are considered to be multicausal. According to the 1980 article, "Craniomandibular (TMJ) Disorders-The State of the Art", "Etiological factors are multicausal and include genetic, developmental, physiological, traumatic, pathological, environmental and behavioral factors. Etiologies can be divided into predisposing, precipitating and perpetuating factors[10]."

One only has to read past and current dental literature and/or to attend several "TMJ courses" to realize that a great deal of confusion and controversy exists in nearly every conceivable aspect of etiology, evaluation, treatment and symptoms of the TMJ. A recent paper, "Report of the President's Conference on the Examination, Diagnosis and Management of Temporomandibular Disorders", stated that ". . . few, if any, organized or standardized approaches to the examination, diagnosis or treatment of the TMJ disorders exist[11]."

It is this author's opinion that the following are the possible reasons for such confusion, controversy and mystique that have shrouded the TMJ:

1. Failure of the practicing clinician to understand the fundamental aspects of anatomy, physiology, function and dysfunction of the TMJ and adjacent areas.

2. Failure to realize that, when present in combination and interpreted properly, signs of dysfunction and a positive response to various diagnostic tests constitute a TMJ affliction; it is not diagnosed by symptoms alone.

3. Misused terminology, as well as theoretical and impractical definitions, further breeds alienation among clinicians of the same field and makes for difficult communication between other fields.

4. Inadequacies in clinical and scientific research designs.

5. Accepting the findings of various epidemiological studies too easily without first raising critical questions regarding their validity[12].

6. Failure in understanding various referred pain mechanisms that will mimic those of TMJ origin. Treatment that is mistakenly thought to be specific to the TMJ may actually be helping or aggravating symptoms originating from the adjacent areas.

7. Failure to accept that with every patient, but to varying degrees, there is a complex interaction of structure and function among the occlusion, TMJ and cervical spine.

8. Failure to acknowledge the significant influence that posture has on mandibular mobility and positioning — not only during growth and development, but also in the adult.

The previously mentioned failures exist, not only in patient care, but also in clinical and scientific studies. These failures must be addressed, or at least acknowledged, in order to further the progress that Costen and others of his era made.

Since there is an unstable foundation for every angle of approach to the TMJ disorder one should avoid, or at least keep an open mind when listening to those clinicians who offer "the only way", "the best way" and "the proven way" to treatment of the TMJ problem. Iatrogenically induced problems and their symptoms may occur in the patient, unbeknownst to both the treating clinician and the patient. The best clinician is one who recognizes his own weaknesses and strengths concerning the understanding and treatment of a problem. One should approach the patient with reversible treatment techniques unless contraindicated and should realize that it will take a team effort with the majority of these patients. The treatment coordination of various team efforts, however, should be approached in a logical, progressive manner and not by the "shot gun method."

Although basic, extensive and clinical research have provided some insight to some of these problems, the scope of such research and the associated literature has become so broad that it is nearly impossible for any single individual to integrate all of this information into a useful, meaningful and practical whole. Certainly, there will be no attempt here to do so. The objective in this synopsis is to present, in the fewest words possible, currently accurate and dependable information concerning: 1) functional anatomy of the TMJ; 2) TMJ function; 3) TMJ affliction; 4) TMJ evaluation and 5) TMJ treatment.

The following material contains guidelines for the initial steps toward the understanding of the TMJ, but by no means does it represent the total and complete solution to the TMJ dilemma.

TMJ ANATOMY

The literature on the anatomy of the TMJ is so profuse that to approach the subject with originality is nearly impossible. The purpose of this section will be to familiarize the reader with the significant anatomy of the TMJ which will enhance the understanding of its function, dysfunction, examination and treatment.

OSSEOUS STRUCTURES

Temporal Bone

The roof of the TMJ consists entirely of the squamous part of the temporal bone, and is divided into four descriptive parts (Fig. 7-1). Starting posteriorly, one will find the post-glenoid spine, the mandibular fossa, the articular eminence and the articular tubercle[13]. In the area of the post-glenoid spine, there is no posterolateral osseous structure of the temporal bone. This allows easy access for palpation of the structures situated posterolaterally to the condyle via the external auditory meatus. Externally, structures such as the lateral capsule, the temporomandibular ligament and the retrodiscal tissue in the posterolateral aspect of the joint can be easily palpated in the pre-auricular area, especially with the mouth open. The mandibular fossa is made up of very thin, compact bone; consequently, condylar function does not occur there. The slope of the articular eminence is between 30-60°. Slopes

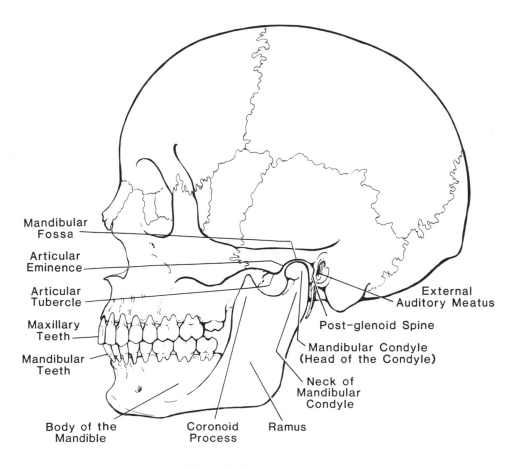

Mandibular
Fossa

Articular
Eminence

Articular
Tubercle

Maxillary
Teeth

Mandibular
Teeth

External
Auditory Meatus

Post-glenoid Spine

Mandibular Condyle
(Head of the Condyle)

Neck of
Mandibular
Condyle

Body of the
Mandible

Coronoid
Process

Ramus

Fig. 7-1. Skeletal anatomy.

of less than 30° are considered flat and slopes of greater than 60° are considered steep.

Mandibular Condyle

The ends of the mandible are composed of condyles which form the floor of the TMJ. The shapes of the frontal projection of thousands of mandibular condyles have been studied, resulting in four basic shapes to be considered[14]. The majority of human condyles (58%) are slightly convex superiorly. The next largest portion (25%) of condyles are flat superiorly. Approximately 12% are pointed or angular in shape, and approximately 3% are bulbous or rounded in shape (Fig. 7-2)[14].

Important landmarks of the condyle include the medial and lateral poles because of their ligamentous attachments. The lateral pole provides an anatomical landmark during tests of palpation and mobility (Fig. 7-3)[15] and can be easily palpated, even though its tip is approximately 13mm beneath the skin.

Lines drawn through the medial and lateral poles represent the long axes of the condyles. The

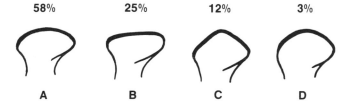

58%   25%   12%   3%

A   B   C   D

Fig. 7-2. Four shapes of mandibular condyles viewed in the frontal plane: A) convex condyle; B) flat condyle; C) angular condyle and D) rounded condyle (adapted with permission from Yale.)[14]

long axes of the condyles are usually orientated in a posteromedial plane so that lines extended through them will intersect at the anterior margin of the foramen magnum. Because of this axial orientation, a simple hinge movement during full opening does not exist (Fig. 7-4).

The condyles merge inferiorly with the neck and the neck merges inferiorly with the ramus of the mandible. These three specific regions are not clearly delineated (Fig. 7-1). The ramus continues superiorly to become the coronoid process for the attachment of the temporalis muscle. Inferiorly, the

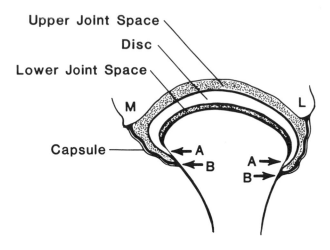

Fig. 7-3. Schematic drawing showing a frontal view of the left TMJ indicating: A) attachments of the disk to the medial and lateral poles; B) the medial and lateral attachments of the capsule to the neck. Note that there are no attachments of the disk to the medial and lateral poles of the mandibular condyle

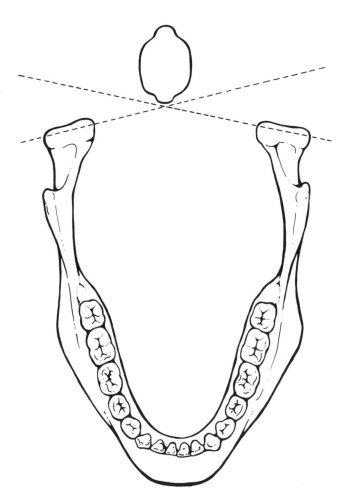

Fig. 7-4. This drawing shows that extensions of the long axes of the condyles would intersect near the anterior margin of the foramen magnum.

ramus becomes the body of the mandible, which joins the temporomandibular joints together. The mandible also houses the mandibular teeth, which articulate with the maxillary teeth.

INTRACAPSULAR STRUCTURES

Articular Disc

The temporal bone is separated from the mandibular condyle by the articular disc[16]. The disc (not a meniscus) separates the TMJ into a larger upper joint space and a smaller lower joint space (Fig. 7-3)[15]. The disc is composed of fibrocartilagenous tissue and is thereby pliable, being able to support, protect and aid in the lubrication of the articulating surfaces.

The articular disc is divided into three bands or zones: anterior (pes meniscus), intermediate (pars gracilis) and posterior (pars posterior.) The posterior band is thicker than the anterior band, and the intermediate band is the thinnest of the three (1-2mm thick) (Fig. 7-5)[17].

The intermediate band of the articular disc is positioned between the pressure bearing articulating surfaces of the temporal bone and mandibular condyle. It is this intermediate band which is both avascular and aneural with its fibrous tissue being most dense. The anterior and posterior bands have both vascular and neural elements present.

The articular disc has the following attachments (Fig. 7-5)[17]:

1. Posterior attachments

Posterior attachments of the disc are complicated.

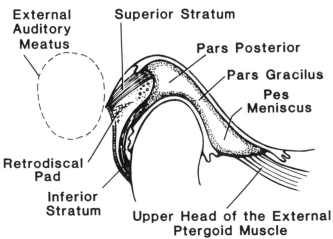

Fig. 7-5. Schematic drawing of a sagittal view of the TMJ (adapted with permission from Mahan.)[17]

The posterior-superior disc attaches to the superior stratum, which then attaches to the post-glenoid spine. The posterior-inferior disc attaches to the inferior stratum which then attaches to the neck of the mandibular condyle. The disc also attaches to the posterior capsule.

2. Anterior attachment

Anteriorly, the disc is attached to the capsule. At this point, fibers from the upper head of the external pterygoid muscle attach through the capsule into the medial part of the anterior edge of the disc.

3. Medial and lateral attachments (Fig. 7-3)[15]

Medially and laterally, the disc inserts into the corresponding roughened poles of the mandibular condyle, via the medial and lateral collateral ligaments.

Important characteristics of the attachments of the articular disc:

1. The superior stratum is comprised of elastic fibers rather than collagen fibers. Therefore, this stratum has a true modulus of elasticity.

2. The inferior stratum is comprised of collagen fibers with the elastic fibers being absent.

3. The upper head of the external pterygoid muscle contracts during closing movements of the mandible[19].

4. The capsule is not attached to the disc medially or laterally, nor to the medial and lateral collateral ligaments (Fig. 7-3)[15].

Retrodiscal Pad (Fig. 7-5)[17]

The superior and inferior stratum or laminae enclose an area termed the bilaminar zone[20]. This bilaminar zone consists of loose neurovascular connective tissue referred to as the retrodiscal pad[21]. Since the retrodiscal pad consists of both vascularized and innervated tissue within the capsule, non-arthritic intracapsular inflammation can occur. In addition, the retrodiscal pad may be the source of edema, hematoma and arthralgia.

CAPSULAR AND EXTRACAPSULAR STRUCTURES

Capsule

A fibrous capsule surrounds the TMJ. Superiorly, it is attached to the medial and lateral boundaries of the mandibular fossa and articular eminence. It arises posteriorly from the anterior surface of the post-glenoid spine and anteriorly, it attaches at the junction of the anterior disc/upper head of the external pterygoid muscle. Laterally, it is reinforced by the temporomandibular ligament. It attaches inferiorly to the neck of the mandible. Medially, the capsule has no attachments, other than what have been previously described as its superior and inferior attachments (Fig. 7-3)[15].

The synovial membrane, a highly vascularized layer of connective tissue, lines the fibrous capsule as well as the upper and lower surfaces of the retrodiscal pad. The synovial membrane does not cover any of the pressure bearing areas of the TMJ. Synovial fluid, synthesized by the synovial membrane, is the medium for metabolic exchange for the avascular joint tissue and lubricates the joint surfaces.

The clinical importance of the TMJ capsule is the sequela of a tight capsule (periarticular tissue.)[23,23]. A tight capsule can occur secondary to varying degrees of immobilization, which is sometimes seen with post-orthognathic surgery, TMJ surgery or use of rubber bands during orthodontic treatment. Capsular trauma, even without hemarthrosis or macrotrauma, will cause various areas of the capsule to undergo biomechanical and biochemical changes[24]. Various disease processes will also influence the extensibility of the periarticular tissue[25]. A tight capsule will then result in varying degrees of restrictions in mandibular dynamics and/or altered activity of the mechanoreceptors. The examination and treatment of a tight capsule will be discussed later.

Ligaments

The most prominent ligament of the temporomandibular articulation is the temporomandibular ligament. This ligament provides support to the lateral wall of the capsule with which it is associated. One end of the temporomandibular ligament is inserted into the posterior and lateral margins of the condylar neck; the other end is inserted into the zygomatic process and tubercle of the temporal bone (Fig. 7-6).

The other ligaments often associated with the TMJ, the stylomandibular and sphenomandibular ligaments, may be mentioned here. They do not contribute significantly to the temporomandibular unit, and are only important to function in that they limit jaw movement at maximum opened and protruded positions (Fig. 7-7).

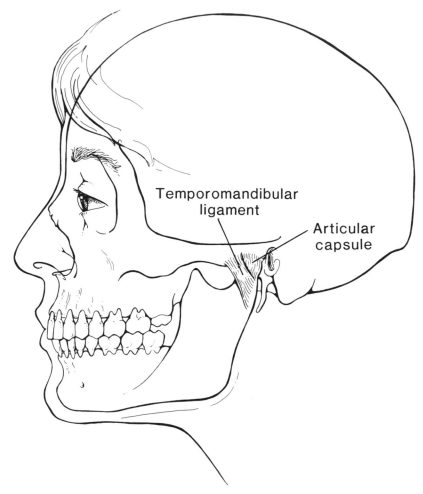

Fig. 7-6. Lateral view of ligamentous-capsular support of the TMJ.

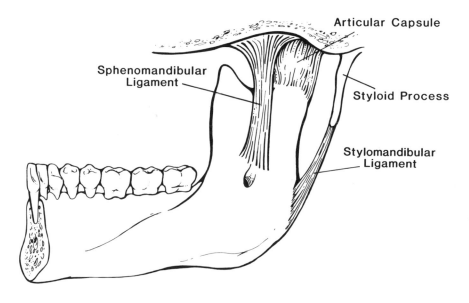

Fig. 7-7. Medial view of ligamentous-capsular support of the TMJ.

TMJ INNERVATION

The innervated tissues of the TMJ are supplied by three nerves which are part of the mandibular division of Cranial Nerve V. The posterior deep temporal and masseteric nerves supply the medial and anterior regions of the joint and the auriculotemporal nerve supplies the posterior and lateral regions of the joint. The auriculotemporal nerve also sends a few branches to the tympani membrane, the external auditory meatus, the superior one-half of the auricle on its lateral aspect and to the skin of the temple and scalp[28, 29].

The auriculotemporal nerve is the major nerve innervating the capsular blood vessels, the retrodiscal pad, the posterolateral capsule and the TMJ ligament of the temporomandibular joint. These tissues have an abundant supply of Type IV receptors (articular pain receptors.) This is of clinical significance as the auriculotemporal nerve crosses posterior to the neck of the mandibular condyle and anesthestizing the nerve at this point will usually block TMJ pain. The posterior deep temporal and masseteric nerves which supply medial and anterior regions of the joint contain fibers that are larger than C and A-delta fibers that subserve pain[30]. Assimulating this testing procedure with other evaluation findings makes this a good differential diagnostic test. In other words, if one anesthetizes the TMJ via the auriculotemporal nerve and pain still persists, then one may assume that the pain is probably coming from some structure other than the TMJ because the deep temporal and massenteric nerves contain very few, if any, pain fibers.

In addition to the Type IV receptor system, other receptors in which the three nerves terminate are Type I, II and III mechanoreceptors. For detailed understanding of their morphological and functional characteristics, articles by Klineberg, Clark and Wyke are recommended[31, 32].

The general characteristics of Type I, II and III mechanoreceptors for all synovial joints are 1) postural and kinesthetic perception; 2) reflexive influence on motor neuron pool activity and 3) inhibition of nociceptor mechanoreceptor activity.

Of clinical importance is the fact that intracapsular pressure changes (hemiarthrosis, edema), capsular tightness (trauma, immobilization) and strained positions of the mandibular condyles (various dental procedures, some cervical traction devices) will cause abnormal activity of these receptors[33]. As a result there will be altered muscle activity of those muscles innervated by Cranial Nerve V and altered perception of mandibular movement and positioning.

TMJ HISTOLOGY

The TMJ is one of the few synovial joints which does not have articular surfaces composed of hyaline cartilage. This joint has a fibrous type of articular tissue which is converted postnatally into fibrocartilage in pressure bearing areas. Fibrocartilage has the capacity to undergo a great deal of remodeling. These remodeling changes will be, to a certain extent, dependent upon the functional demands placed on the joint. Remodeling will occur throughout life and is significant enough to alter the growth contours of the joint. The location of the fibrocartilage on the osseous structures indicates where function takes place. Fibrocartilage is located most abundantly on the articular tubercle and eminence of the temporal bone and on the anterior-superior surface of the mandibular condyle[26, 27]. Any treatment procedure that is performed to the TMJ must keep the functional requirements of this joint in mind. Function of the TMJ occurs with the condyle translating along the slope of the articular eminence, with the non-innervated portion of the disc between the two articulating surfaces.

MUSCLES

Movements of the mandible are a result of the action of the cervical and jaw muscles. The cervical muscles stabilize the head to increase the efficiency of the mandibular movements. Therefore, the function and method of examination for all muscles of the upper quarter area (cephalad to the mid-thoracic area) need to be understood because of their impact on TMJ function/dysfunction.

Altered muscle activity, with or without associated active or latent myofascial trigger points of the muscles in the head, jaw and neck regions, can be the result of a TMJ affliction. Conversely, these same muscles may be the cause of various TMJ afflictions. Combinations of other predisposing, precipitating and perpetuating etiological factors can influence muscle activity of the head, jaw and neck regions. Such factors include stress, malocclusion and altered head/neck posturing[34, 35, 36]. It would be naive to assume that normalization of muscle activity will occur through treatment of the TMJ only. The involved adjacent areas must be considered in any treatment plan. Those who claim success with normalizing muscle activity and decreasing pain through treatment of the TMJ alone may inadvertently be treating adjacent areas which helps to decrease pain and normalize muscle activity. One cannot separate one physiological area from the other when it comes to function, dysfunction and the actual reasons for the success or failure of certain treatment procedures.

For the above reason, this author prefers not to consider muscles under the topic of TMJ affliction, simply because there is no intracapsular muscle of the TMJ (with the possible exception of the upper head of the external pterygoid.) However, muscles of the upper quarter area will always need to be examined. This examination should include palpation for an increased or decreased muscle tone, and any associated active or latent myofascial trigger points should be noted[37]. The initial examination usually will not test for muscle strength or coordination due to false positives which may occur until other means of restoring function are initiated. To this end, one should progress with muscle strengthening or coordination exercises if necessary[38].

The functions of only those muscles which have a close neurophysiological relationship to the TMJ will be mentioned here. These muscle include those innervated by Cranial Nerve V. It can be assumed that each of the muscles innervated by the fifth cranial nerve will be involved with a TMJ affliction. The primary functions of those muscles innervated by Cranial Nerve V are (Figs. 7-8 through 7-12):

1. Temporalis — elevation of the mandible.
2. Masseter — elevation of the mandible.
3. Internal pterygoid muscle — elevation of the mandible.
4. External pterygoid muscle — the upper head contracts on closing, influencing the relationship of the disc to the condyle; the lower head protrudes and deviates the mandible to the opposite side; bilateral contraction will protrude the mandible in midline.
5. Anterior digastric muscle — depresses the mandible.

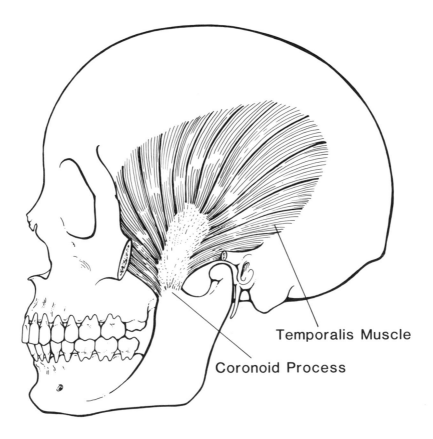

Temporalis Muscle

Coronoid Process

Fig. 7-8. Temporalis muscle.

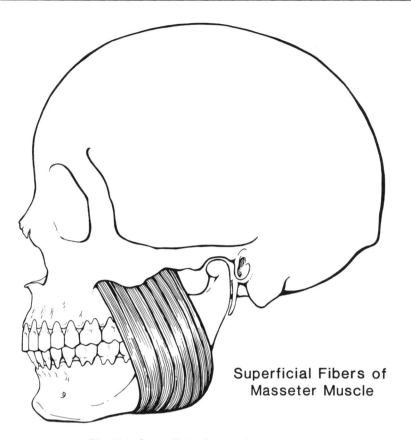

Superficial Fibers of Masseter Muscle

Fig. 7-9. Superficial fibers of masseter muscle.

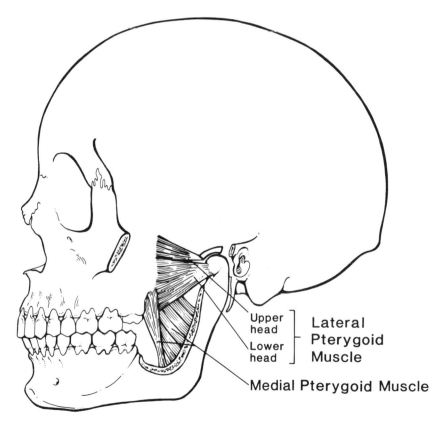

Upper head
Lower head
] **Lateral Pterygoid Muscle**

Medial Pterygoid Muscle

Fig. 7-10. Medial and lateral pterygoid muscles.

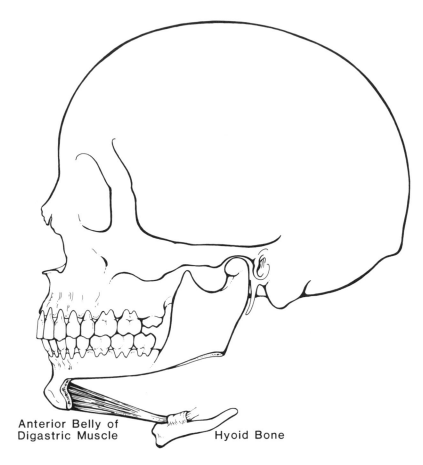

Fig. 7-11. Anterior belly of the digastric muscle.

6. Mylohyoid muscle — depresses the mandible

7. Tensor tympani muscle — controls movement of the tympanic membrane.

8. Tensor veli palatini muscle — controls diameter of the eustachian tube.

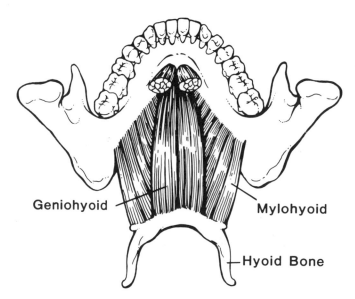

Fig. 7-12. Mylohyoid and geniohyoid muscles viewed from above and behind the floor of the mouth.

For more detail regarding origin, insertion and secondary functions of these and other muscles of the upper quarter area, the reader should refer to any anatomy text. It should be remembered that when one finds a muscle or a group of muscles that have altered muscle tone and/or myofascial trigger points, one should not treat the TMJ without first considering the other etiological factors which may be contributing to muscle imbalances.

TMJ FUNCTION

The TMJ is described as a ginglymo-arthrodial articulation. Ginglymo means a simple hinge joint, and arthodial refers to a form of joint in which the articular surfaces glide over or slide against each other during movement[39]. The TMJ allows the mandible to perform opening and closing movements, retrusive and protrusive movements and lateral movements. During such activities as chewing and talking, a variety of movements is possible, combining the conventional arthro-kinematic movements of rotation, translation and spin of the TMJ[40]. These basic arthrokinematic movements which occur during normal activity will be described as well as the movements of the disc and its relationship to the joint surfaces. By understanding these movements and relationships, the reader will be able to determine dysfunction through observations and measurements.

MOVEMENT OF THE CONDYLE IN RELATIONSHIP TO THE TEMPORAL BONE

In the absence of any TMJ afflictions and the presence of "normal" osseous structures, one should be able to observe normal range of motion. One needs to realize that genetic factors such as the shapes of the mandibular condyle, changes in the longitudial axis of the mandibular condyles and the slopes of the articular eminence will also influence mandibular dynamics. Altered mandibular dynamics in the absence of other signs and symptoms may be "normal" for an individual patient.

Mandibular Opening

Posterior rotation of the condyle occurs from a closed position of the mandible (tooth-to-tooth contact) to approximately 11mm of opening. This movement is measured from the tip of a middle upper incisor to the tip of a lower middle incisor. At this point of opening, anterior translation begins and continues with rotation until a functional opening of approximately 40mm is achieved. During mandibular closing, the reverse occurs.

Mandibular Protrusion

During protrusive movements the condyles translate anteriorly. It is not necessary to measure the actual distance of protrusion, but contact between the upper and lower incisors is necessary to form certain phonetic sounds (hiss, house, church, etc. . .) and incise certain foods.

Mandibular Lateral Movements

During lateral movements there will be translation of the condyle on the contralateral side and spin of the condyle on the ipsilateral side. Normal lateral movements are present when the inferior frenulum moves at least the width of one full upper middle incisor (approximately 8mm.) The inferior frenulum can be seen by pulling the patient's lower lip down slightly (Fig. 7-13).

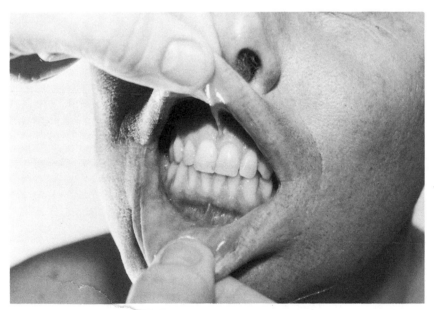

Fig. 7-13. This photograph shows both upper and lower frenulums. In mandibular testing, one should observe the frenulums stay in midline during opening and protrusive movements. During lateral movements, one should observe the bottom frenulum move the width of one full upper middle incisor.

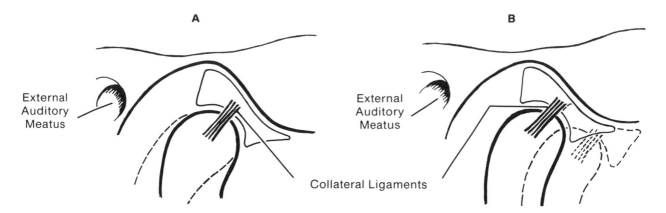

Fig. 7-14. A) This drawing shows rotation occurring in the lower joint space. B) This drawing shows translation occurring in the upper joint space (adopted with permission from Bell.)[41]

MOVEMENT OF THE DISC IN RELATIONSHIP TO THE HEAD OF THE CONDYLE

During the initial phase of opening, which involves only posterior rotation of the mandibular condyle, the disc basically remains stationary. Rotation thus occurs between the disc and the mandibular condyle (lower joint space.) Due to the firm attachment of the disc on the mandibular condyle via the collateral ligaments, the condyle and disc move as a unit during translation. Translation must then occur between the disc and the articular eminence and tubercle (upper joint space) (Fig. 7-14)[41].

During the first 11mm of opening, the disc remains stationary as the condyle rotates under the disc. After this approximately 11mm of opening, the disc and the mandibular condyle begin to translate anteriorly together in relation to the articular eminence of the temporal bone. The disc is rotated posteriorly relative to the mandibular condyle by the pull of the superior stratum [41, 42]. This keeps the non-innervated middle part of the disc between the articulating surfaces during opening. During closing, the reverse occurs. The head of the condyle and the disc translate posteriorly together in relation to the temporal bone. The disc is then rotated anteriorly relative to the mandibular condyle by the contraction of the upper head of the external pterygoid muscle. During this time, the superior stratum progressively relaxes as closing occurs. Once again, the non-innervated part of the disc is maintained between the articulating surfaces (Fig. 7-15)[42].

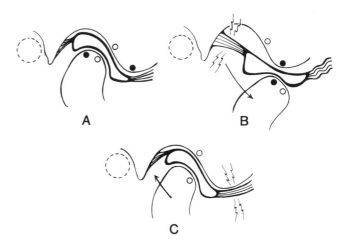

Fig. 7-15. A) Position of the disc with the teeth together. B) Position of the disc during mandibular opening. The disc is rotated posteriorly to the head of the condyle by the tension produced in the superior stratum. This occurs after the condyle has entered into the translation phase. C) Position of the disc during mandibular closing. The disc is rotated anteriorly to the head of the condyle by contraction of the upper head of the external pterygoid.

Note: White dots indicate location of maximum pressure on the articular surfaces with the teeth together and black dots indicate location of maximum pressure with the teeth apart (adapted with permission from Mahan.)[42]

The disc can be viewed as a passive structure that is attached to the mandibular condyle. During movement, the disc is kept in proper position between the mandibular condyle and the articular eminence and tubercle by the non-contractile tissue, the superior stratum and the contractile tissue, the upper head of the external pterygoid muscle. Proper coordination between these two types of tissues and intact collateral ligaments are essential for normal functioning to occur.

TMJ AFFLICTIONS

Throughout this chapter, the phrase "TMJ afflictions" has been repeatedly mentioned. TMJ afflictions will be broadly classified as:[43]

1. Developmental Abnormalities

These include such abnormalities such as hypoplasia, hyperplasia and chondromas of the TMJ.

2. Diseases

Diseases such as degenerative, rheumatoid and psoriatic arthritis, as well as osteochondritis and infections of the TMJ are included here.

3. Macrotrauma

This classification includes injury resulting in fractures and dislocations of the TMJ.

4. Dysfunction

A dysfunction is an abnormal condition that is neither a developmental abnormality nor a disease, and any trauma was such that a fracture or dislocation of the TMJ did not occur.

There is such a complex interrelationship of developmental abnormalities, diseases and dysfunctions with or without macrotrauma, that in a clinical situation it is entirely possible for a patient to have a combination of TMJ afflictions. Fortunately, the patient who is seeking help for a painful TMJ affliction will usually present a problem of the dysfunctional type in the typical clinical setting[44]. This chapter will concern only the examination and treatment of those types of TMJ afflictions which are dysfunctional in nature.

EXAMINATION FOR TMJ DYSFUNCTION

GENERAL COMMENTS

The TMJ examination will be divided into two parts. Part I will address the signs of dysfunction, and Part II will address the symptoms of dysfunction as illicited by tests of provocation.

Dorland's Medical Dictionary[45] defines a *sign* as "an indication of the existence of something; any objective evidence." A *symptom* is what the patient subjectively states as being wrong. If a patient has various signs of TMJ dysfunction present, but complains of no local symptoms, or if no symptoms can be illicited by special tests of provocation, the clinician should look elsewhere for the patient's source of pain. This is not meant to de-emphasize the importance of signs which are present and are not symptomatic. Rather, it implies that treatment of the TMJ in the absence of pain becomes a matter of clinical judgement. Since it has yet to be established that certain types of therapy are prophylactic for TMJ problems, a "Pandora's Box" may be opened for both the patient and therapist. Thus, the therapist must be well versed in the total treatment concept for TMJ patients.

If no signs of dysfunction are present with the TMJ but the patient complains of pain, one should consider the possibility of referred pain or pain coming from adjacent tissues. The clinician runs the risk of being misled by the patient and needs to carefully assess the responses by the patient. This is particularly true of the patient who does not respond to tests of provocation painfully and shows no signs of dysfunction. Initiation of treatment in this case would be inappropriate. It is very difficult to selectively test only one tissue without involving adjacent tissues. A single test reveals little, but several comparable tests may reveal much. Realistically, there is no ideal way to examine functional disorders of the TMJ.

An evaluation form used in examination for TMJ dysfunction is shown in Fig. 7-16.

SIGNS OF DYSFUNCTION

Disc-Condyle Derangements

A. Anterior Disc Dislocation That Reduces (Fig. 7-17)[43]

This is the most common disc-condyle derangement which presents itself clinically. With the teeth together, the disc is anterior to the condyle with the condyle in a more posterior-superior position relative to the disc. The classical signs of this dysfunction are:

— A distinguished, sometimes loud click during mandibular opening, signifying that the disc has relocated itself with respect to the condyle.

— During mandibular closing, a more subtle click usually occurs signifying that the disc has displaced itself anterior to the mandibular condyle.

— The jaw position at the moment of the opening click is usually a different jaw position at the moment of the closing click.

— Once the patient opens and experiences the opening click, if he then closes to an edge-to-edge

TMJ EVALUATION FORM

I.   History[11]

— Do you have difficulty opening your mouth? _____

— Do you hear noises from the jaw joint? _____

— Does your jaw get "stuck", "locked", or "go out"? _____

— Do you have pain in or about the ears or cheeks? _____

— Do you have pain on chewing or yawning or wide opening? _____

— Does your bite feel uncomfortable or unusual? _____

— Have you ever had an injury to your jaw, head, or neck? _____

— Have you ever had arthritis? _____

— Have you previously been treated for a temporomandibular disorder? _____

— If so, when, what, how, and by whom? _____

II.   Mandibular Dynamics

MANDIBULAR DYNAMICS

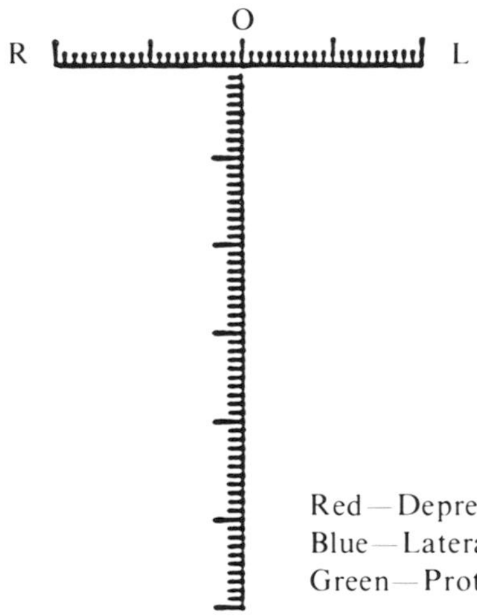

Red—Depression
Blue—Lateral Deviation
Green—Protrusion

III.   TMJ Joint Noises Present: Yes_____, No_____, Describe _____

IV.   TMJ Loading:

     A.   Pain with retrusive overpressure   L _____   R_____

     B.   Forced biting on left, pain   L _____   R_____

        Forced biting on right, pain   L _____   R_____

V.   TMJ Palpation:

     A.   Around the lateral pole mouth closed, pain   L _____   R_____

     B.   Around the lateral pole mouth open, pain   L _____   R_____

     C.   Palpation via the external auditory meatus, pain   L _____   R_____

Fig. 7-16. TMJ evaluation form.

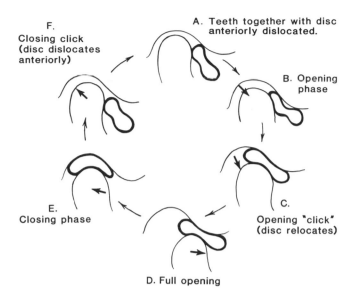

Fig. 7-17. Anterior disc dislocation that reduces. A) The disc is displaced anteriorly in the closed position. B) As the condyle translates forward, the disc remains in front of the condyle until the opening click occurs. C) Coincident with the opening click, the condyle snaps downward beneath the thick posterior band of the disc. D) Condylar translation proceeds normally. E) During retrusion, the disc and condyle remain normally positioned until the last instant of retrusion. F) When the closing click occurs, the condyle is suddenly displaced posterior-superiorly and the disc is displaced anteriorly (adapted with permission from Farrar and McCarty.)[43]

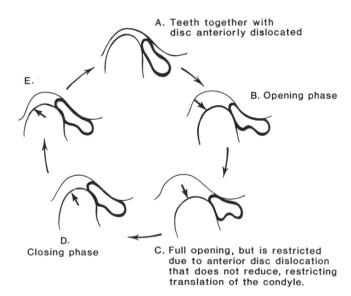

Fig. 7-18. Anterior disc dislocation that does not reduce. The range of condylar translation is limited by the anteriorly dislocated disc. The disc thickens or becomes folded and reciprocal clicking does not occur (adapted with permission from Farrar and McCarty.)[43]

position with his anterior incisors, and opens and closes in this position, no reciprocal click will be heard. If, however, the reciprocal click is still heard in this position, the dysfunction may not be able to be helped by conservative care.

The only structure which can possibly relocate the disc during opening is the superior stratum. This normally occurs once the condyle begins to translate. If it has sufficient integrity, tension develops in the superior stratum and "snaps" the disc into place. One can reason that if the opening click occurs late in the opening that this indicates a decrease in the elastic properties in the superior stratum. A loss of elasticity renders the superior stratum ineffective in relocating the disc.

The clinician needs to be aware of "trick" movements which produce no joint noises that the mandible can make to subtly "recapture" the disc. These movements are usually lateral movements during opening, presenting as an "S" curve or a side-to-side movement. If this is suspected, the patient should be encouraged to open widely, keeping the jaw in midline. This will usually expose the reciprocal click.

B. Anterior Disc Dislocation That Does Not Reduce (Fig. 7-18)[43]

When this condition is present in its early phase, no joint noises will be heard. Instead, there will be a series of reproducable restrictions during mandibular movements. These restrictions are due to the disc blocking translatory glide. Examples of such altered mandibular dynamics due to an anterior disc dislocation that does not reduce (right TMJ) are:

— Deviation to the right during mandibular opening and less than functional opening (40mm.)

— Deviation to the right during protrusive movements.

— Decrease in left lateral movements.

The patient's history may suggest one or a combination of the following, which may have preceded the restrictions in mandibular movement:

— Trauma to the mandible

— The patient states that his TMJ(s) "used to click and pop, but now do not" (went from a disc that dislocated-relocated to one that is now staying dislocated.)

— Iatrogenically induced[46].

In the early phase, some individuals are able to tolerate the disc dislocation that does not reduce.

Over time, these individuals may literally push the disc further anteriorly, and end up with no restrictions in mandibular movement. The key to identifying this condition is the patient's history, in that in the absence of trauma and iatrogenically induced problems, the majority of the patients will recall that their jaw "used to click and pop."

Capsule

The involvement of the capsule as described here will be a capsule that has undergone bio-chemical and biomechanical changes resulting in a "tight" capsule. The history that may be associated with capsular tightness is:

— Immobilization of the joint(s). This is seen post-orthognathic surgery where the maxillary and mandibular arches were wired shut for an extended period (usually six to eight weeks.)

— Trauma to the mandible.

— Post TMJ surgery with incision of the capsule.

The capsular pattern of limitation of motion for the right TMJ during mandibular movements is:

— Deviation to the right during opening, with less than functional opening.

— Deviation to the right during protrusive movements.

— Decrease in the left lateral movement.

These restrictions in mandibular movement are the same for an anterior disc dislocation that does not reduce in its early phase. History is the key to the differential diagnosis. In the absence of trauma or iatrogenically induced problems, mandibular re-strictions due to an anterior disc dislocation that does not reduce are classically preceded by a reciprocal click. If trauma is involved, both conditions could exist. In this case, the patient should be asked if he used to have joint noises with movement of the mandible. If this provides no insight, then a trial treatment of distraction to the TMJ is indicated (see Treatment.) During the dis-traction techniques, if a "snap, pop" is heard, followed by immediate restoration of normal mandibular dynamics, then an anterior disc dis-location was the problem and it has now been reduced.

Subluxation (Too Much Translation)

The TMJ can sublux itself through its own muscular dynamics. Subluxation occurs when the condyle translates onto the articular tubercle and then back to the articular eminence. There may be some predisposing factors to allow the subluxation to occur more easily in some individuals more than others, such as a decrease in the slope of the articular eminence or a flattened condylar head. Even though a large percentage of the "normal" population can sublux their TMJ(s), such subluxation should be controlled for reasons that will be mentioned later.

Subluxation can be evaluated by observing:

— Excessive mandibular opening (greater than 40mm.)

— Palpation of the lateral poles during opening to see if they move too far anteriorly.

— If unilateral subluxation occurs, there will be a quick deviation from midline to the contra-lateral side at the end of opening.

— Typically there will be no opening noise heard, but instead a noise at the beginning of closing.

Some clinicians mistake a subluxation condi-tion for an anterior disc dislocation that reduces, treating it based only upon the finding of joint noises.

Translation Occurring Too Soon in Opening (Within the First 11mm of Opening)

By observing mandibular opening and/or palpating the lateral poles with the middle fingers and the thumbs lightly touching the tip of the chin, early translation may be appreciated. What the clinician will feel is a jutting of the jaw forward at the onset of opening. Such a movement is contrary to the normal arthrokinematic movements (translation beginning only after the first 11mm of opening.) This dysfunction places more stress on the intra-capsular tissues and collateral ligaments.

Both subluxation and translation occurring too soon in opening are conditions that involve muscle imbalances. There may be no actual TMJ dys-function present with these two conditions (disc-condyle derangements, tight capsule, etc. . .) and they may occur separately or together in the same individual. These two conditions are placed under the category of TMJ dysfunction for the reason of their immediate or long range effect on the TMJ. If either or both of these conditions are observed, it is important to control them to: 1) minimize the stress placed upon the intracapsular tissues and 2) prevent the perpetuation of a TMJ dysfunction which is present and may be a hindering factor to the treatment.

These two conditions represent muscle imbalances which can be controlled initially through neuromuscular re-educational exercise. Other means of controlling muscle imbalances, such as looking at the occlusion and its interrelationship to head/neck posturing, will also need to be considered.

SYMPTOMS OF TMJ DYSFUNCTION AS ILLICITED BY TESTS OF PROVOCATIONS

When examining for TMJ dysfunction, one always has to remember that one physiological area cannot be divorced from another with respect to functional interrelationships. Pain arising from muscles related to TMJ dysfunction or to the cervical spine and occlusion needs to be considered as well as pain arising from the cervical spine which is being referred into the head, facial and jaw areas.

It is advisable that the patient be evaluated by other health professionals, such as a neurologist, otolaryngologist, or optomologist when correlation of signs and symptoms is difficult. If no structural and/or pathological involvement is found by these specialists, then the therapist can base his treatment or recommendation on the findings of the physical therapy examination.

The following tests of provocation are designed to illicit pain (altered sensation) from the patient and require the patient's testimony as to whether the tests increased, decreased or did nothing to the perception of his pain. The results of these tests will be compared with the signs of dysfunction in order to determine the degree of TMJ involvement. With little agreement in the literature as to the symptoms which arise from a TMJ dysfunction, the following tests of provocation, based on this author's clinical experience, are those most frequently found to reproduce the patient's symptoms. The patient with a TMJ dysfunction may complain of: 1) pain in the immediate area of the TMJ with mandibular movement during acts of chewing, talking and yawning; 2) referred pain occurring around the ear and eyes, along the zygomatic arch and in the temple areas. The following tests are done with the clinician seated or standing facing the patient:

A. **Palpation**
B. **Loading (Forced Biting)**
C. **Loading (Forced Retrusion)**

A. Palpation

1. With the patient's mouth closed, palpate over the lateral pole, behind it, and along the course of the temporomandibular ligament. Some patients may have a palpable swelling about the TMJ.

2. With the mouth open, palpate as described in #1. The mandibular condyle will have translated anteriorly giving more access to the tissues in the posterior-lateral aspect of the joint cavity.

3. With the patient's mouth open, insert the fifth fingers into the external auditory meatuses with the fleshy part of the fingers facing anteriorly. Have the patient close slowly (Fig. 7-19).

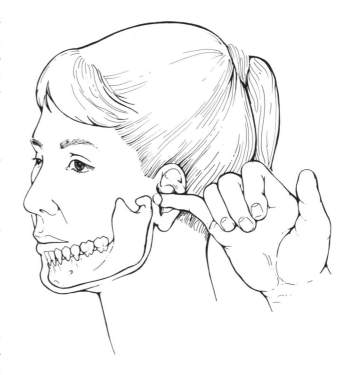

Fig. 7-19. Palpation of tissue in the area posterolateral to the mandibular condyle.

The above tests are for palpation of the lateral capsule, temporomandibular ligament and the retrodiscal tissue in the posterior-lateral aspect of the joint. They also test the ability of these tissues to tolerate additional mechanical stresses placed upon them by the palpation.

B. Loading (Forced Biting)

Studies indicate that, when placing a fulcrum such as a cotton roll on the posterior teeth and having the patient bite, there will be distraction of the condyle from the mandibular fossa on the ipsilateral side and compression of the condyle into the mandibular fossa on the contralateral side.[47] The following conclusions can be made from the patient's response to this test:

1. Forced biting on the side of complaint with no increase in pain indicates that the load is reduced on the involved tissues (retrodiscal tissue.) This should be confirmed by forced biting on the contralateral side of the pain which should increase the patient's original complaint of pain.

2. Forced biting on the side of the complaint with an increase in pain indicates a tensional force on the involved tissues (capsule and ligament.) This should be confirmed by forced biting on the contralateral side of the patient's pain which should not increase the patient's original complaint.

C. Loading (Forced Retrusion)

The clinician should support the patient's head by resting him in the supine position or by sitting or standing him against a wall. The clinician then presses on the tip of the mandible (chin) in a posterosuperior direction; first in midline, then to the right and left. This compresses the more central and medial structures to the TMJ, testing primarily the retrodiscal tissues. If this test is negative even when others are positive for involved intercapsular tissues (retrodiscal tissue), this may be because the muscles of mastication are powerful and may resist any posterosuperior motion applied to the mandible.

Since any combination of signs and symptoms may be present, it is difficult to give a clear-cut example of TMJ dysfunction. With study of physiology and function of the TMJ, the clinician's interpretation of the findings from the examination will improve with time and experience. Treatment will be based upon a continuing re-evaluation of the patient's condition prior to each treatment session.

In summary, a patient will be considered to be experiencing a TMJ dysfunction if a combination of following are present:

1. Altered mandibular dynamics.
2. TMJ joint noises.
3. Significant findings on x-rays.
4. Patient's positive pain response to loading of the temporomandibular joints.
5. Patient's positive pain response to palpation of the temporomandibular joints.

TMJ IMAGING

When presented with a suspected TMJ affliction, an x-ray examination should be included if the evaluation findings are questionable or if one wants to rule out pathological involvement. However, treatment based solely on x-ray findings is not justifiable. Madsen, Copp and Rockler found no positive correlation between radiological findings and the severity of pain and dysfunction in the TMJ[48]. However, others believe TMJ radiography plays a primary role in the diagnosis of such dysfunctions[49, 50]. There are many who believe that any description of what appears on a radiograph is only a description of what no one else but the describer sees.[47, 48] In summary, the primary goal of TMJ x-rays is to rule out specific pathology and to ascertain the osseous structural integrity of the joints prior to treatment. For further reading on radiological investigations of the TMJ, refer to the bibliography.

ARTHROGRAPHY OF THE TMJ

Arthrography is the injection of contrast material into a synovial space followed by radiography of the joint. Arthrography of the TMJ is used to identify disc dislocation. The objective is to opacify the joint synovial space (inferior joint space) so that radiography may provide images of the articular disc and its attachments. TMJ arthrography is usually not necessary to confirm the diagnosis with patients experiencing a disc dislocation. It is a beneficial diagnostic tool if there are doubts about disc dislocation being present and the integrity of the posterior attachments of the disc. It provides scientific documentation of a dislocation prior to any surgery if conservative treatments fail. Disadvantages of the procedure are: 1) it may be painful; 2) the risk of infection; 3) hypersensitive reaction to the dye. For further reading regarding technique and normal vs. abnormal arthrograms, the reader is referred to the bibliography, numbers 53, 54 and 55.

TREATMENT FOR TMJ DYSFUNCTION

Treatment is based upon the initial evaluation and subsequent re-evaluation of the patient's condition before each additional treatment session. Since every patient has a different degree of functional and pathological involvement, duration of involvement and perception of pain, it would be most difficult to discuss in detail the progression of treatments.

Therefore, a discussion of isolating a single involved tissue will ensue, but one should realize that clinically, things do not occur singularly, but plurally. Once again, the clinician must rely upon the basic knowledge of functional anatomy and clinical experience.

INTRACAPSULAR INFLAMMATION (RETRODISCAL TISSUE)

Immediate treatment for this condition would involve the use of modalities. The guidelines for using modalities are the same as those followed for any other joint inflammatory conditions of the extremities or spine. If muscle imbalances are present, which contribute to subluxation or to translation occurring too soon with opening, they need to be controlled. If the imbalances are not controlled, these conditions will perpetuate intracapsular inflammation.

If present, certain imbalances of the bite (malocclusion) can perpetuate intracapsular in-

flammation. In this situation, the patient will require an occlusal adjustment (irreversible treatment) and/or the use of a removable intra-oral appliance (reversible treatment.) Discussion of occlusion, its evaluation and the specifics in the use and design of intra-oral appliances is beyond the scope of this chapter.

ANTERIOR DISC DISLOCATION THAT REDUCES

Intra-oral mouth appliances will need to be fitted to the patient by a dentist who has a working knowledge of disc displacements, the use of certain mouth appliances and the progressive use of the mouth appliances. These appliances will typically reposition the mandible in a more forward position to help in maintaining the proper disc-condyle relationship until "healing has taken place" (Fig. 7-20). Once again, controlling for any muscle imbalances will need to be done to avoid perpetuating this problem.

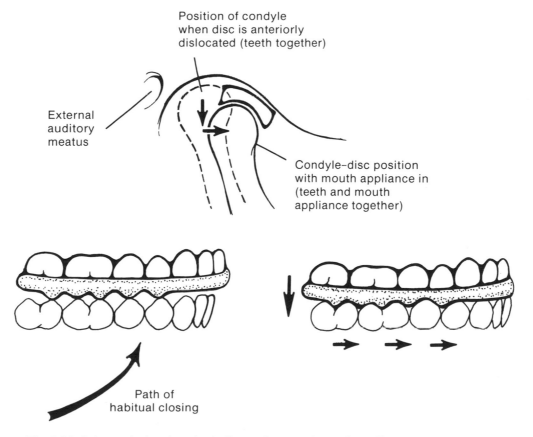

Fig. 7-20. Schematic drawings including an intra-oral mouth appliance used to maintain a proper disc-condyle relationship until "healing has taken place." During habitual closing, the design of the mouth appliance will cause the muscles to immediately dictate the jaw to close more forward, thereby preventing the condyle from going too far posteriorly. Therefore, the disc is not able to dislocate anteriorly.

ANTERIOR DISC DISLOCATION THAT DOES NOT REDUCE

Intra-oral distractional techniques with or without anterior glide will be applied, in order to attempt to recapture the disc (Fig. 7-21)[56]. Before doing these techniques, patient preparation is important. Use of modalities to help relax the adjacent muscles is indicated. Medication and/or injections will be beneficial to further relax the musculature. Once the disc is relocated (confirmed by restoration of normal mandibular dynamics), an intra-oral mouth appliance will be used to help maintain proper disc condyle positioning. If a physical therapist is performing the distractional techniques and is successful, he should place cotton rolls between the back teeth and refer the patient to a dentist who is knowledgeable in the application of such mouth appliances.

TIGHT CAPSULE

The same intra-oral techniques as were used for the anterior disc dislocation that does not reduce

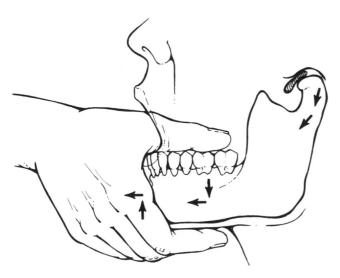

Fig. 7-21. An intra-oral distraction technique used to relocate a disc that does not relocate itself during opening (an anterior dislocation that does not reduce.) The thumb is extended to cover the occlusal surfaces of the mandibular teeth. The fingers are positioned to grasp the inferior border of the mandible. On the side of the dislocated disc, pressure is applied by the thumb to torque the condyle downward while pressure is applied upward with the fingers. Then, the condyle of the affected side is pulled anteriorly and medially. When this procedure is successful, the condyle is pulled downward under the thick posterior band of the disc and the disc snaps back to its normal position above the condyle (adapted with permission from Farrar and McCarty.)[56]

will be used for this condition, as well as joint play techniques (Fig. 7-22, 7-23). Patient preparation utilizing modalities is indicated. The patient will also be placed on a home treatment program of heat-ice combination while using tongue blades for constant stretch. He should build up a stretching tolerance of 6 to 10 minutes, 4 to 6 times per day. The patient can work on protrusive movements so as to encourage normal translation, but only after he can open at least 11mm (approximately seven tongue blades stacked and placed between the anterior teeth as a gauge.) When the patient is treated clinically, the use of a heat-ice combination followed by ultrasound, applied while on stretch using the tongue blades, will be beneficial. This can then be followed by the intra-oral techniques as previously described. If the tight capsule is due secondary to surgery on the TMJ, the aggressiveness of the intra-oral techniques should be tailored to the patient's tolerance and rate of healing.

MUSCLE IMBALANCES

A simple and effective exercise that can be done for immediate control of mandibular movement for the patient with muscle imbalances contributing to too much translation (subluxation), or translation occurring too soon is as follows:

Have the patient touch the lateral pole of the condyle on the most involved side with the middle index finger. Have him lightly touch his chin with the other hand. Then have the patient place the tongue flat against the palate. Ask the patient to open his mouth, keeping the tongue against the palate while palpating the lateral pole. This will allow the condyle to rotate only (Fig. 7-24). Once the patient can do this, have him do the same exercise with the tongue away from the palate. This will allow translation to occur along with rotation, restoring normal arthrokinematics, but translation will still be controlled by the proprioceptive feedback from the palpating fingers. As with any neuromuscular re-educational exercise, repetition and the patient's conscious effort will determine the success of this form of treatment.

CLOSING REMARKS

It is imperative that all clinicians who are involved with the treatment of patients experiencing upper quarter pain and dysfunction have a good

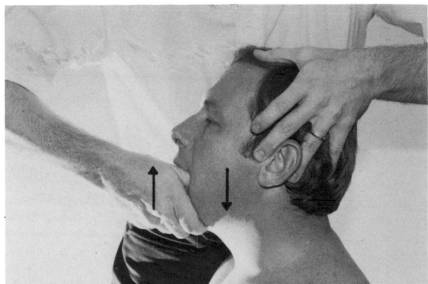

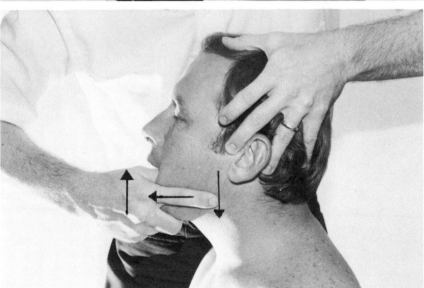

Fig. 7-22. Distraction without (top) or with (bottom) anterior glide. The hand placement is the same as described in Fig. 7-21.

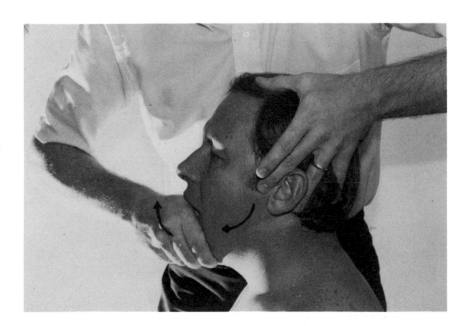

Fig. 7-23. Lateral glide (joint play technique.) This photo depicts a lateral glide technique to the left TMJ. The thumb is placed on the inside of the left posterior mandibular teeth. The fingers are positioned to grasp the tip of the mandible. The thumb applies pressure to the left as the fingers pull the tip of the mandible to the right.

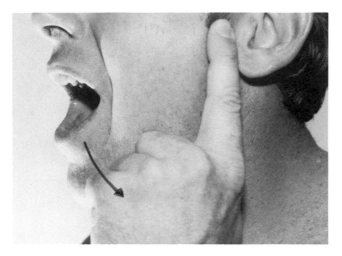

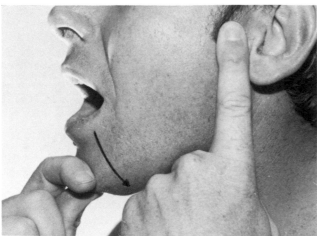

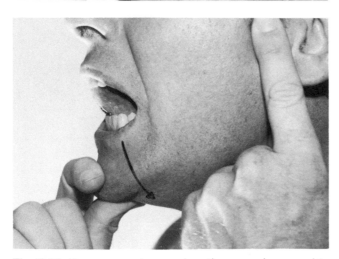

Fig. 7-24. Neuromuscular re-education exercises used to help correct conditions such as too much translation (subluxation) or translation occurring too soon.

working knowledge of the TMJ. Emphasis in this chapter was placed on TMJ dysfunction. An understanding in the anatomy, mechanics, and physiology is essential in the examination of TMJ dysfunction and in properly interpreting the findings of the examination.

Advancements relative to the etiology, symptoms, standardization of examination and the treatment of TMJ dysfunction will occur when there is a better understanding or at least an acknowledgement of the influence of adjacent areas on the TMJ and their functional interdependency. These adjacent areas include but are not limited to the occlusion and the cervical spine. Appropriate examination to determine the extent of interdependent involvement and appropriate treatment is indicated. If one attempts to treat TMJ dysfunction independently of the occlusion and cervical spine, thinking that such treatment will help the occlusion or cervical spine, less than satisfactory results will be achieved.

The clinician also needs to be aware that in the absence of any TMJ afflictions there still can be involvement in the posturing and movement of the mandible as it relates to the cervical spine and occlusion. The important relationship that exists between the cervical spine, movement and positioning of the mandible, and the occlusion, is their combined performance during the physiological functions of respiration and maintenance of the head, mandible, tongue and hyoid bone positionings. During movement of the head and neck, mastication, deglutition, speech, yawning, coughing and moistening of the lips, these physiological functions are increased. If these physiological functions are to occur with a minimum amount of muscular effort, the cervical spine, movement and positioning of the mandible and the occlusion need to be examined and treated appropriately.

By following the guidelines as presented in this chapter and by being open to other possible adjacent areas of involvement, the therapist will initiate steps towards decreasing the TMJ dilemma.

References:

1. Ruffer, A: Study of Abnormalities and Pathology of Ancient Egyptian Teeth. Am Joul Phys Anthropol 3:355, 1920.
2. Breasted, J: Edwin Smith Surgical Papyrus. University of Chicago Press, Chicago 1930.
3. Annandale, T: On Displacement of the Interarticular Cartilage of the Lower Jaw and Its' Treatment by Operation. Lancet 1:411, 1887.
4. Lanz, W: Discitis Mandibularis. Zentralbl Chir 36:289, 1909.
5. Costen, J: Syndrome of Ear and Sinus Symptoms Dependent Upon Disturbed Function of the Temporomandibular Joint. Ann Otol 43:1, March 1934.
6. Sicher, J: Temporomandibular Articulation in Mandibular Overclosure. JADA 36:131, Feb 1948.

References: (Continued)

7. Zimmerman, A: "Evaluation of Costen's Syndrome From An Anatomic Point of View",The Temporomandibular Joint (B. Sarnat,ed.) Springfield, Illinois 1951.

8. May, W: Reduction of Stress in the Chewing Mechanism. Basal Facts, Vol 3, No 3.

9. Fonder, A: The Dental Distress Syndrome. Basal Facts, Vol 6, No 1.

10. McNeill, C, et al: Craniomandibular (TMJ) Disorders-The State of the Art. J Prosthet Dent, Vol 44, No 4, October 1980.

11. Report of the President's Conference on the Examination, Diagnosis and Management of Temporomandibular Disorders. JADA, Vol 106, Jan 1983.

12. Greene, C: Epidemiologic Studies of Mandibular Dysfunction: A Critical Review. J Prosthet Dent, Vol 48, No 2, Aug 1982.

13. Choukas, N and Sicher, H: The Structure of the Temporomandibular Joint. Oral Surg 13:1203, 1960.

14. Yale, S; Allison, B and Hauptfuehrer, J: An Epidemiological Assessment of Mandibular Condyle Morphology. Oral Surg 21:169, 1966.

15. Kreutziger, K and Mahan, P: Temporomandibular Degenerative Joint Disease. Oral Surg 40:165, Aug 1975.

16. Griffen, C; Hawthorn, R and Harns, R: Anatomy and Histology of the Human Temporomandibular Joint. Monogr Oral Sci. Vol 4, 1975.

17. Mahan, P: "Temporomandibular Problems", Biologic Diagnosis and Treatment (Solberg and Clark, ed.) p. 35. Quintessence Publishing, Chicago, 1980.

18. Griffen, C and Sharpe, C: The Structure of the Adult Human Temporomandibular Meniscus. Aust Dent Jour 5:190, 1960.

19. Mahan, P; Wilkinson, T; et al: Superior and Inferior Bellies of the Lateral Pterygoid Muscle, EMG Activity at Basic Jaw Position. J Prosthet Dent, Vol 50, No 5, p. 710, Nov 1983.

20. Rees, L: The Structure and Function of the Temporomandibular Joint. Brit Dent J 96:125-133, 1954.

21. Griffen, C: A Neuro-myo-arterial Glomus in the Temporomandibular Meniscus. Med J Austr 48:113-116, 1961.

22. Donatelli, R and Owens-Burkhart, H: Effects of Immobilization on the Extensibility of Periarticular Connective Tissue. JOSPT Vol 3, No 2, Fall 1981.

23. Glineburg, R, et al: The Effects of Immobilization of the Primate Temporomandibular Joint. J Oral Maxillofac Surg 40(1):3-8, Jan 1982.

24. Cotta, J and Puhl, W: The Pathophysiology of Damage to Articular Cartilage. Progress in Ortho Surg, Vol 3, pp. 15-31, 1978.

25. "Biology of Connective Tissue and the Joint". In: Primer on the Rheumatic Diseases. The Arthritis Foundation Conference, Atlanta, 1973.

26. Moffett, B Jr: Articular Remodeling in the Adult Human Temporomandibular Joint. Am J Anat 115:119-142, July 1964.

27. Blackwood, J: Vascularization of the Condylar Cartilage of the Human Condyle. J Anat 99:551-563, London 1965.

28. Davis, D: Gray's Anatomy, Descriptive and Applied, 34th ed., pp. 1049, Longmans, Green, London 1967.

29. Greenfield, B and Wyke, B: Reflex Innervation of the Temporomandibular Joint. Nature 211:940-941, London 1966.

30. Thilander, B: Innervation of the Temporomandibular Joint Capsule In Man. Trans T Schools 7:1, Stockholm 1961.

31. Klineberg, I: Structure and Function of Temporomandibular Joint Innervation. Ann Roy Coll Surg, Vol. 49, England 1971.

32. Clark, R and Wyke, B: Contributions of Temporomandibular Articular Mechanoreceptors to the Control of Mandibular Posture: An Experimental Study. Joul of Dent, Vol 2, No 3, 1974.

33. Kawamura, Y, et al: Physiologic Role of Deep Mechanoreceptors in Temporomandibular Joint Capsule. J Osaka Univ Dent School 7:63-76, 1967.

34. Laskin, D: Etiology of the Pain Dysfunction Syndrome. JADA 79(1):147-153, 1969.

35. Weinberg, L, et al: Clinical Report on the Etiology and Diagnosis of TMJ Dysfunction-Pain Syndrome. Joul of Prosthet Dent 44:642, 1980.

36. Halbert, R: Electromyographic Study of Head Position. Joul of Can Dent Assoc, Vol 24, pp. 11-23, 1958.

37. Symposium Report on Myofascial Trigger Points. Arch of Phys Med and Rehab, Vol 62, No 3, March 1981.

38. Vladimir, J: "Muscles, Central Nervous Motor Regulation and Back Problems", The Neurobiologic Mechanisms in Manipulative Therapy (Irvin Korr, ed.) Plenum Press, New York, 1978.

39. Sicher, H: "Functional Anatomy of the TMJ", The Temporomandibular Joint (B Sarnat, ed.) Charles Thomas, Springfield, 1964.

40. Brown, T: Mandibular Movements. Monogr Oral Sci 4:126, 1975.

41. Bell, W: Synopsis; Oral and Facial Pain and the Temporomandibular Joint, 1967.

42. Mahan, P: "Anatomic, Histologic and Physiologic Features of the TMJ", Current Advances in Oral Surgery (V. Irby, Ed.) C.V. Mosby, 1980.

43. Farrar, W and McCarty, W Jr: Outline of Temporomandibular Joint Diagnosis and Treatment, 6th ed. Normandy Study Group, Montgomery, Alabama, Feb 1980.

44. Guralnick, W, et al: Temporomandibular Joint Afflictions. New Engl Joul of Med 299(3):123-129, 1978.

45. Dorland's Illustrated Medical Dictionary, 24th ed. Saunders, 1965.

46. TMJ Symposium Through the Eyes of the Editor. Am J Orthod, Vol 80, No 1, pp. 98, July 1981.

47. Hylander, W: An Experimental Analysis of Temporomandibular Joint Reaction Forces In Macaques. Am J Phys Anthrop 51:433-456, 1979.

48. Hansson, L, et al: A Comparison Between Clinical and Radiologic Findings in 259 Temporomandibular Joint Patients. Joul of Prosthet Dent, Vol 50, No 1, July 1983.

49. Mongini, F: The Importance of Radiography in the Diagnosis of TMJ Dysfunctions. Joul of Prosthet Dent, Vol 45, No 2, Feb 1981.

50. Weinberg, L: What We Really See in a TMJ Radiograph. Joul of Prosthet Dent, Vol 30, No 6, Dec 1973.

51. Berrett, A: Radiology of the Temporomandibular Joint. Dent Clin of N Am, Vol 27, No 3, July 1983.

52. Weinberg, L: An Evaluation of Asymmetry in TMJ Radiographs. Joul of Prosthet Dent, Vol 40, No 3, Sept 1978.

53. Blaschke, D, et al: Arthrography of the Temporomandibular Joint: Review of Current States. JADA, Vol 100, March 1980.

54. Dolurck, M, et al: Arthrotomyographic Evaluation of the Temporomandibular Joint. J Oral Surg, Vol 37, Nov. 1979.

References: (Continued)

55. Farrar, W and McCarty, W: Inferior Joint Space Arthrography and Characteristics of Condylar Paths in Internal Derangements of the TMJ. Joul of Prosthet Dent, Vol 41, No 5, p. 548, May 1979.
56. Farrar, W: Characteristics of the Condylar Path in Internal Derangements of the TMJ. Joul of Prosthet Dent, Vol 39, No 3, Mar 1978.

CHAPTER 8
JOINT MOBILIZATION

HISTORY

Joint mobilization is an art which has been practiced since prehistoric times. The first documentation of mobilization was made by Hippocrates (460 BC to 375 BC.) He taught his students to apply a vertical manipulative thrust on a gibbus (prominent vertebra) and to give exercises afterward. Galen made reference to the manipulation of the spine for misalignment in a patient following trauma to the neck[1].

For many centuries in England, bonesetters practiced manipulation as a family tradition. People consulted them to have their joints manipulated because they were causing pain. Bonesetters still exist today in many European countries. In 1876, Sir James Paget (1814 to 1899), the renowned British surgeon, published his famous lecture, "Cases That Bonesetters Cure," in the British Medical Journal. Paget delineated the types of cases which were responsive to manipulative therapy. He exhorted his readers to "Learn them...imitate what is good and avoid what is bad in the practice of bonesetters." Paget's words fell on deaf ears. Orthodox medicine of the day found the rationale behind bonesetting untenable, an attitude probably justified in part even though patients who had visited bonesetters attested to their skill[1].

Two major schools of thought of mobilization/manipulation are osteopathy and chiropractic. Superficially, these two schools bear certain resemblances to each other with regard to the mechanistic approach to illness but beyond that, their scope and philosophies are quite different[1].

The history of osteopathy is intimately connected with Andrew Taylor Still (1828-1917.) He studied medicine at the College of Physicians and Surgeons in Kansas City, Missouri. Still lost three of his sons in an epidemic of spinal meningitis, even though they had the best medical treatment available. Still became disillusioned with orthodox medicine as it was practiced during his day. A deeply religious man, the idea of osteopathy came to Still like a "revelation". He concluded that the human body possessed self-healing properties, that efficient functioning was dependent on unimpaired structure and that proper nerve and blood supply to the tissues was necessary for health maintenance. These concepts were contained in his "Rule of the Artery" which he proclaimed in 1874 and which became the basic concept of osteopathy. He founded the American School of Osteopathy in 1892 in Kirksville, Missouri[1].

Today, osteopathic physicians (D.O.'s) may be found in virtually every field of medicine and surgery as their backgrounds expanded to encompass both osteopathic and allopathic knowledge.

Chiropractic began in Davenport, Iowa with Daniel David Palmer, a grocer. Palmer, having read some of Still's work, reported in 1895 that he "cured" the deafness of a janitor after he "adjusted" the latter's misaligned vertebra. Palmer's belief was that the spinal column was the controller of the human machinery and that all diseases could be traced to it. He formulated "The Law of the Spinal Nerve" as the basis for chiropractic. Palmer founded the first chiropractic school in Davenport in 1897. His adolescent son was its first graduate. Today there are 14 chiropractic colleges in the United States recognized by the two major chiropractic professional associations — the National Chiropractic Association (N.C.A.), founded in 1910, and the International Chiropractic Association (I.C.A.), founded in 1926.

The basis of chiropractic philosophy is the theory of "subluxation". Chiropractors claim that subluxation in the spinal column interferes with nerve function and that this is the significant factor in disease causation. Manipulation of the appropriate area of the spine restores the natural alignment of the spine which, in turn, relieves the symptoms. Statements regarding the adjustment of the spine for disorders such as diabetes, various intestinal disorders, heart trouble and cancer are quite common in chiropractic literature[1].

There is still no consensus as to the rationale behind spinal manipulations, but there exists a wealth of theories. Each school of thought has advanced its own rationale and has evolved manipulative techniques consistent with it.

The number of allopathic physicians (M.D.'s) who have recognized and used manipulative principles is few, but these physicians have made remarkable contributions to its conceptualization.

James Mennell, M.D., who was once in charge of the Physical Medicine Department at St. Thomas' Hopital in London, published a book in 1952 entitled *The Science and Art of Joint Manipulation*. He pointed to the facet joints, postural strain and adhesions as causative factors in back pain. Later, his son John enunciated the concepts of "joint play" and "joint dysfunction[1]".

James Cyriax, M.D. was the orthopaedic physician at St. Thomas' Hospital in London after James Mennell. More than any other physician, he has done a great deal to bring the usefulness of manipulation to the medical profession. His book, *Textbook of Orthopaedic Medicine*, first published in 1954, is invaluable. Because of his ardent belief in the disc as a source of back pain problems, most of Cyriax' manipulative techniques are designed for the reduction of disc herniation. He claims that his rotatory maneuvers apply a torsional stress on the spine, which exerts a centripetal force which reduces the bulging disc material if the longitudinal ligaments are intact[1].

The driving force behind a school of thought which has flourished in Scandinavia is Freddie Kaltenborn, who is a physiotherapist, a chiropractor and an osteopath. His philosophy is a synthesis of what he considers to be the best in chiropractic, osteopathy and physical medicine. He uses some of Cyriax's methods to evaluate the patient and mainly employs specific osteopathic and sometimes chiropractic techniques for treatment[1]. His refinement and development of treatment techniques has made a vast contribution to our understanding of mobilization therapy.

In 1964 Geoffery Maitland published his book, *Vertebral Manipulation*. He distinguishes between mobilization and manipulation and puts heavy emphasis on mobilization. His techniques are fairly similar to the "articulatory" techniques used by osteopaths. These involve oscillatory movements performed on a chosen joint in which the movement induced by the therapist is within the patient's available range of movement tolerance in order to release a fixed synovial joint. Because his techniques are of a gentle nature and are easier to learn, they have appealed to physical therapists and have gained much recognition, especially in Australia (where Maitland is a private practitioner in physiotherapy and a part-time instructor at the University of Adelaide) and in the United Kingdom. By using the word mobilization instead of manipulation, he has successfully eliminated the emotional aspects surrounding the subject, which has led to its better acceptance among members of the medical profession[1].

RATIONALE/APPLICATION

Mobilization/manipulation techniques are passive movements applied to a joint (or soft tissue) in a specific manner in order to restore the full, free, painless active range of motion of a joint. Such techniques must observe the biomechanics of the joint in question as well as laws of physiological motion (spine) and component motions (extremities) in order to be safe and effective.

As previously discussed, **the indications for the use of mobilization techniques are in those joints assessed as being hypomobile.** A discussion of the muscle-joint relationship has already been given with regard to adaptive shortening and lengthening of muscle/ ligamentous structures in the face or hyper/hypomobility of joints. Obviously, a muscle cannot be fully rehabilitated if its joint is not free to move, and conversely, a muscle cannot move a joint which is not free to move. This creates a paradoxical situation. Thus, there are clear reasons to employ such mobilization techniques.

The effects of mobilization/manipulation are both neurophysiological and mechanical. The work of Wyke and others [2-4] in the area of joint mechanoreceptors indicates that mobilization techniques can be used to relieve pain, cause reflex inhibition of muscles and promote relaxation (Fig. 8-1)[5]. Mobilization techniques are mechanical in that when they are employed into the range of restriction, they are moving into the area of plastic deformation of the soft tissue (collagen.) An example of a stress-strain curve (hysteresis loop) appears in Fig. 8-2. Simply stated, if a tissue is stretched only in its elastic range, no permanent structural change will occur. It is only when the tissue is stretched into the plastic range and beyond that permanent structural changes occur. Obviously, if stretched beyond the plastic range to the fatigue point, fracture will occur. For example, imagine bending the handle of a toothbrush back and forth rapidly. At first, there is much resistance, but as the bending continues, there is less resistance and the handle begins to bend further. Finally, it will break. Judiciously applied, mobilization/manipulation techniques can stretch tissue and break adhesions effectively. Indiscriminately applied, they can tear tissue and cause sprains or strains of the joints.

Type	Location	Receptor Appearance	Sensory Unit	Physiologic Function
I	Stratum fibrosum of capsule; ligaments Higher density in proximal joints	Laminated Ruffini-like corpuscle 300 μm wide 300–800 μm long	Myelinated parent axon and 2–6 corpuscles	Active at rest and during movement Low threshold for activation Slowly adapting
II	Junction of synovial and fibrosum of capsule; intra-articular and extra-articular fat pads Higher density in distal joints	Laminated, pacinian-like, conically shaped corpuscle 150–250 μm long 20–40 μm wide	Myelinated parent axon and 1–5 corpuscles	Active at onset and termination of movement Low threshold for activation Rapidly adapting
III	Collateral ligaments Not found in interspinous ligaments of cervical region	GTO-like corpuscle 800 μm long 100 μm wide	Myelinated parent axon and 1 corpuscle	Active at end of joint range High threshold for activation Slowly adapting
IV	Ligaments, capsule, and articular fat pads Absent in synovial tissue	Free nerve endings or lattice type endings	Thinly myelinated parent axon and terminal endings	Active only to extreme mechanical or chemical irritation High threshold for activation Slowly adapting

Composite of sources: Freeman and Wyke,[2] Polacek,[3] and Halata.[4]

Fig. 8-1. Characteristics of joint receptors (reprinted with permission from Newton)[5].

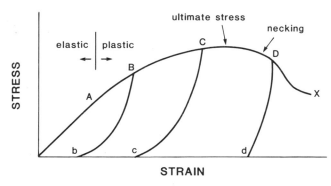

Fig. 8-2. Stress strain curve for collagen (hysteresis loop).

One must have a basic appreciation of joint mechanics in order to effectively employ mobilization techniques, especially in the extremity joints. Two terms have been coined to describe the relationship of joint surfaces as they move with respect to each other. These terms are arthrokinematic and osteokinematic. Simply put, arthrokinematics are those movements taking place between the joint surfaces, namely, roll, glide and spin. Osteokinematics are the directions in which the long bone is moving (up, down, etc.) These concepts apply to the convex-concave relationship found in most synovial joints (more obvious in the extremities than in the spine.) Two rules of motion result:

1) When the convex surface is fixed and the concave surface is moving upon it, the arthrokinematics and the osteokinematics are *in the same direction*. Take, for example, flexion/extension of the MCP joints of the hand — the osteokinematics (movement of the proximal phalanx in an up and down motion) and the arthrokinematics (mostly roll and glide between the joint surfaces) are in the same direction (up or down) (Fig. 8-3A.)[6]

2) When the concave surface is fixed and the convex surface is moving upon it, the arthrokinematics and the osteokinematics are *in opposite directions*. Take, for example, abduction/adduction of the shoulder — the osteokinematics (movement of the humerus in an up and down motion) and the arthrokinematics (mostly roll and glide between the head of the humerus and the glenoid fossa) occur in opposite directions (Fig. 8-3B.)[6]

The application of these rules will be explained more fully when extremity joints are discussed.

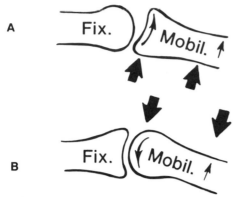

Fig. 8-3. Drawing showing the direction mobilization should be performed to increase mobility. The small arrows indicate the direction the bone is moving and the large arrows indicate the direction of the mobilizing force. A) If mobilizing a concave bone on a stabilized convex bone, the mobilizing force is in the same direction as the desired movement. B) If mobilizing a convex bone on a stabilized concave bone, the mobilizing force is in the opposite direction of the desired movement (adopted from Kaltenborn.)[6]

Joint play motions, first described by Mennell[7], are *involuntary*, interarticular motions which are present in all synovial joints. Joint play is necessary for painless, unrestricted, voluntary motion. Joint play movements occur by an external force (a therapist passively moving a joint) and include long axis distraction, tilts, glides and rotations. For example, distraction and A-P glide of the MCP joint of the hand would be joint play motions. They do not occur in voluntary active motions. However, the range of movement in these particular planes must exist (passively) in order for the full, unrestricted, voluntary motion to take place. Some refer to this concept as normal joint laxity or "slack".

Component motions are generally thought of as extra-articular movements which normally accompany active motions. They are not usually recognized, but are nonetheless necessary for full range of movement. Examples of component motions include spreading of the mortise of the ankle in dorsiflexion or the sliding of the radius along the ulna during elbow extension[8].

Articular position of the joint as described by MacConaill and Basmajian[9] must be considered when performing joint mobilization. The close-packed position is at the extreme of one of the most habitual movements of the joint. It is the position in which the concave surface (smaller area) is in complete congruence with the convex surface (larger area.) The capsule and ligaments are maximally taut and the two bones of the articular unit cannot be separated by traction across the joint surface. Joint

mobilization should not be performed or attempted in the maximal close-packed position. If joint motion is to be avoided, this position can be used. For example, the spinal segments above and below a segment to be mobilized may be "locked" into a close-packed position in order to isolate the mobilizing force to the desired level. Any position other than that of close-packed is called loose-packed. The articular surfaces are not totally congruent and some parts of the capsule are lax. The maximum loose-packed position is the best position for early mobilization. In this position, the capsule is most relaxed. The bones of the articular unit can be drawn apart to the greatest extent by traction. This position is often described as the resting position of the joint. All examinations and the first treatment for restricted joint movement are performed from this position or from a position as close as possible to this. Subsequent treatments may be performed in positions nearer the close-packed position, but they are never performed in the maximum close-packed position. Generally speaking, rotation will cause a close-packed position. Likewise, extremes of all motions will tend to place the joint into more of a close-packed position, whereas mid-range of a joint movement will be closer to the loose-packed position. Extension is the maximum close-packed position of the spine[9].

The joint capsule is a richly innervated structure that is made up of two layers — the synovial lining on the inside and an external layer of dense, irregular collagen connective tissue. This outer layer of collagen fiber is somewhat thickened and immobile in joints that have a capsular pattern of hypomobility. This may be caused by increased collagen fiber that is laid down in response to injury or inflammation, or it may be caused by a binding together of the individual collagen fibers. These collagen fibers cannot be stretched like yellow elastic fibers; rather, they must be mobilized in a more subtle manner and allowed to rearrange and loosen over a period of time. Articulating, stretching and traction techniques are more appropriate than manipulation to help rearrange and loosen the fibers[6]. If, on the other hand, joint hypomobility is due to joint impingement (articular pattern), manipulation may be more effective[10, 11].

Soft tissue massage, contract-relax techniques, passive stretching and active and passive range of motion exercises all increase the mobility of soft tissue in general. However, their effectiveness in mobilizing the joints is limited to stretching the contractile (muscle-tendon) tissue. Specific and general joint mobilization techniques are generally more effective in restoring mobility of the joints because they act specifically on the inert structures (capsule, ligament, cartilage and intervertebral disc.) They can often be done with the joint in a comfortable mid-range position rather than at the often painful limit of range of motion[3].

Because of pain, mobilization cannot always be performed in the most restricting direction. In this case, it is performed in directions other than, or possibly opposite to the direction of restriction. Restoration of mobility in one direction will usually increase mobility in other directions as well. For example, a rotational mobilization is likely to increase range of motion in all other planes of motion. Therefore, if mobilization in one direction is particularly painful, one may still achieve beneficial results by mobilizing in less painful directions initially. Many times, the first mobilization treatment given consists of gentle tractions applied to the joint structures with five to ten second holds. The purpose is to relieve the pain. Gradually, the mobilization may be increased.

Treatment to increase joint mobility is of primary importance. As soft tissue injuries and inflammations heal, stiffness is inherent. Left alone, the joints may become hypomobile. The untreated hypomobile joint will soon begin to show signs of joint degeneration. To avoid this pathological chain of events, mobilization techniques must be used. The earlier they are started in the treatment regime, the more benefit obtained, provided they are not aggravating to the soft tissue pathology with which one is dealing.

Joint mobilization is not a panacea. It does, however, have a place in the armamentarium of the physical therapist. It has a place among the modalities aimed at reducing human suffering and increasing man's quality of life. It is unfortunate that practitioners of mobilization have made exaggerated claims and that orthodox medicine finds it difficult to admit it's own ignorance of the subject. Both the advantages and shortcomings of mobilization should be investigated before judgement is made.

METHODS

Joint mobilization is a form of passive movement done to restore joint play, component motion and/or range of motion. Most of the mobilization techniques shown in this text for the spine involve passive range of motion techniques and most of those shown for the extremities involve joint play and component motion techniques.

Joint mobilization includes the following:

Articulations are graded, oscillating movements done to restore joint play, component motion or range of motion to a hypomobile joint. They are graded as follows:

Grade 1 — Gentle movements of small amplitude done at the beginning of available range.

Grade 2 — Gentle movements of larger amplitude done into available mid-range of a joint.

Grade 3 — Moderate movements of large amplitude done thru the available range of the joint and into the restricted range.

Grade 4 — Oscillating movements of small amplitude done at the end of range and into the restriction.

Grade 5 — Thrusting movements done to the anatomical limit of the joint.

A *progressive articulation* is done in a progressive step-wise manner from the beginning of the range into the restriction, with a quick release.

A *stretch articulation* is done in a smooth manner from the beginning of the range into the restriction, with a quick release (Fig. 8-4).

Grade 1 and 2 articulations are done to maintain joint mobility and relieve pain. They are primarily neurophysiologic in effect. Grade 3 and 4 and progressive articulations are done to increase joint mobility. For example, Grade 1 and 2 articulations are often indicated in the subacute stage of a joint sprain or inflammation to guard against the development of joint hypomobility, to relieve pain, and promote healing whereas Grade 3 and 4 and progressive articulations are indicated in the more advanced stages of joint hypomobility such as seen in frozen shoulder or other joint contractures that have been present for an extended period of time. Grade 5 mobilizations are thrust techniques used to gain full joint mobility.[12]

The rules of mobilization are as follows[7]:

1. Patient and therapist must be relaxed.

2. The procedure must be relatively pain free.

3. When possible, stabilize one bone and move or mobilize the other.

4. The first treatment must be done gently to get a chance to observe the patient's reaction.

5. Always compare and observe the "good" side (extremity) or the level above or below (spine)

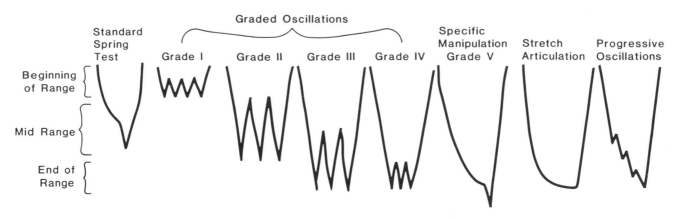

Fig. 8-4. Grades of mobilization.

to gain knowledge of individual patient differences.

6. When possible, examine one joint and one movement at a time.

7. Do not examine for joint mobility if active joint inflammation/active traumatic injury is present.

8. Keep lever arms of force as short as possible.

Mobilization, like any other evaluative or treatment skill, cannot be learned or developed entirely by the reading of a textbook. There is no substitute for clinical practice and experience. It is reasonable to assume that the beginner will feel some insecurity and uncertainty when attempting these techniques for the first time. With perserverance, these techniques can be perfected.

The techniques which follow are the ones this author has found to be the most satisfactory. The arrows indicate the directions of the mobilizing forces.

SPINAL MOBILIZATION

CERVICAL SPINE

Before attempting to test or mobilize the upper cervical spine, the therapist should perform the vertebral artery test to ensure that the movements performed during mobilization will not embarrass vertebral artery circulation. The therapist instructs the patient to keep his eyes open throughout the procedure, focusing on the tip of the therapist's nose. Seated at the patient's head, the therapist first fully backward bends the patient's cervical spine, especially the upper segments. He

then rotates the head to one side and holds this position for approximately 30 seconds. The therapist questions the patient as to any symptoms of tinnitis, dizziness, nausea, throbbing or unusual sensation. The therapist is observing the patient's pupils for constriction/dilation and continues to do so for a few seconds after the head is brought back to the neutral position. The opposite side is then tested in a like manner (Fig. 8-5).

Eight basic cervical mobilizations are presented in this text. Five of the techniques are similar to the passive cervical mobility tests described in Chapter 3. Of the remaining three techniques, one involves manual traction with passive range of motion, one is

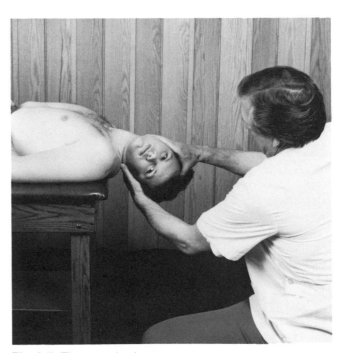

Fig. 8-5. The vertebral artery test.

for manual traction-relaxation and one is a self-mobilization.

The five mobilization techniques patterned after the passive cervical mobility tests are: forward bending, backward bending, rotation, side bending and side gliding. For these techniques, the patient is

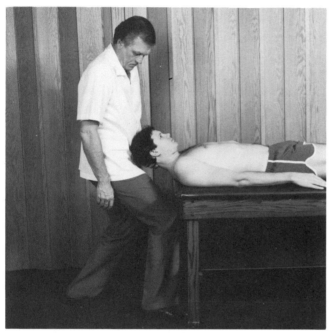

Fig. 8-6. The patient's head rests against the therapist's anterior hip for cervical passive mobility testing.

positioned supine with his head extending over the end of the treatment table, resting it on the therapist's hip (Fig. 8-6). The therapist's hands are placed to cradle the patient's head and neck with the index fingers supporting the articular pillar superior to the segment to be mobilized (Fig. 8-7). The patient's head and neck are held in 30° of forward bending when doing the forward bending technique. In the other techniques, the head and neck are held in a neutral, mid-range position.

The **forward bending** mobilization is done by lifting the head and neck straight upward with both hands. To start, the therapist's knees should be somewhat flexed. The therapist then alternately extends and flexes his knees slightly to keep the patient's head in correct position as the mobilization force is applied (Fig. 8-8). The mobilizing force is applied and directed through the index fingers, but maximal hand contact is maintained with the neck and head so they are carried along with the movement. Using the proximal interphalangeal joints (PIP's), the principle contact is made with the index fingers against the articular pillars of the neck. One should be careful not to use the fingertips with these techniques as this will cause discomfort.

Backward bending is done in similar fashion as forward bending except that the head and portion of the neck superior to the point of contact of the index fingers is not carried along with the movement.

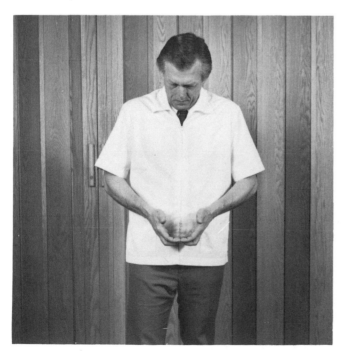

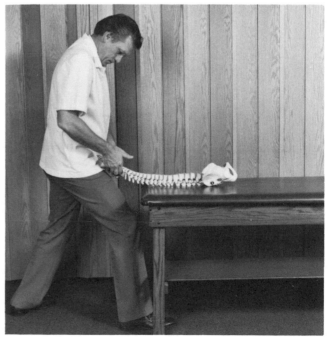

Fig. 8-7. Position of hands for cervical mobilization.

Rather, as the mobilizing force is applied upward onto the posterior aspect of the articular pillars by the index fingers, the head and portion of the neck superior to the force are allowed to fall into backward bending. Thus, a backward bending force is effected to the cervical joints superior to the contact, especially to the segment immediately superior to the contact point (Fig. 8-9).

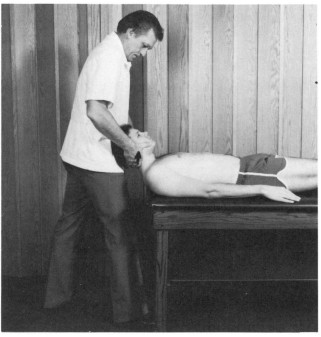

Fig. 8-8. Forward bending cervical mobilization.

The cervical **rotation** mobilization is similar to the forward bending technique described above except that it is done to only one side at a time with the head and neck held in a neutral, mid-range position. For example, to do left rotation, the right hand with PIP contact lifts upward to perform the mobilization while the left hand supports the head and neck. The head and neck are carried along with the movement (Fig. 8-10).

The cervical **side bending** mobilization utilizes the same positioning. The point of contact by the index finger using the radio-palmar surface near the metacarpophalangeal joint (MCP) is against the lateral aspect of the articular pillar. The mobilization force is applied in a medial and slightly inferior direction causing the segment below the point of contact to side bend to the same side as the mobilizing force. The opposite hand supports the head and neck (Fig. 8-11).

The cervical **side gliding** mobilization also utilizes the same basic position. The mobilizing force is applied in a medial direction through the index finger as it contacts the lateral aspect of the articular pillar, causing movement to occur at the segment below the contact. The point of contact on the index finger is on the palmar surface of the MCP joint. The main difference between this technique and that of cervical side bending is that in this technique, the patient's head is carried to the side with the movement. In order to do this, the therapist

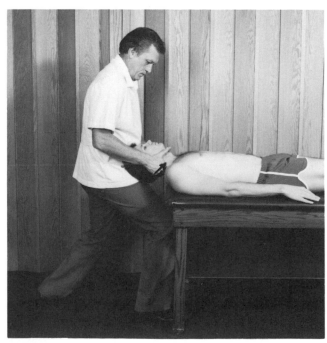

Fig. 8-9. Backward bending cervical mobilization.

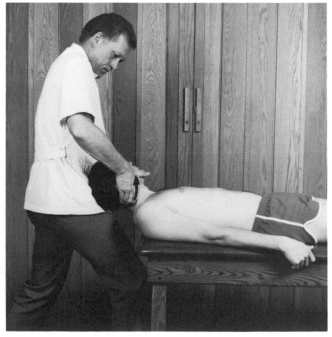

Fig. 8-10. Rotational cervical mobilization.

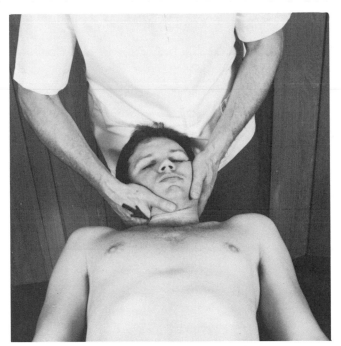

Fig. 8-11. Side bending cervical mobilization.

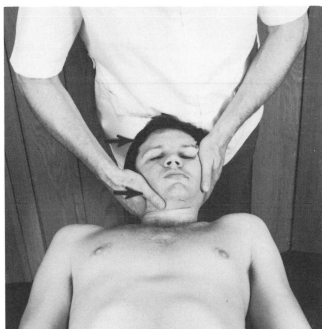

Fig. 8-12. Side gliding cervical mobilization.

must shift his hips in the direction of the mobilization (Fig. 8-12).

Graded passive movements (articulations) and stretching techniques are most effective with the five techniques described above. Hold-relax and contract-relax muscle stretches are also effective.

The **manual traction** mobilization technique shown in Fig. 8-13 may be done as a straight midline pull, or may be done in combination with passive range of motion in any plane. The ulnar border of the mobilizing hand makes contact with the base of the occiput, while the palmar surface

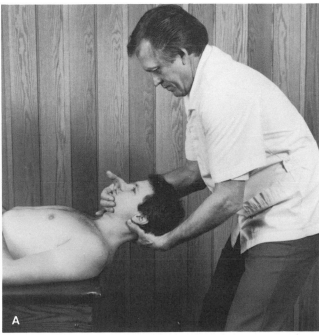

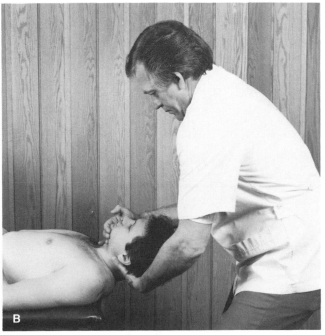

Fig. 8-13. Manual cervical traction: A) Straight; B) Side bending; C) Rotation; D) Side bending and rotation; E) Backward bending; F) Axial extension (head back, chin in). Traction is first applied with the hand holding the occiput, then the passive movement is performed throughout the range. (Fig. 8-13 is continued on next page.)

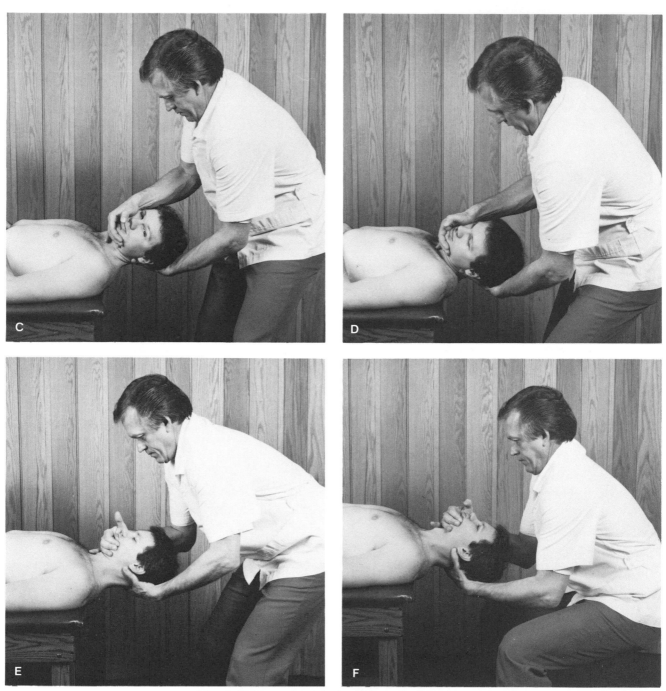

Fig. 8-13 Manual cervical traction. (Continued)

supports the neck. The thumb and middle finger grasp inferior to the occipital bone. The weight of the head is also balanced by this hand. The other hand cradles the chin to provide stabilization. The operator is cautioned to neither squeeze the neck with one hand nor apply force through the chin. Range of motion of the neck may be done while traction is being applied. Movements should be carried out slowly and may be held for a few seconds as a stretching technique.

Inhibitive manual traction is a mobilization technique which applies mild traction to the cervical muscles and spine and incorporates a muscle relaxation technique through direct pressure on muscle/tendon insertions at the base of the skull. The therapist rests the back of his hands on the treatment table with the fingers extending upwards. The "balance" is maintained with a slight amount of traction for up to several minutes (Fig. 8-14).

Self-mobilization of the cervical spine is done

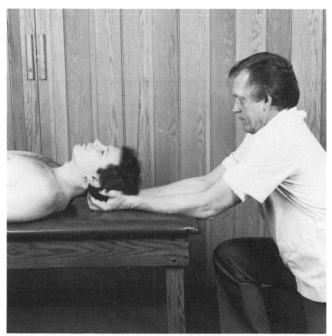

Fig. 8-14. Inhibitive manual traction.

ing, rotation and/or side bending are done. The greatest mobilizing force is concentrated at the level just superior to the stabilization. The patient may change the segment to be mobilized by moving the stabilization superiorly or inferiorly.

UPPER THORACIC SPINE

Three upper thoracic mobilizations are presented in this text. Two are rotational techniques and one is a side bending technique.

The **rotational** technique shown in Fig. 8-16 may be done either with the patient prone with pillows under his chest or with the patient seated resting his head and arms forward on a treatment table. Lateral pressure in opposite directions is applied to the spinous processes at two adjacent levels. The inferior segment, or base, is the segment stabilized, with the mobilizing force applied to the spinous process of the superior segment. This spinous process is moved in the opposite direction of the rotational movement desired (the spinous process moving right imparts left rotation into the segment.) Graded passive movements (articulations) and stretches can be used with this technique. Thumb contacts are effective when mild or moderate specific mobilization is desired. However, thumb contacts are sometimes uncomfortable if strong pressure is

by having the patient grasp and stabilize the cervical spine as shown in Fig. 8-15. The points of stabilization are the vertebrae below the segment to be mobilized. For example, if level C2,3 is to be mobilized, the patient stabilizes the C3 vertebra and does not allow movement to occur from that point inferiorly. Then, active forward and backward bend-

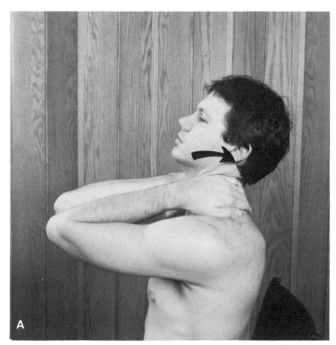

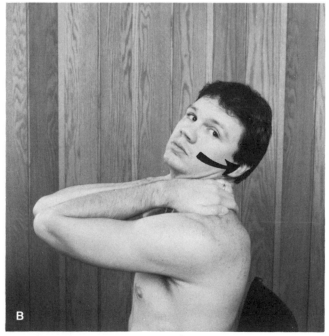

Fig. 8-15. Cervical self-mobilization: A) backward bending and B) rotation.

exerted because of the small contact area of the thumbs. Therefore, pisiform (mobilizing) and/or thenar eminence (stabilizing) contacts are more effective if vigorous mobilization is desired. For maximum effect the patient's head should be turned in the same direction as the desired mobilization.

When the head and neck are rotated, the spinous processes move in the direction opposite to the movement. For example, as the head and neck are rotated to the left, each spinous process is observed to move to the right on its base. If a specific segment is manually blocked from moving, the rotational movement is prevented from occurring below that point and a greater **rotational** force can be directed to the segment above the point of stabilization. Such a technique is done with the patient sitting and with the hands positioned as shown in Fig. 8-17. The thumb is held against the lateral aspect of the spinous process to stabilize while the opposite hand rotates the patient's head and neck to the opposite side to take up slack. The mobilizing force is then directed through the thumb. Graded passive movements and stretches can be utilized with this technique.

The **side bending** mobilization technique for the upper thoracic spine is similar to the rotational technique shown above. With the patient seated, the therapist side bends the head and neck while blocking movement of the spinous process at the selected level with his thumb (Fig. 8-18). Normally the spinous processes move in the same direction as the movement being performed. The thumb prevents this movement from the point of stabilization inferiorly

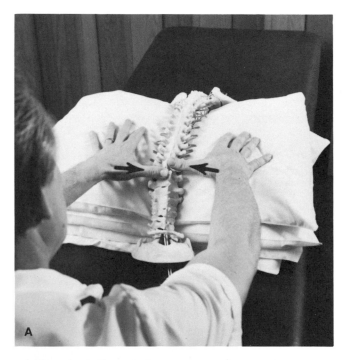

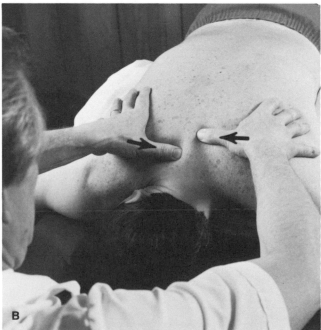

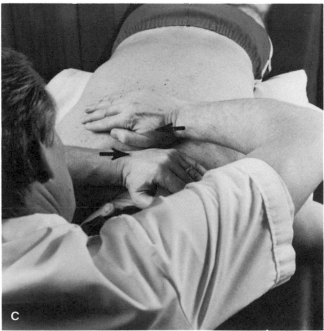

Fig. 8-16. A) Contact positions for rotational mobilization of the upper thoracic spine. B) The inferior thumb stabilizes as the superior thumb directs a lateral force against the spinous process. C) The pisiform bone contacts the superior spinous process (mobilization) and the thenar eminence contacts the inferior spinous process (stabilization.) A right rotation technique is shown.

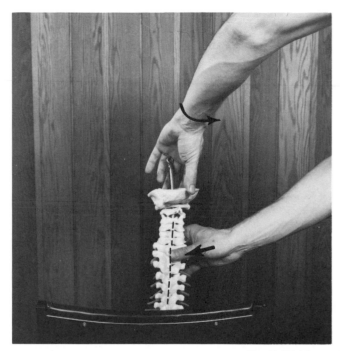
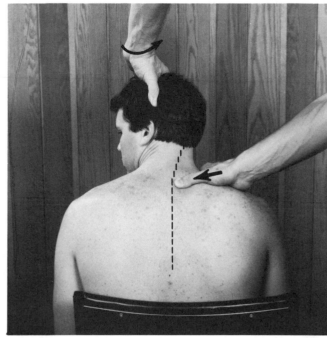

Fig. 8-17. Upper thoracic rotation.

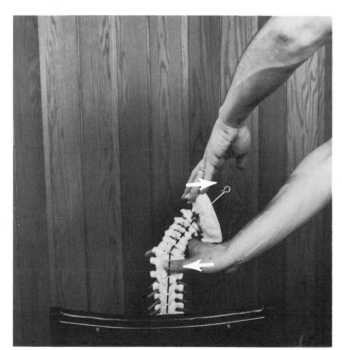
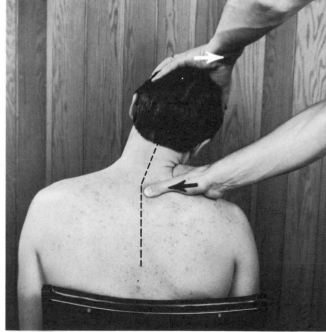

Fig. 8-18. Upper thoracic side bending.

and directs an increased side bending force to the segment above the point of stabilization. This technique should be done in three distinct steps as follows: 1) Stabilize with the thumb; 2) Take up slack by passively side bending the head and neck; and 3) Mobilize with the thumb. Graded passive movements and stretches can be utilized with this technique.

The two previous techniques can be modified by changing the hand hold on the patient's head to one in which the therapist cradles the patient's head in his arm and against the chest (Fig. 8-19). This

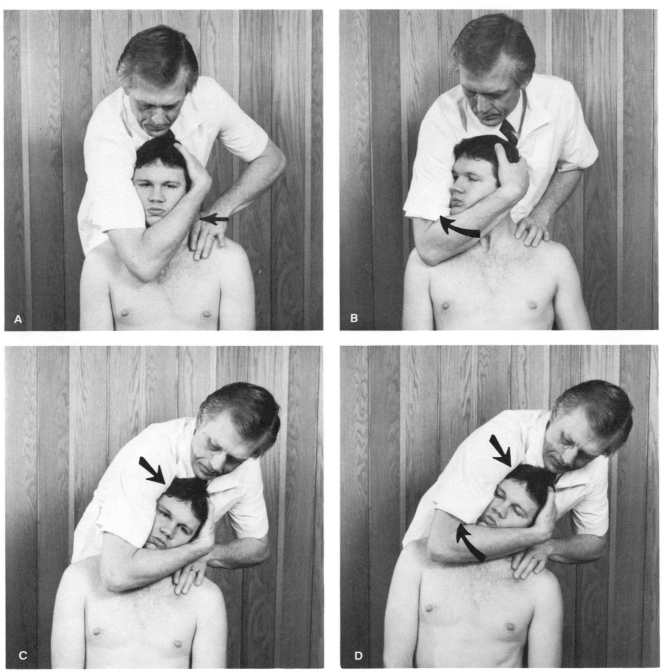

Fig. 8-19. Alternate method of holding the patient's head for upper thoracic mobilization: A) Therapist cradles the patient's head to gain more control. The therapist's thumb stabilizes against the spinous process inferior to segment to be mobilized; B) Rotation; C) Side bending; and D) Rotation and side bending combined.

affords more head control and enables greater force to be applied. Side bending in one direction with rotation in the opposite direction may be combined to increase the effectiveness of these techniques. An obvious disadvantage to this technique is that an uncomfortable stress may be applied to the cervical spine as the slack is taken up. If this occurs, the technique shown in Fig. 8-16 should be substituted.

MID AND LOWER THORACIC SPINE

Five techniques appropriate for the mid and lower thoracic spine are shown here. One is for forward bending, two are rotational techniques, one is for backward bending and one is a traction-backward bending technique.

The **forward bending** technique is shown in Fig.

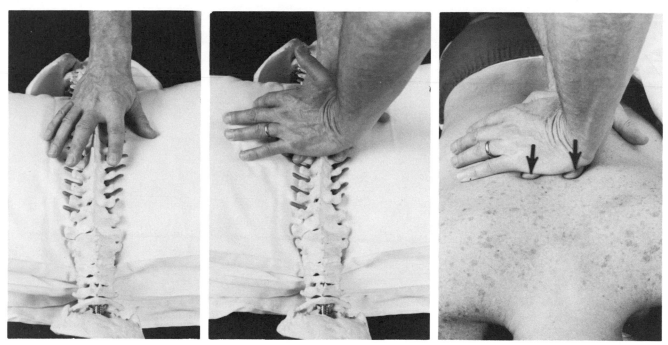

Fig. 8-20. Forward bending, mid and lower thoracic spine.

8-20. When anterior pressure is directed to the transverse processes of a vertebra, it causes that vertebra to forward bend on the vertebra inferior to it. Such a force may be imparted by the hypothenar eminence of one hand, through the fingertips placed over the transverse processes of a segment. The pisiform bones may also be used as contacts (Fig. 8-21). The transverse processes are located approximately one level higher than the spinous processes of their corresponding segments. The transverse processes can only be palpated indirectly so their approximate position must be determined in relation to the spinous processes. Thus, the transverse processes of a vertebra can be found at one level

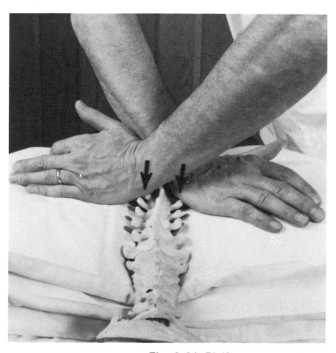 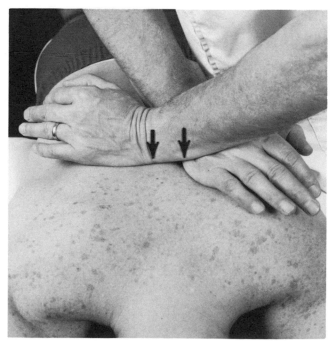

Fig. 8-21. Pisiform contact for mid and lower thoracic mobilization.

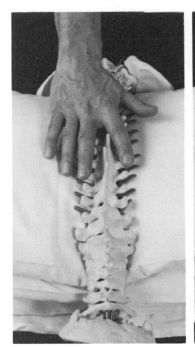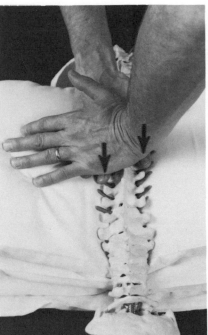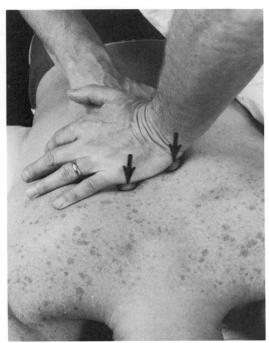

Fig. 8-22. Rotation, mid and lower thoracic spine. A left rotation technique is shown.

higher and approximately one inch lateral to the midline. Graded passive movements, stretches and thrusts may be utilized with this technique.

The forward bending techniques can be modified to produce **rotation** by placing the fingertip contacts on the transverse processes at adjacent levels. The rotation produced is in the direction of the more inferiorly placed finger. This technique is shown in Fig. 8-22. If a more forceful mobilization is required, this technique can be modified utilizing pisiform contacts as shown in Fig. 8-21.

The **rotational** technique shown in Fig. 8-23 also utilizes contact with the transverse processes at two adjacent levels. In this technique, the therapist makes a fist and places it so that the thenar eminence makes transverse process contact on one side while the flat surfaces of the middle phalanges make transverse process contact at the opposite adjacent level. The spinous processes lie in the hollow created between the fingers and the thenar eminence. Thus, a fulcrum has been produced. This contact is maintained as the therapist applies a mobilizing thrust through the patient's arms and chest as he rolls the patient over the fulcrum. Rotation is in the direction of the thenar eminence.

A **backward bending** mobilization force can be given by direct pressure on a spinous process with a pisiform contact as shown in Fig. 8-24. The mobiliza-

tion occurs at the segment inferior to the spinous process being contacted. Graded passive movements, stretches and thrusts can be utilized with this technique.

A **traction-backward bending** technique is shown in Fig. 8-25. It is done with a rolled bath towel or pillow stabilizing the level above the segment to be mobilized. Depending upon the level being mobilized and the height of the therapist and the patient, it may be necessary for the therapist to stand on a stool to obtain the correct position. The patient holds his arms crossed with his hands on opposite shoulders. The therapist reaches around the patient with both arms and grasps the patient's elbows and lifts upward and slightly backward. The amount of backward bending can be varied. The technique is often effective when done as a slow stretch and may involve a thrust at the end of the stretch. The thrust can be done by the therapist raising on his tiptoes then dropping suddenly onto his heels. The patient's weight is totally or partially being held as this is being done. This technique can also be done sitting on a stool. Mennell describes an alternate method of doing this technique by standing back to back with the patient to effect the mobilization at the lumbar level. In this instance, the therapist's hip acts as a fulcrum as the patient is lifted into extension with traction[13].

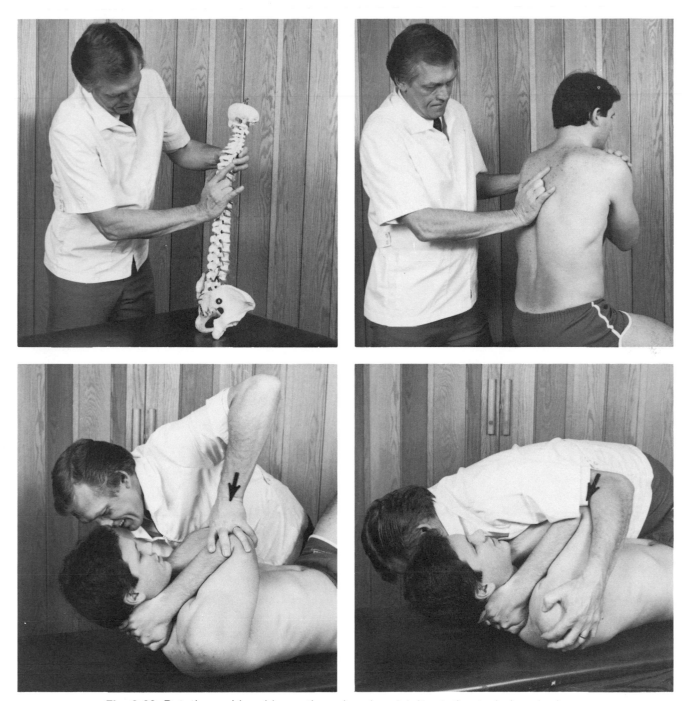

Fig. 8-23. Rotation, mid and lower thoracic spine. A left rotation technique is shown.

RIBS

The **rib mobilization** shown in Fig. 8-26 is done with the patient lying prone with pillows under his chest. The transverse processes are stabilized with the hypothenar eminence placed parallel to the spine on the opposite side of the rib to be mobilized. The forearms are crossed and the mobilization force is directed anteriorly and laterally through the hypothenar eminence that is contacting the postero-medial aspect of the rib. Graded passive movements, stretches or thrusts may be utilized with this technique.

LUMBAR SPINE

Six basic techniques for the lumbar spine are presented. Four are rotational techniques, one is a side bending technique and one involves side bending and may also incorporate rotation. The back-

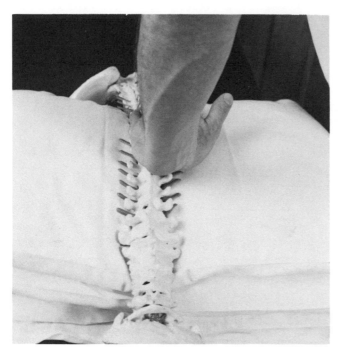 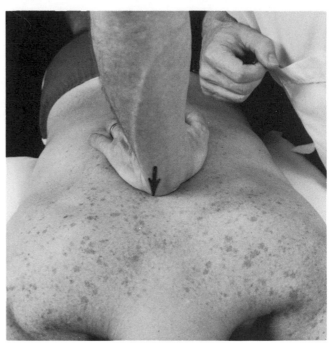

Fig. 8-24. Backward bending, mid and lower thoracic and lumbar spine.

ward bending technique shown in Fig. 8-24 and the backward bending and traction technique shown in Fig. 8-25 are also effective mobilization techniques for the lumbar spine.

The **rotational** technique shown in Fig. 8-27 is performed with the patient lying prone. The lateral aspect of the MCP joint of the thumb is used to stabilize the lateral aspect of the selected spinous process. The thenar eminence and heel of the hand also stabilize along the lateral aspect of the spinous processes superior to the MCP stabilization. Slack is taken up by rotating the pelvis and spine with the hand grasping the anterior rim of the ilium of the side opposite the stabilization and lifting upward and medially. The mobilizing force is then given with the hand that is stabilizing against the lateral aspect of the spinous processes. This technique is specific to the L5-S1 segment if the L5 spinous process is being mobilized. Although this technique becomes less specific as the mobilization force is moved superiorly, the greatest mobilizing force is always directed to the segment just inferior to the contact point of the MCP joint of the thumb. For example, if the third lumbar spinous process is contacted, the mobilization force is directed to the three segments between L3 and S1 with the L3,4 segment receiving the greatest force. Graded passive movements and stretches are effective with this technique. Thrusting is usually not utilized with this

technique. This technique can also be effective in the lower and mid-thoracic spine. It is most effective when done in three distinct steps: 1) Stabilize against spinous processes; 2) Take up slack by rotating the pelvis and 3) Mobilize with the hand that was previously stabilizing against the spinous processes. The **rotational** technique shown in Fig. 8-28 is also done with the patient lying prone. The mobilizing force is directed on the transverse process with a pisiform contact. The transverse process of L1 is smaller and partially shielded by the 12th rib and the L5 transverse process is usually shielded by the iliac crest. Three hand placements for L2,3 and 4 are shown as only these transverse processes are prominent enough to be contacted by the hypothenar eminence. The transverse processes can only be palpated indirectly through soft tissue, therefore the contact is sometimes only approximate to the level desired. This technique is thus semi-specific to the level described and may be used when general hypomobility is present rather than hypomobility at one specific level. The L4 transverse process is contacted by placing the hypothenar eminence parallel and slightly medial and superior to the posterior rim of the iliac crest. The L2 transverse process is contacted by placing the hypothenar eminence parallel and slightly inferior to the 12th rib. The L3 transverse process is contacted by placing the hypothenar eminence perpendicular to

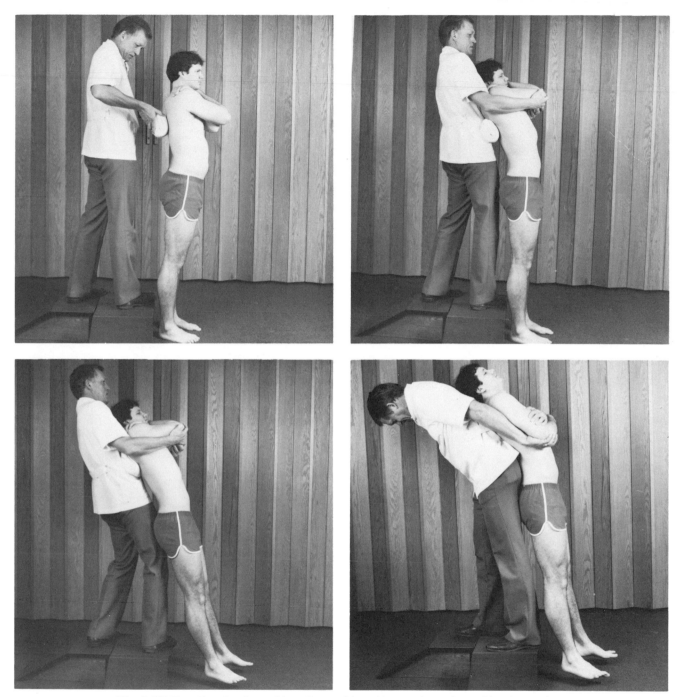

Fig. 8-25. Traction/backward bending, mid and lower thoracic and lumbar spine.

the spine midway between the L4 and L2 contacts. The pisiform contact should always be as close to the spinous process as possible with the mobilizing force directed posteroanteriorly. This causes the vertebra to rotate on its base. For example, when the L4 transverse process is contacted, the mobilization is effected primarily to the L4,5 segment. If the contact is on the left side, the direction of the mobilization is right rotation. Only graded passive movements and stretches are effective with this technique and it is an

especially useful technique when gentle, semi-specific mobilization is indicated.

The **rotational** technique shown in Fig. 8-29 is a non-specific technique which can be effective in the mid and lower thoracic spine as well as in the lumbar spine. It can also be utilized as an effective self-mobilization or home treatment technique. The patient is positioned supine with the knees and hips flexed as the pelvis is laterally rotated. The degree of knee and hip flexion determines the general level of

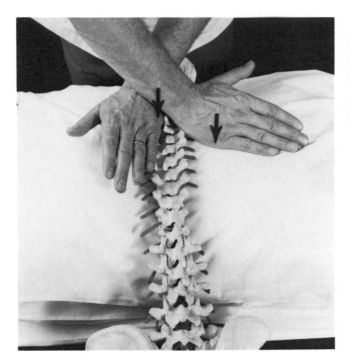
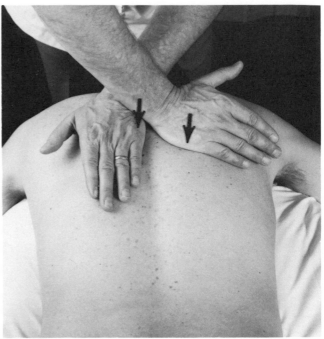

Fig. 8-26. Rib mobilization.

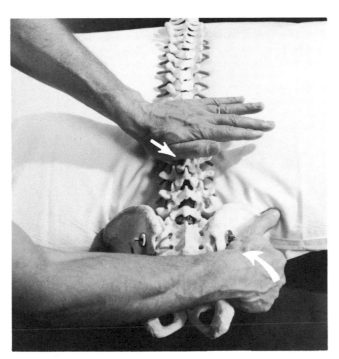
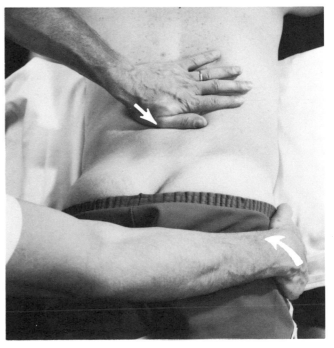

Fig. 8-27. Lumbar rotation technique showing stabilization with the left hand against the spinous processes. The right hand takes up slack then the mobilizing force is applied with the left hand. A left rotation technique is shown.

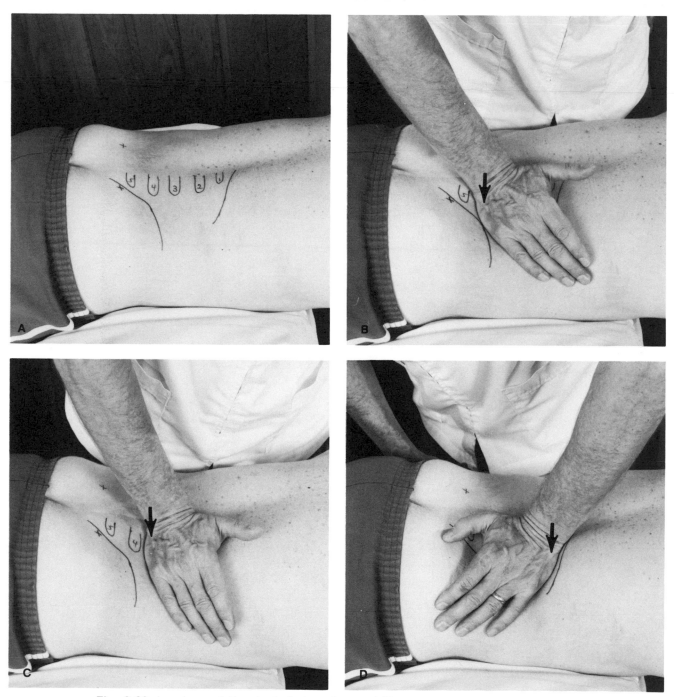

Fig. 8-28. Lumbar rotation technique using a pisiform contact to mobilize on the transverse process: A) Approximate location of the transverse processes; B) Contact of the L4 transverse process; C) Contact of the L3 transverse process and D) Contact of the L2 transverse process. A left rotation technique is shown.

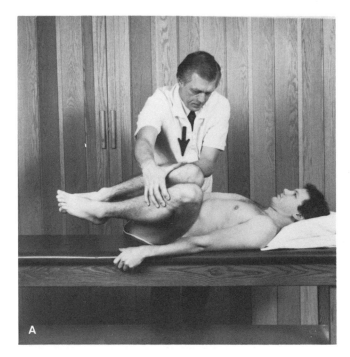

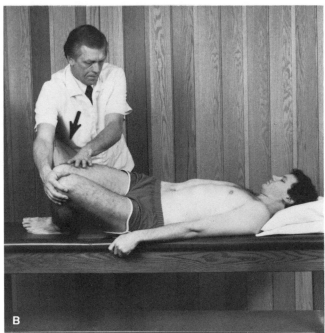

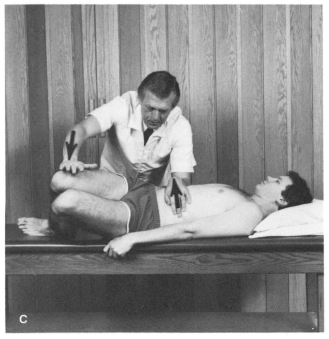

Fig. 8-29. Rotation technique showing: A) Mid and lower thoracic mobilization; B) Lumbar mobilization; C) Lumbar mobilization with added stabilization across the lower rib cage. A right rotation technique is shown.

spinal mobilization. If the knees and hips are flexed completely to the chest, the mobilization is directed into the mid-thoracic spine. As the amount of flexion is decreased, the level of the mobilization moves lower into the thoracic and the lumbar spine. If the patient's lower rib cage is stabilized, the mobilization becomes specific to the lumbar spine.

Graded passive movements and stretching techniques are most effective with this technique. Hold-relax and contract-relax muscle stretches are also effective.

The **rotational** technique shown in Fig. 8-30 is the classic "lumbar roll" mobilization which can be effective for articulation, stretch and manipulation. It is a specific technique in that it can be isolated to one segment and utilizes principles of ligamentous locking and facet apposition to gain specificity. The patient is positioned on the side opposite the desired direction of mobilization. As the therapist faces the patient, he places his cephalad hand over the patient and palpates between spinous processes at the desired level for mobilization. With his caudal hand, he gains a secure hold on the lower portion of the patient's top leg. He then passively flexes the patient's hip and knee using his own hip as a balance point for the patient's knee. Flexion is thus passively imparted into the lower lumbar spine as the therapist performs a side-gliding movement with his pelvis parallel to the patient. He palpates for the arrival of flexion at the segment. When he feels the inferior spinous process begin to move, he stops and lowers the leg to the table, "locking" the spine in flexion to that point. He then imparts rotation down to the segment by rotating the trunk. This is done by pulling the patient's inferior arm toward the therapist. Rotation is stopped when movement is palpated at the superior spinous process of the desired

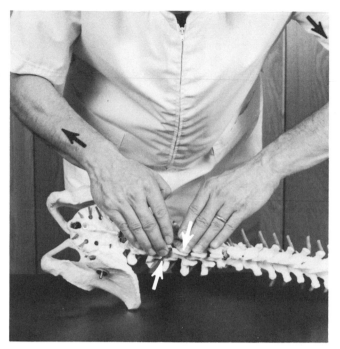 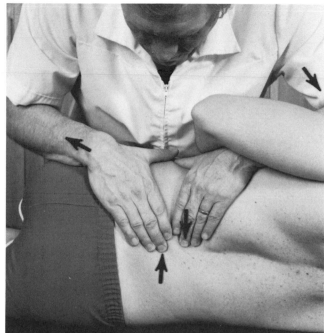

Fig. 8-30. Lumbar rotational mobilization technique using finger pressures on the spinous processes as well as force through the operator's forearms to effect a rotational force to one specific level. A left rotation technique is shown.

segment. In effect, this "locking" of the lower segments in flexion and upper segments in rotation causes the mobilizing force to be focused at the one desired level. The actual mobilization is accomplished by rotating the pelvis and lower segments in a direction toward the therapist and the shoulder and upper segments in a direction away from the therapist. Some of the mobilizing force is directed through the therapist's forearms to the patient's pelvis and shoulder, but it is important to concentrate as much force in the fingers as possible when doing this mobilization, thus following the rule of short lever arms. The fingers are placed on the lateral aspects of the spinous processes to produce the rotational force. The fingers in contact with the inferior spinous process are to the lateral aspect of that spinous process on the down side. The fingers in contact with the superior spinous process are on the top side. The therapist pulls the pelvis and inferior spinous process toward himself and pushes the superior spinous process and shoulder away. The thumb may be used instead of the fingers for the superior contact.

The **side bending** technique shown in Fig. 8-31 is done with the patient lying prone. As the hip is abducted, the lumbar spine side bends. If a stabilizing force is placed against the lateral aspect of the spinous process, side bending is prevented from that

point superiorly. The technique is done in three steps similar to those described for the first rotational technique (Fig. 8-27). The lateral aspect of the MCP joint, the thenar eminence and the heel of the hand stabilize along the lateral aspect of the spinous processes, the hip is abducted to take up slack and the mobilization force is then effected against the spinous processes. This technique concentrates the greatest side bending force at the segment just inferior to the point of contact of the MCP joint. If the patient is large or if vigorous mobilization is necessary, it may be necessary to utilize one therapist to stabilize and mobilize and an assistant to maintain abduction of the patient's leg. Placement of the other hand on top of the mobilizing hand can impart greater force when necessary. Occasionally, both legs must be carried to the side to achieve the desired amount of side bending.

Positional stretch is a mobilization technique that involves **side bending** and may also incorporate **rotation** (Fig. 8-32). The patient is positioned on his side over a six to eight inch roll. The roll is positioned between the crest of the ilium and rib cage in order to achieve the maximum side bend to a specific area. As the spine bends over the roll, the facet joints are separated and the muscles and ligaments are stretched on the superior side. If the pelvis is allowed to roll forward and the shoulder

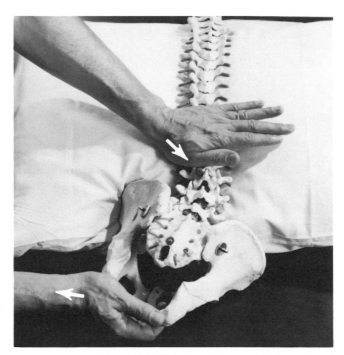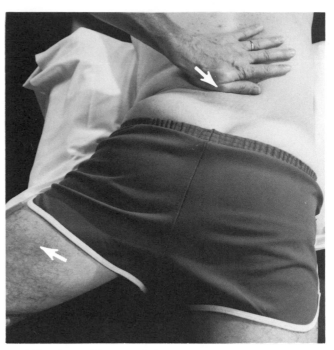

Fig. 8-31. Side bending technique showing stabilization with the left hand (step 1), abduction of the hip to take up slack (step 2), and mobilization of the hip with the left hand (step 3.)

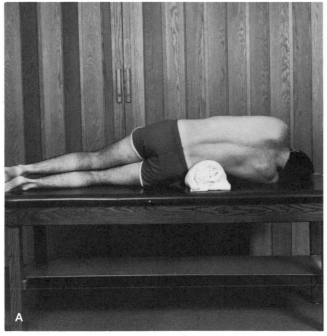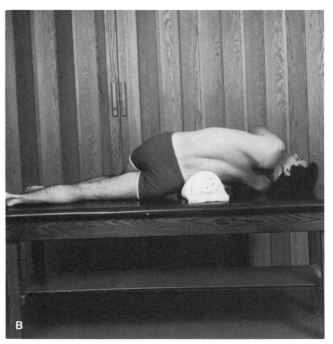

Fig. 8-32. Positional stretch: A) Side bending and B) Side bending and rotation.

backward, a rotational component is added and even more separation and stretching is achieved. Even more stretch can be obtained if the patient's top leg is allowed to hang over the edge of the treatment table.

This technique may be used for nerve root impingement problems as well as for joint hypo-mobility and muscular tightness. When used for nerve root impingement, one must distinguish between an impingement arising from a disc pro-trusion with a lateral shift and an impingement caused by narrowing, thickening, osteophyte forma-tion or a disc fragment in the intervertebral foramen.

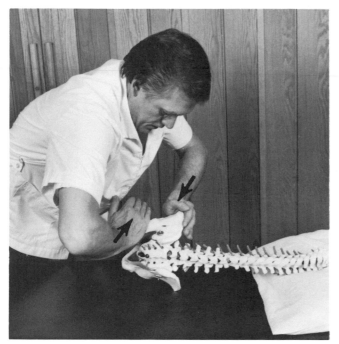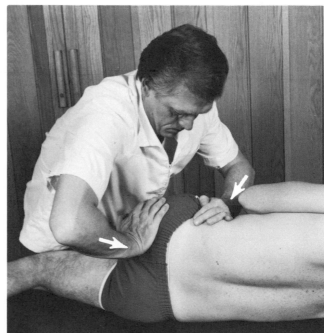

Fig. 8-33. Posterior rotation of the ilium on the sacrum.

In the latter instance, the patient should be placed with the side of the impingement up. In the former instance, one would desire to correct the lateral shift. This would be accomplished by placing the patient on the side of pathology. This technique to correct a lateral shift should be done only if centralization of the patient's symptoms occurs (see discussion of disc herniation with protrusion in Chapter 5.) Positional stretch is usually done up to a maximum of ten minutes. It is also an effective home or self-treatment.

SACROILIAC

The sacroiliac mobilization shown in Fig. 8-33 is a **posterior rotational** technique of the innominate on the sacrum. This technique can be utilized when the ilium is subluxed in an anteriorly rotated position on the sacrum. The patient is positioned sidelying with the joint to be mobilized on the top side. One hand is placed on the ASIS and the other is on the ischial tuberosity. The anterior rim of the ilium is pushed posteriorly while the ischial tuberosity is pushed anteriorly, producing a force couple. This action results in a posterior rotational movement of the ilium on the sacrum. Additional force may be added to this technique by stabilizing the bottom-side hip in extension and flexing the top-side hip. Additional force may be gained if the top-

side knee is extended and allowed to hang over the edge of the treatment table. This action tethers the hamstring muscles and helps pull the innominate posteriorly. Graded passive movements, stretches and thrusts may be utilized with this technique.

The sacroiliac mobilization shown in Fig. 8-34 is an **anterior rotational** technique of the innominate on the sacrum and is appropriate for a posterior subluxation. The patient is positioned prone, the hip is passively extended on the side to be mobilized and a pillow is placed under the thigh to achieve a mild prolonged stretch. If additional force is desired, direct pressure may be placed on the inferior portion of the sacrum which in effect accomplishes the same force by posteriorly rotating the sacrum on the stabilized right innominate. Further force may be imparted by direct pressure on the PSIS in an anterior and slightly superior direction. The hip on the affected side should be maximally extended by reaching around and lifting at the knee. This maneuver takes up all slack and helps stabilize for these stronger mobilizations. If still more force is desired, the patient's hip on the unaffected side may be allowed off the side of the table while the leg on the affected side remains on the table as the direct pressure techniques are applied to inferior sacrum and the PSIS. Stretching and/or thrusting mobilizations may be utilized.

Figure 8-35 shows a mobilization technique used to: 1) reduce a posterior rotation subluxation

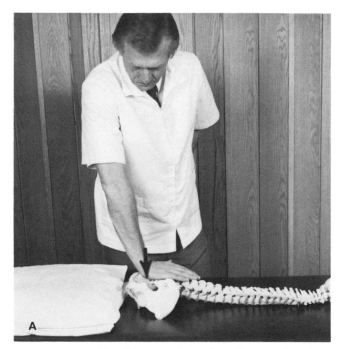

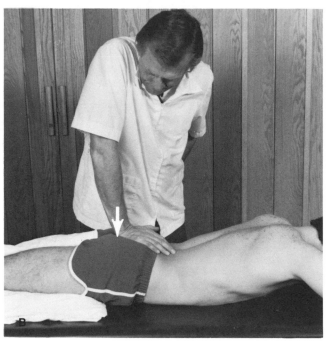

Fig. 8-34. Rotation of the ilium on the sacrum. The photograph shows the technique for a right sacroiliac joint: A) Hand position on inferior sacrum; B) Mild mobilization with a pillow under the thigh and downward pressure on inferior sacrum. Added force may be accomplished by placing the leg on the unaffected side off the side of the table for added stabilization and by lifting the right hip into full extension.

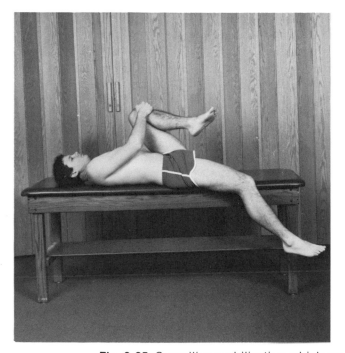

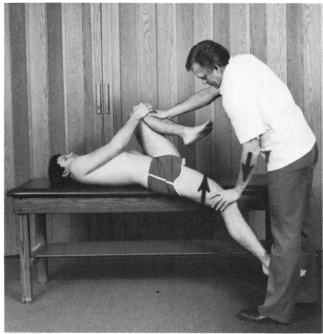

Fig. 8-35. Sacroiliac mobilization which causes: 1) an anterior rotational force of the right innominate on the sacrum or 2) a posterior rotational force of the left innominate on the sacrum.

(innominate on the sacrum) of the right sacroiliac joint or 2) increase anterior rotation mobility of the right innominate on the sacrum. As the weight of the right leg pulls the right innominate into anterior rotation, the left innominate is stabilized by holding the left knee toward the chest. Active contraction of the right hip flexors against resistance is an effective adjunct to this technique. This technique is actually applying a mobilizing force in the opposite direction to the left sacroiliac joint; therefore, as shown, it is also an effective mobilization technique for reducing an anterior rotation subluxation (innominate on sacrum) on the left or increasing posterior rotation mobility of the left innominate on the sacrum.

COCCYX

The position for coccyx mobilization is shown in Fig. 8-36. The patient is prone with one or two pillows under the pelvis to raise the pelvis into a position accessible for mobilization. The mobilization is done with the index finger inserted internally into the rectum and the thumb placed externally to grasp the coccyx. Anterior-posterior glide and long axis extension (traction) are the two mobilization techniques used for the coccyx. Graded passive movements are effective with these techniques.

EXTREMITY MOBILIZATION

Many of the evaluative techniques used on the extremities can be easily modified into mobilization

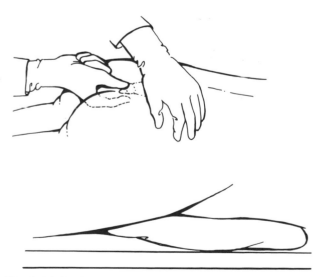

Fig. 8-36. Position for coccyx mobilization.

techniques. In order to determine normalcy for a given patient, the uninvolved extremity is tested first and serves to demonstrate to the patient what will be done on the involved extremity. Most of the testing techniques require only mild or moderate force to demonstrate joint mobility. The examining techniques often must be done quickly in order to see or feel joint play. The beginner often makes the mistake of taking up all the joint play (slack) before performing test movements. He is thus unable to demonstrate normal joint play. He must remember that the slack in the joint **is** the joint play movement. Many of the joint play movements test ligamentous stability.

The following rules apply to mobilization and testing of joint play movements in the extremities: 1) The therapist must consider the concave-convex rules of joint motion when evaluating or treating the joints of the extremities; 2) The joint play movements are tested with the joint in a neutral or mid-range position; 3) The therapist's grip should be firm but not painful; 4) The forces applied should be as close to the joint line as possible as long lever arms may cause excessive force and 5) Subsequent treatments may be done with the joints at the end of their available ranges in order to stretch capsules and ligaments where indicated.

UPPER EXTREMITY

JOINTS OF THE HAND AND WRIST (FIG. 8-37)

Metacarpophalangeal and Interphalangeal Joints (Fig. 8-38)

All of the techniques for the MCP and IP joints can be performed with the patient's hand palm down and stabilized against the therapist's chest or thigh as they sit next to each other at an oblique angle. An alternative method may have the therapist and patient facing each other across a table with the forearm resting on the table for stability. Most of the techniques are done with the joints in the mid-range position.

    a. Anterior-posterior (volar-dorsal) glide is performed with the thumbs as close together as possible on the dorsal surface on either side of the joint line. The more distal hand provides the mobilizing force on the proximal phalanx in a direction parallel to the joint line. When performed as a testing

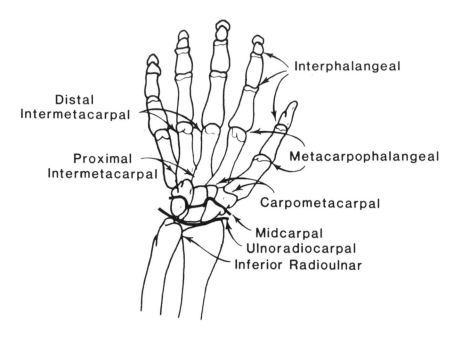

Fig. 8-37. Joints of the hand and wrist.

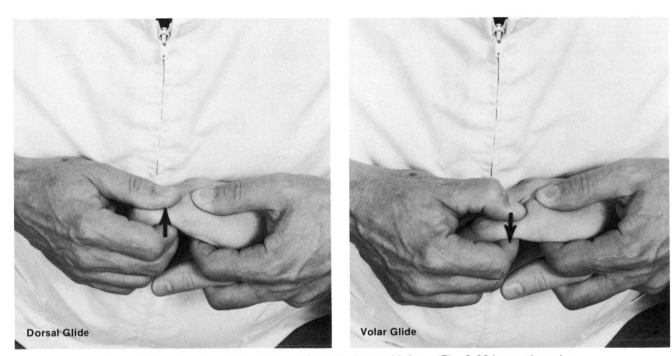

Dorsal Glide

Volar Glide

Fig. 8-38. Metacarpophalangeal and interphalangeal joints. (Fig. 8-38 is continued on next page.)

procedure, these volar-dorsal movements are done alternately. Remembering the concave moving on convex rule, mobilizations done for treatment are applied in the direction of limitation. For example, an MCP joint limited in flexion would be mobilized volarly. Volar-dorsal glide for the IP joints is

done with the same technique.

b. Medial-lateral glide for the MCP joint is performed by simply changing the grip of the mobilizing hand to the radial and ulnar sides of the proximal phalanx. Stabilization remains the same with the mobilization applied at the proximal joint line in a

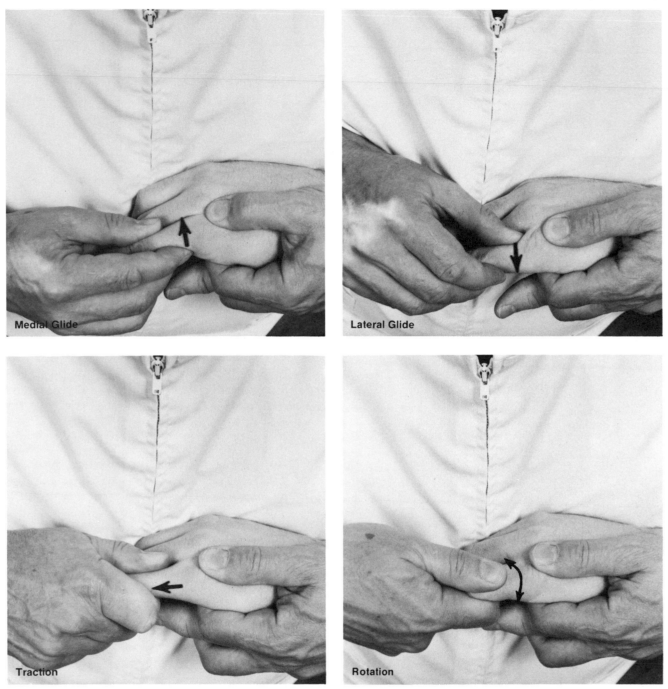

Fig. 8-38. Metacarpophalangeal and interphalangeal joints. (Continued)

medial-lateral direction. This technique may be modified into one of side bending rather than one of gliding in order to test the collateral ligaments at the MCP's and IP's.

c. Traction or long axis distraction may be performed utilizing the same grips as are used for dorsal-volar glide or medial-lateral glide. The IP joints should be flexed in order to provide a better grip when doing the MCP joints.

d. Rotation also uses the same grips as described for the other MCP and IP techniques. The mobilization is given by rotating the more distal segment about its long axis. The IP joints may be flexed to provide a better grip when doing the MCP joints.

Intermetacarpal Joints (Fig. 8-39)

The distal intermetacarpal techniques are best performed with the patient and therapist seated facing each other. The patient's elbow and forearm may be stabilized on a flat surface. The forearm is supinated. The therapist is now facing the dorsum of the patient's hand. The therapist, using thumb/index finger grips, grasps the heads of two adjacent metacarpals. Volar-dorsal glides are employed for this technique. The head of the third metacarpal is stabilized while the head of the second metacarpal is mobilized. Then, in turn the fourth is stabilized while the fifth is mobilized and, finally, the third is stabilized as the fourth is mobilized.

Rotation of the metacarpals is done by grasping the head of the metacarpal and rotating it about its long axis. Stabilization at the patient's wrist may be necessary. The movement is accomplished correctly when the therapist utilizes his shoulder for the mobilization as his grip is held fixed to avoid rolling the skin on the underlying bone. Approximately 30° of rotation is present at each of these joints.

Carpometacarpal (CMC) Joint — Thumb (Fig. 8-40)

The CMC joint of the thumb is convex distally and concave proximally. The CMC joint techniques are performed with the patient's hand stabilized against the therapist's chest, thigh or the treatment table. The stabilization for all four techniques is the same. The patient's wrist is held by grasping the dorsal surface of the hand and wrist with the therapist's thumb pointing toward the patient's elbow. The therapist's fingers are curled around to the volar surface of the patient's wrist, thus stabilizing all of the carpal bones. Volar-dorsal glides, medial-lateral glides, traction and rotational mobilizations are applied in the same manner to the CMC joint as to the MCP and IP joints. The mobilizing grip is as close to the joint line as possible.

Midcarpal Joint (Fig. 8-41)

The midcarpal joint is a functional joint formed by the articulation of the distal and proximal carpal rows. The distal carpal row, made up of the trapezium, trapezoid, capitate and hamate, is tightly bound by the dorsal and volar ligaments and tends to move as a group on the proximal carpal row. The proximal carpal row is comprised of the navicular (scaphoid), lunate, triquetrum and pisiform. The majority of wrist extension takes place at the midcarpal joint. This joint is convex distally and concave proximally.

a. Traction is done by placing the stabilizing hand against the distal end of the patient's humerus (elbow flexed to 90°). The mobilizing force is given by grasping the patient's hand distal to the mid-carpal joint, palm-to-

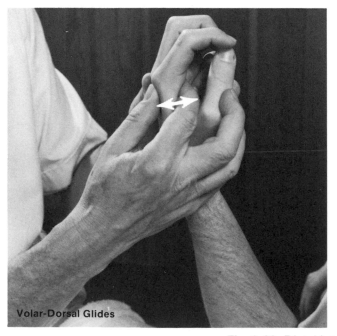

Volar-Dorsal Glides

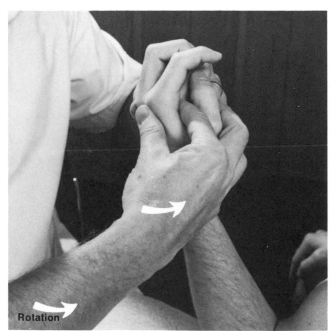

Rotation

Fig. 8-39. Distal intermetacarpal joints.

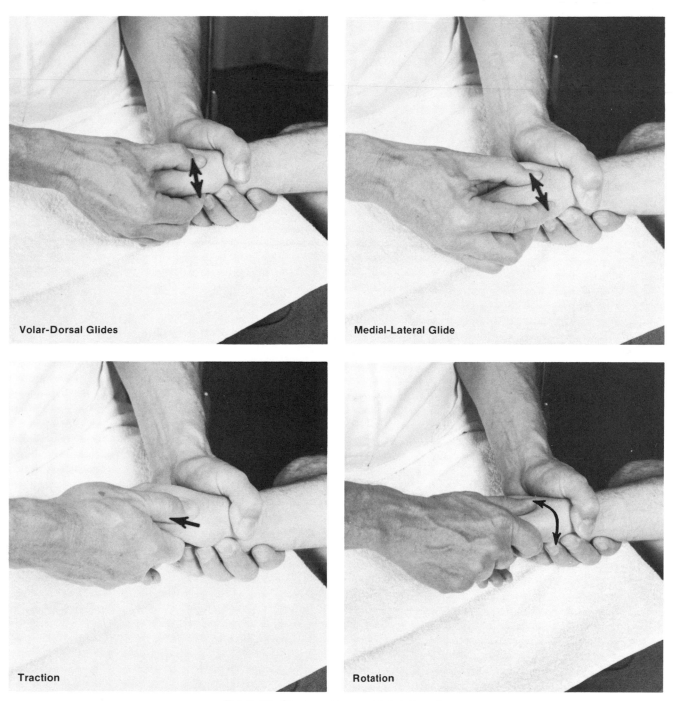

Fig. 8-40. Carpometacarpal joint-thumb.

palm as in shaking hands, and pulling parallel to the forearm. This force is being directed across the radiocarpal joint and also serves as a mobilization technique for that joint. Distal glide of the radius on the ulna is also accomplished with this force. A technique such as this which involves more than one joint is usually poor for examination as it is difficult to determine at which of the joints movement is occurring. Distal glide of the radius on the ulna can be eliminated from this technique by positioning the stabilizing hand around the patient's forearm rather than at the distal humerus. The technique may be further modified by stabilizing around the distal forearm and radiocarpal joint in an attempt to isolate the traction to the midcarpal joint.

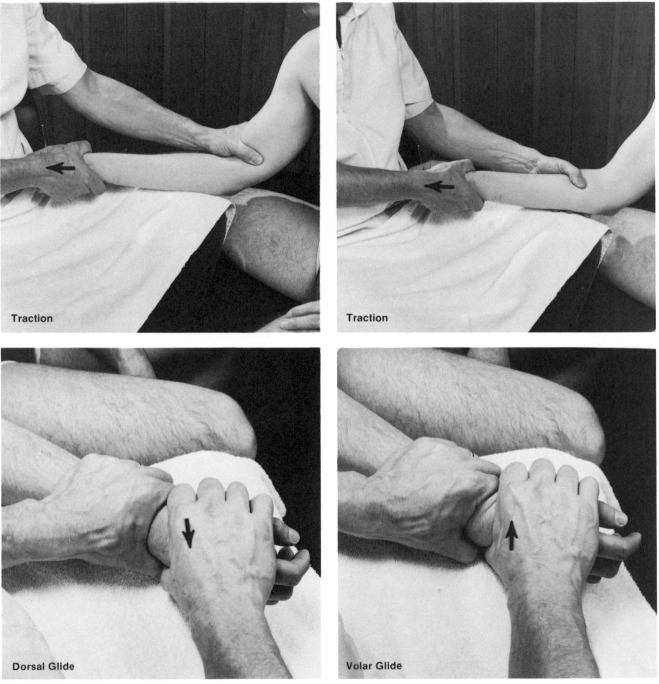

Fig. 8-41. Midcarpal joint. (Fig. 8-41 is continued on next page.)

b. Volar-Dorsal glide is performed with the dorsum of the patient's hand facing the therapist. The proximal row of carpal bones is stabilized and the distal row is mobilized. The therapist's thumbs and index fingers are adjacent to each other. The examining or the mobilizing forces are at a 45° angle to the stabilizing force. It is critical that the proximal row of carpal bones be well stabilized or the movement will not be isolated to the midcarpal joint. There is often one-fourth to one-half inch of joint play present with this movement. The midcarpal joint may also be mobilized by squeezing the joint between the two thenar eminences. The therapist interlocks his fingers around the radial border of the patient's hand. The thenar eminence of the volar side hand stabilizes the proximal

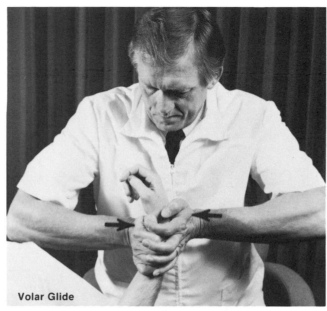

Fig. 8-41. Midcarpal Joint. (Continued)

carpal row. The thenar eminence on the dorsal side is placed against the distal carpal row. A very powerful gliding action can be produced as the therapist squeezes his palms together. Volar glide is shown in Fig. 8-41. Hand positions can be reversed to perform dorsal glide.

Radiocarpal Joint (Fig. 8-42)

The radiocarpal joint is actually comprised of the scaphoid and lunate articulating on the distal

radius. The triquetrum is involved during ulnar deviation and the pisiform articulates only with the hamate. The distal radius is concave and the proximal carpal row is essentially convex. The majority of wrist flexion, radial deviation and ulnar deviation occurs at the radiocarpal joint.

a. Volar-dorsal glide techniques for the radiocarpal joint are best applied with the therapist's hands encircling the wrist from the radial side. The more proximal hand stabilizes at the level of the distal radius and the more distal hand provides the mobilization force at the level of the carpal row. It is essential that the index fingers of the therapist be nearly touching at the joint line for best results. Large amounts of force can be generated with this technique, so care must be exercised in its application.

b. Medial (ulnar) and lateral (radial) tilts are performed by using the same positioning as described for anterior-posterior glide. The therapist simply tilts the wrist medially (ulnar deviation) and laterally (radial deviation.) During medial tilt the thumbs are the fulcrum and the scaphoid and radius are tilted apart. During the lateral tilt the index fingers become the fulcrum and the triquetrum and ulna are tilted apart.

c. Backward tilt of the scaphoid and lunate on the radius is done with the patient sitting or standing with his arm hanging relaxed. The

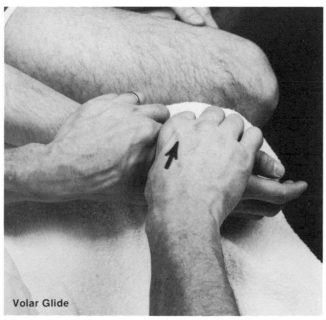

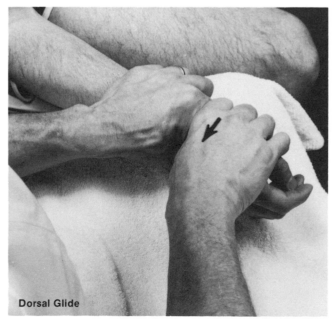

Fig. 8-42. Radiocarpal joint. (Fig. 8-42 is continued on next page.)

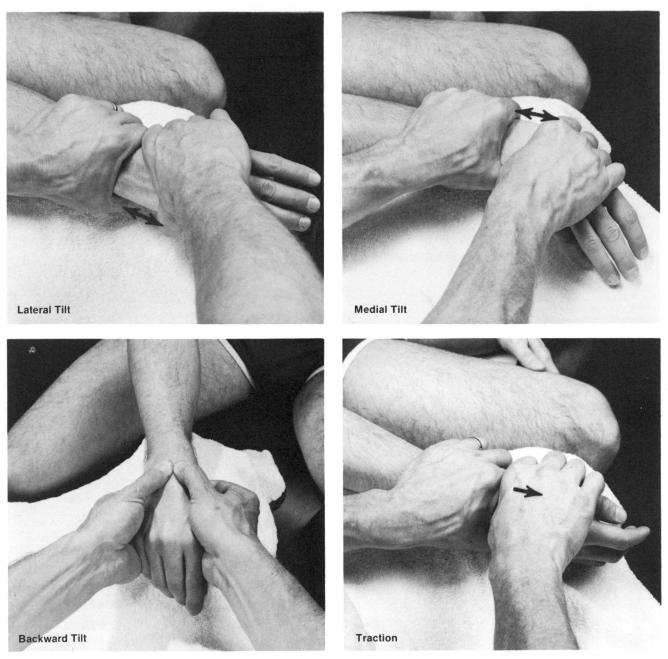

Fig. 8-42. Radiocarpal Joint. (Continued)

therapist grips the scaphoid between the thumb and index finger of one hand and the lunate between the thumb and index finger of the other hand. Then, while holding tight to the two bones, he tilts them backward (extension) on the radius. If the normal joint play is present, a "grating" or "grinding" sensation is felt. Although this is a slightly unpleasant sensation, it is a necessary joint play movement.

    d. Traction, or long axis distraction of the radiocarpal joint utilizes the same hand positionings as in the volar-dorsal tech-

nique. The therapist simply stabilizes with the proximal hand and separates the joint with a distractive force with the distal hand. Traction may be incorporated with any of the gliding techniques described.

Ulnomeniscotriquetral Joint

    The triquetrum, as part of the proximal carpal row, does not articulate with the radius except perhaps with ulnar deviation. Its primary articulation is with the ulna. A fibrocartilagenous meniscus covered with hyaline cartilage forms the proximal joint surface. The triquetrum will be mobilized when performing any of the techniques for the radiocarpal joint. The triquetrum may be mobilized against the ulna with the therapist employing the thumb-index finger grips previously described, stabilizing the distal ulna and mobilizing the triquetrum.

Inferior Radioulnar Joint (Fig. 8-43)

Pronation and supination are the principal movements at this joint. The inferior radioulnar joint is examined and mobilized with the patient and therapist seated facing each other. The patient's elbow and shoulder are flexed with the forearm supinated. Resting the elbow against a table top may be helpful. The therapist is facing the dorsum of the patient's forearm and hand. The therapist stabilizes the radius and carpals of the wrist by grasping them along the dorsum of the patient's hand. The thumb and index and middle fingers of the other hand grip the distal ulna.

a. Volar-dorsal glides may be applied in a straight front-to-back movement.

b. Rotation is done by grasping the distal ulna and rotating it around the radius. The therapist's hand is held fixed as the movement is accomplished with shoulder motion. This helps avoid rolling of the skin over the underlying bone.

JOINTS OF THE ELBOW (FIG. 8-44)

Superior Radioulnar Joint (Fig. 8-45)

Pronation and supination are the principle movements of this joint, but long axis glide along the ulna is an important component motion. The superior radioulnar joint is examined and mobilized with the patient and therapist seated facing each other.

a. Anterior-posterior glide of the radius on the ulna is done with the patient's forearm resting across the therapist's lap. The proximal ulna is stabilized with one hand while the radial head is held with the thumb and index and middle fingers of the other hand. The fingers are positioned directly on the proximal end of the radial head on the dorsolateral aspect of the forearm where the radial head is palpable. The thumb is positioned ventral to the radial head, squeezing

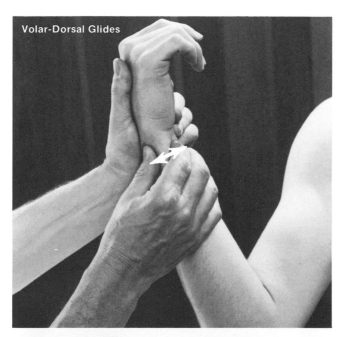

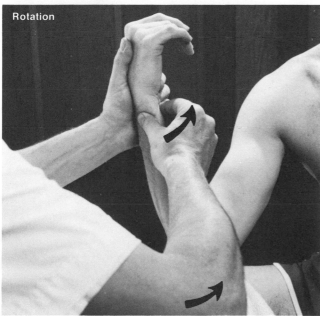

Fig. 8-43. Inferior radioulnar joint.

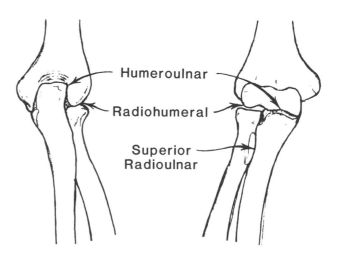

Fig. 8-44. Joints of the elbow.

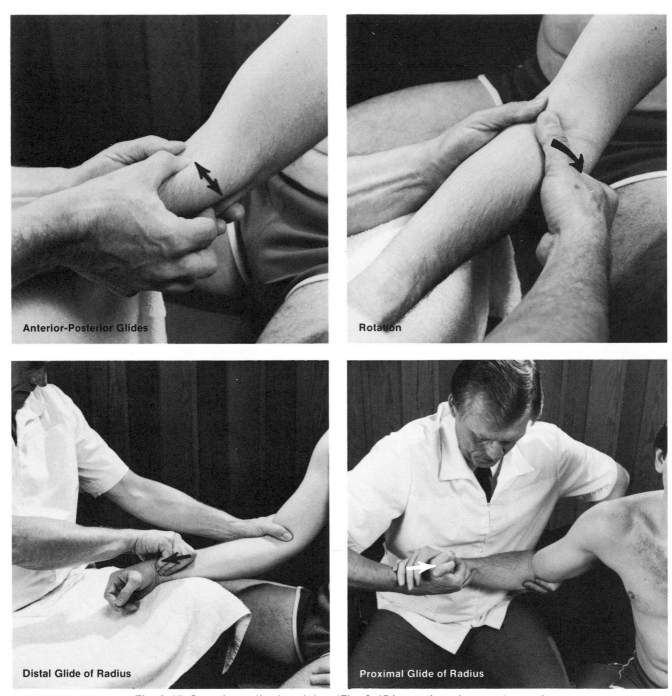

Fig. 8-45. Superior radioulnar joint. (Fig. 8-45 is continued on next page.)

the forearm musculature against the radial head. The mobilizing force is directed dorsoventrally. Joint play may be difficult to feel because of the soft tissue involved with the grip.

b. Rotation of the radius on the ulna is done in the same position as anterior-posterior glide. The mobilizing grip is changed slightly by bringing the radial head further into the web space of the thumb and index finger. The

mobilizing force is directed to the proximal radius in a rotational direction posterolaterally to the ulna.

c. Distal glide of the radius on the ulna may be done as a part of the traction technique described for the midcarpal and radiocarpal joints. If the therapist wants to avoid testing or mobilizing across the wrist joint with this technique, the mobilizing hand should grip the distal radius instead. The radius glides

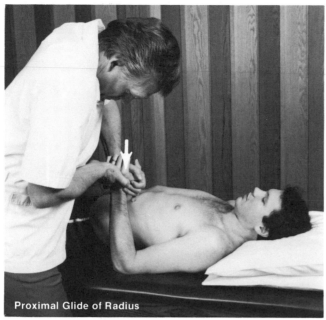

Proximal Glide of Radius

Fig. 8-45. Superior radiocarpal joint. (Continued)

one hand while the other hand is placed palm-to-palm with the patient's hand. The patient's forearm is then brought close to the therapist's chest. In this position, the therapist's forearms are parallel to the patient's forearm. The mobilizing forces are simultaneously directed distally on the ulna and proximally on the radius. It is important that the proximal force be directed to the radius by tilting the wrist slightly to the radial side as the force is given. An alternate way of doing this technique has the patient lying supine with the elbow flexed to 90°. The ulna and humerus are stabilized against the treatment table and the mobilizing force is directed through the wrist to the radius as described above. Since proximal glide of the radius occurs as the elbow is flexed, it is especially important to test this movement when elbow flexion is restricted.

distally on the ulna during elbow extension, so it is especially important to test this movement if elbow extension is restricted.

d. Proximal glide of the radius on the ulna is a force couple technique. When using force couple techniques, no true stabilizing and mobilizing forces exist; rather, one force equals the other in opposite directions. The proximal ulna is stabilized by holding the olecranon and distal humerus in the palm of

Humeroulnar Joint (Fig. 8-46)

Only elbow flexion and extension occur at this joint. The humeroulnar joint is best tested and mobilized with the patient lying supine on a treatment table.

a. Distraction of the humeroulnar joint may be done in one of three positions, depending upon the available range of motion of the joint. The mobilizing force is always directed

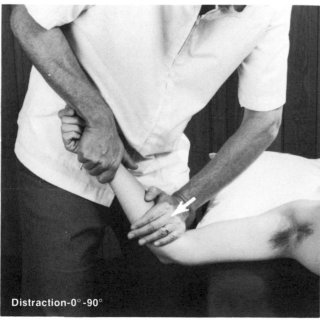

Distraction-0°-90°

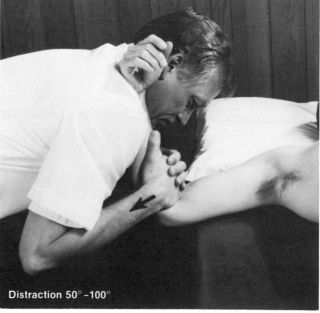

Distraction 50°-100°

Fig. 8-46. Humeroulnar joint. (Fig. 8-46 is continued on next page.)

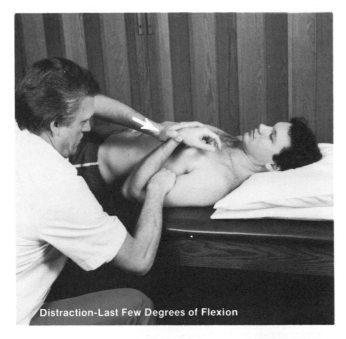

Distraction-Last Few Degrees of Flexion

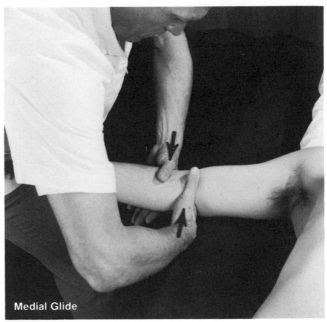

Medial Glide

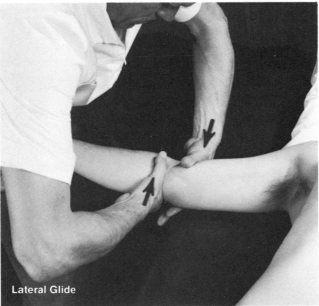

Lateral Glide

Fig. 8-46. Humeroulnar joint. (Continued)

perpendicular to the shaft of the ulna as close to the joint as possible.

From 0° to 90° of range of motion, the technique is done with the shoulder abducted to 90°. The humerus rests against the treatment table with the elbow a few inches over the edge. The therapist stabilizes the forearm at the wrist. The mobilizing force is applied parallel to the humerus with the heel of the hand and directed perpendicular to the shaft of the ulna. Thus, the olecranon is distracted from the humerus. Additional stabilization may be provided by having an assistant hold the shaft of the humerus against the treatment table. This is necessary to avoid any unwanted force at the shoulder joint.

From 50° to 100° range of motion, the patient is positioned as shown with the shoulder abducted and resting against the treatment table. The mobilizing force is applied with both hands around the proximal end of the ulna at the antecubital crease while the distal end of the ulna rests against the therapist's shoulder. The therapist's shoulder acts as a fulcrum as the force is applied perpendicular to the shaft of the ulna. Once again, another person or a strap may be utilized to stabilize the humerus to protect the shoulder joint.

The third distraction technique is done in the last few degrees of flexion. The therapist's fist or a rolled towel is used to make a fulcrum as the patient's elbow is flexed over it. In this technique the patient is supine with the upper arm resting against the treatment table. This technique stretches the posterior portion of the joint capsule. In the two previously described techniques either the ventral or dorsal portions of the capsule may be stretched, depending upon the point in the range of motion in which the technique is performed. If the techniques are performed midway in the available range, the entire capsule is being stretched. If the joint is taken to the end of available extension, the anterior portion will be stretched. Conversely, the posterior portion will be stretched when the joint is taken to the end of available flexion.

b. Medial-lateral glide of the humeroulnar joint is a force couple technique. The web spaces of both hands contact the humerus and ulna as close to the joint line as possible. To perform medial glide of the ulna on the humerus, the web space of one hand is placed just superior to the medial epicondyle of the humerus and the web space of the other hand is placed on the lateral aspect of the forearm at a point over the radial head. The therapist can support the patient's forearm by pressing it against his lateral chest (axilla) with his humerus. The therapist's forearms should be parallel to each other and perpendicular to the joint line. As the forces are applied, the ulna glides medially on the humerus. Lateral glide of the ulna on the humerus is accomplished by using the same technique but with the hand contacts changed so that the web space of one hand contacts the humerus just superior to the lateral epicondyle and the web space of the other hand is placed on the medial aspect of the forearm just inferior to the medial epicondyle.

JOINTS OF THE SHOULDER (Fig. 8-47)

Glenohumeral Joint (Fig. 8-48)

Flexion, extension, abduction, external and internal rotation are the principle movements of the gleno-

humeral joint. The glenohumeral joint surfaces are convex distally and concave proximally. The glenohumeral joint is best tested and mobilized with the patient lying supine on a treatment table. Four test movements and basic mobilization techniques are presented: lateral distraction; posterior glide; anterior glide and inferior glide. The other mobilization techniques shown for the glenohumeral joint are combinations and modifications of these four basic techniques.

a. Lateral distraction of the humeral head in the glenoid fossa is done with the patient's arm in slight abduction. The mobilizing hand is placed in the patient's axilla. A towel may be placed in the axilla for patient comfort and hygiene. The patient's arm is supported at the elbow and the forearm and wrist are cradled between the therapist's hip and elbow of the mobilizing arm. The mobilizing force is directed laterally from the glenoid fossa. It is important that the mobilizing hand be as close to the joint as possible. A mobilizing strap technique as shown in Fig. 8-48 may also be used for lateral distraction.

b. Anterior glide of the humeral head in the glenoid fossa is done in the same position as lateral distraction except that both hands are used to provide the mobilizing force. The therapist grasps the proximal humerus with both hands at the level of the surgical neck of the humerus. The mobilizing force is directed anteriorly by radially deviating the wrists. It is sometimes necessary to have an assistant stabilize the scapula and clavicle or use a stabilization strap during this movement,

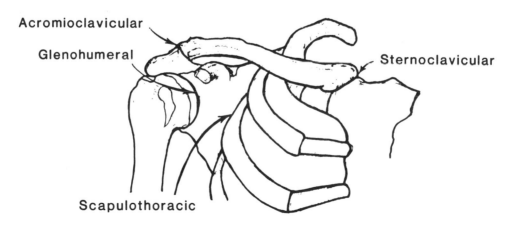

Fig. 8-47. Joints of the shoulder.

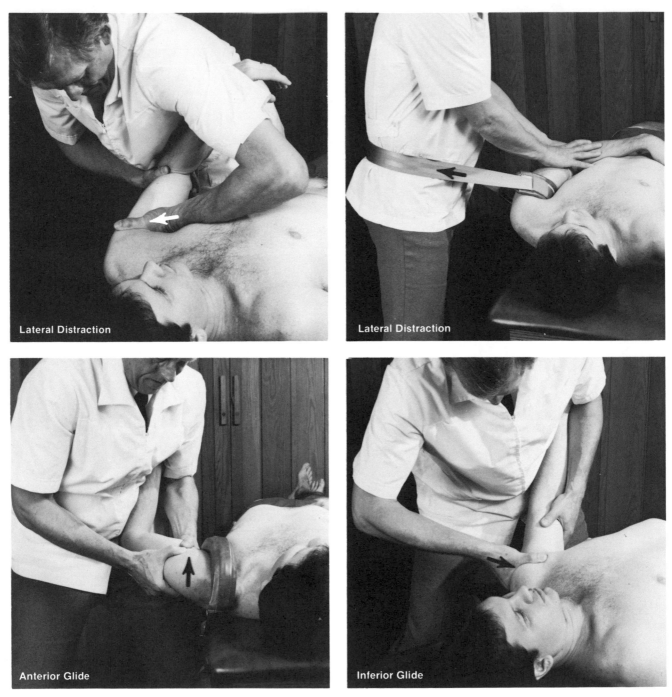

Fig. 8-48. Glenohumeral joint. (Fig. 8-48 is continued on the next two pages.)

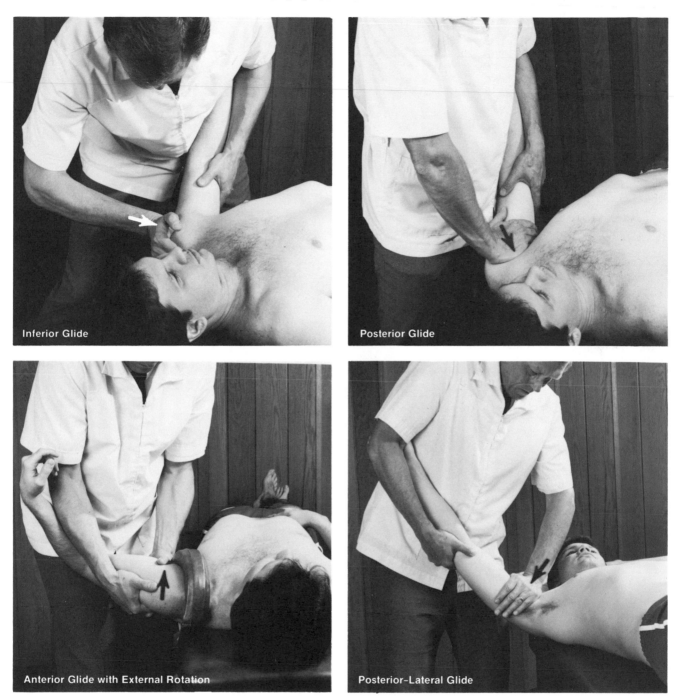

Fig. 8-48. Glenohumeral Joint. (Continued)

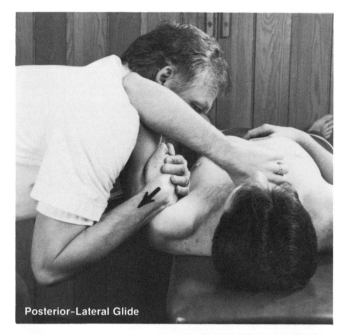

Posterior–Lateral Glide

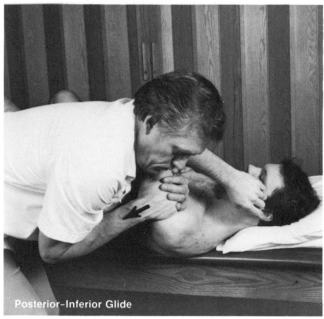

Posterior–Inferior Glide

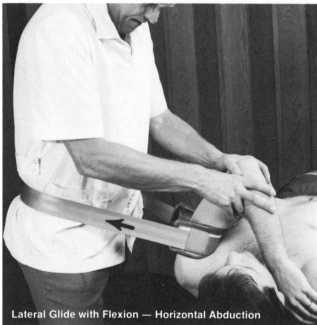

Lateral Glide with Flexion — Horizontal Abduction

Fig. 8-48. Glenohumeral Joint. (Continued)

especially if vigorous mobilization is desired. This technique tests and/or mobilizes the posterior, and more especially, the anterior portions of the joint capsule.

c. Inferior glide of the humeral head in the glenoid fossa is done with the shoulder abducted to approximately 30°. The patient's arm is supported by a hand at the elbow as the forearm and hand are cradled between the therapist's elbow and hip. The mobilizing force is directed inferiorly and medially by placing the web space of the

mobilizing hand against the humeral head and pushing. The therapist must be careful to make contact with the humeral head instead of the acromion. The heel of the hand may be used as an alternate contact for the mobilizing hand.

Since this movement tests and/or mobilizes the inferior portion of the joint capsule, it is perhaps the most important of all of the glenohumeral techniques. The anterior and inferior portions of the capsule most often become restricted when the shoulder is in a resting position or during periods of immobilization. This is because the redundant folds of the capsule which allow normal shoulder motion tend to adhere to each other when in a position of adduction and internal rotation for extended periods of time. Thus, the capsular pattern of limitation of motion results with external rotation (anterior portion) and abduction (inferior portion) most limited in excursion.

d. Posterior glide of the humeral head in the glenoid fossa is done with the shoulder slightly abducted. The patient's arm is supported at the elbow and the patient's forearm can rest across the therapist's forearm for additional support. The hypothenar eminence of the mobilizing hand contacts the humeral head parallel to the joint line with the fingertips in the patient's axilla. The force is directed posteriorly. This technique both tests and mobilizes the anterior, but more especially, the posterior portions of the joint capsule.

e. Anterior glide with external rotation adds a maximal stretch to the anterior portion of the capsule. The technique is done in exactly the same manner as the anterior glide technique except that the joint is taken to the limit of available external rotation before the anterior glide is performed. The therapist may cross his forearm medial to the patient's forearm in such a way as to block the shoulder into external rotation as the anterior glide is performed.

f. Various combinations of posterior, inferior or lateral joint mobilization can be achieved if the shoulder is brought into positions of maximal available flexion, abduction, rotation or horizontal adduction. In ranges less than 45°, the technique for posterior glide may be combined with any of the other desired directions of movement. Above 45°, the technique must be changed such that the therapist grasps the proximal end of the humerus close to the joint line. The therapist puts the patient's elbow against his shoulder (for a fulcrum) and directs the mobilizing force through the ulnar borders of his hands perpendicular to the shaft of the humerus. As the humerus is moved into various positions of flexion, abduction, adduction or rotation, the therapist can mobilize the joint by simply directing the force in the desired direction. For example, if the technique is applied to the shoulder in a lateral direction when the shoulder is brought into horizontal adduction from an abducted-flexed position, the posterior portion of the joint capsule will be stretched. The obvious advantage of this technique is that the joint can be taken to any point of restriction in its range and receive maximal stretch at that point.

Sternoclavicular Joint (Fig. 8-49)

The sternoclavicular (SC) joint is best tested and mobilized with the patient lying supine. It should be remembered that the SC joint has two joint spaces with a meniscus between and a fairly loose capsule. This allows for a rather large range of motion in a joint with a very shallow concave surface on the sternal side. The SC joint is the only point of attachment of the entire shoulder girdle to the axial skeleton. Thus, the joint must allow for elevation, depression, protraction, retraction and rotation of the shoulder. Since the clavicle rotates approximately 55° during shoulder flexion and abduction, the sternoclavicular and acromioclavicular joints should always be tested for mobility when shoulder range of motion is restricted. Joint play for the sternoclavicular joint is tested by gently grasping the medial clavicle near the joint line with the thumb and index fingers and gliding it anteroposteriorly. By changing the grip and placing the thumb under the clavicle, the clavicle can be moved inferosuperiorly. The movement can be palpated with the index finger on the joint line. Mobilizations can be performed in the same manners, except that it may be necessary to utilize both hands in order to exert more force.

Acromioclavicular Joint (Fig. 8-50)

The acromioclavicular joint may be tested and mobilized in several ways. One method has the therapist seated behind the patient whose arms are at his sides. The therapist reaches through the axilla and grasps the humeral head and acromion. The opposite hand palpates the AC joint. The therapist stabilizes by pulling down on the shoulder while the patient attempts to actively elevate the shoulder. If

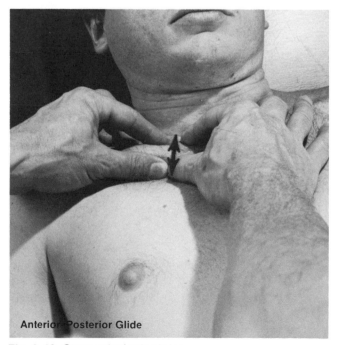

Anterior Posterior Glide

Fig. 8-49. Sternoclavicular joint.

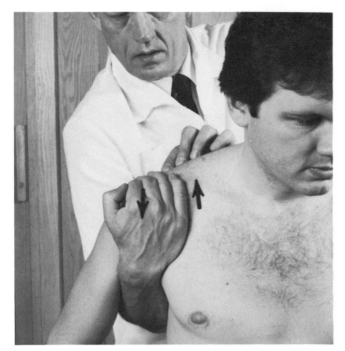

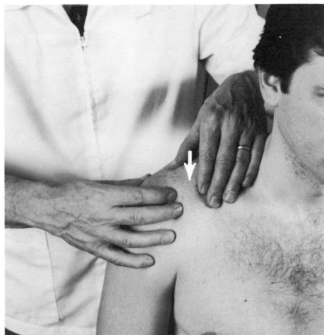

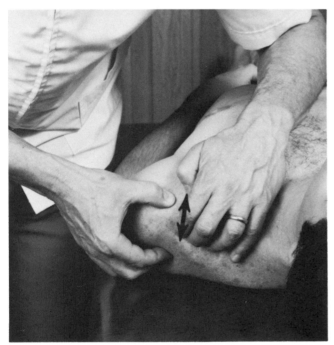

Fig. 8-50. Acromioclavicular joint.

the joint is hypermobile, this will be palpable. A second method for testing hypermobility may be done with the therapist standing behind the patient and applying a springing maneuver to the distal clavicle. A third method for testing and treating has the therapist seated behind the patient or with the patient lying supine. One hand stabilizes the acromion and with the thumb and index finger of the other hand, the therapist grasps the distal clavicle near the joint line and applies anteroposterior glides.

Scapulothoracic Joint (Fig. 8-51)

The scapulothoracic joint is formed by the articulation of the scapula against the rib cage. While it is not a true joint but rather a physiological joint, it should be tested for mobility when limitation of shoulder range of motion or muscular tightness across the upper back is suspected. It should be remembered that the scapula must abduct and upwardly rotate a total of 50-60° in order for the patient to fully flex or abduct the shoulder complex. The patient is positioned either side lying, facing the therapist or prone. The technique is performed by lying the hand flat against the rib cage with the web space around the inferior angle and the border of the index finger just medial to the vertebral border of the scapula. The index finger or web space is gently worked under the inferior angle and vertebral border. The therapist's other hand should gently apply a posteromedial force through the shoulder so that the scapula is moved toward and over the mobilizing hand. It is best to start along the inferior portion of the scapula and move superiorly as the technique is repeated. If normal mobility is present, the therapist will be able to slip at least his index finger under the vertebral border of the scapula. If mobilization is necessary, it is performed in the same manner as described above. This technique is best done slowly and gently in order to avoid muscle guarding and pain.

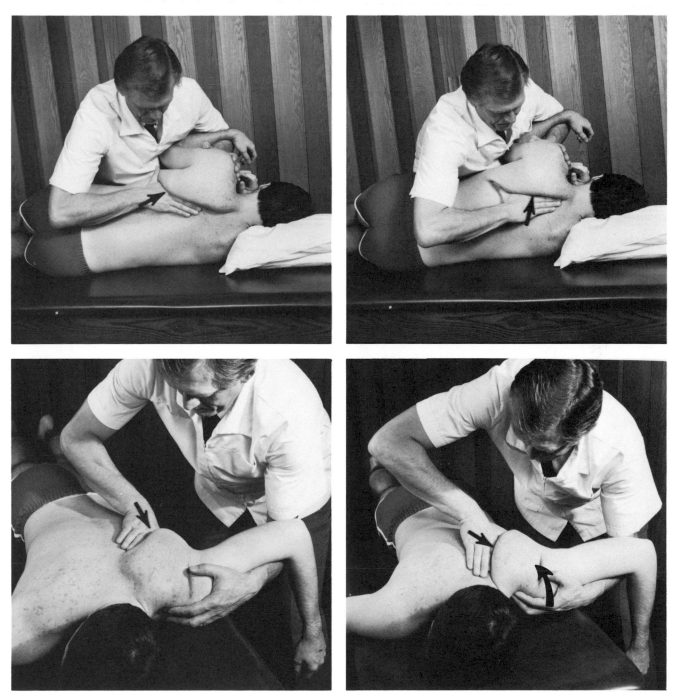

Fig. 8-51. Scapulothoracic joint.

JOINTS OF THE FOOT AND ANKLE (FIG. 8-52)

Metatarsophalangeal and Interphalangeal Joints (Fig. 8-53)

All MTP and IP joints are concave distally and convex proximally. All of the techniques may be performed with the patient sitting on the edge of a treatment table and the therapist sitting with the patient's foot resting in his lap so the lateral border of the patient's foot is toward the therapist. The techniques are similar to those employed for the digits of the hand.

    a. Anterior-posterior glide is performed using thumb-index finger grips with the stabilizing force close to the joint line proximally and the mobilizing force close to the joint line distally. When this technique is done as a testing procedure, the anterior and posterior

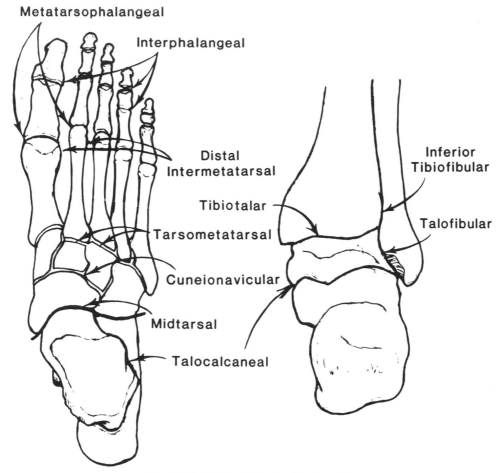

Fig. 8-52. Joints of the foot and ankle.

movements may be done alternately. When they are done as mobilizations, it is often necessary to work in only one direction at a time according to concave-convex rules.

b. Medial-lateral glide for the MTP and IP joints is performed with the stabilization grips at the proximal joint lines as described above. The mobilizing grips are shifted to the medial-lateral aspects of the segment distal to the joint line. The testing and mobilizing forces are given parallel to the joint line.

c. Traction is performed utilizing the same stabilization and mobilization grips as in anterior-posterior glide above. Traction is applied to the distal segment along its long axis.

d. Rotation also utilizes the same stabilization as described in the previous techniques. The mobilization force is given by grasping the distal part and moving in a rotational direction about the long axis of the segment.

Distal Intermetatarsal Joints (Fig. 8-54)

The distal intermetatarsal techniques are performed with the patient sitting on the edge of a treatment table and the therapist sitting with the patient's foot in his lap with the lateral border of the patient's foot directed toward the therapist. Utilizing thumb-index finger grips, the therapist grasps the heads of adjacent metatarsals, stabilizing one and moving the other in relation to it. Straight anterior-posterior and rotational movements are imparted. Each metatarsal joint is mobilized in turn with respect to its adjacent members.

Tarsometatarsal Joints (Fig. 8-55)

The TMT techniques are performed with the patient sitting on the edge of a treatment table and the therapist sitting with the patient's foot in his lap with the lateral border of the patient's foot directed toward the therapist. For all practical purposes, these joints may be regarded functionally as one

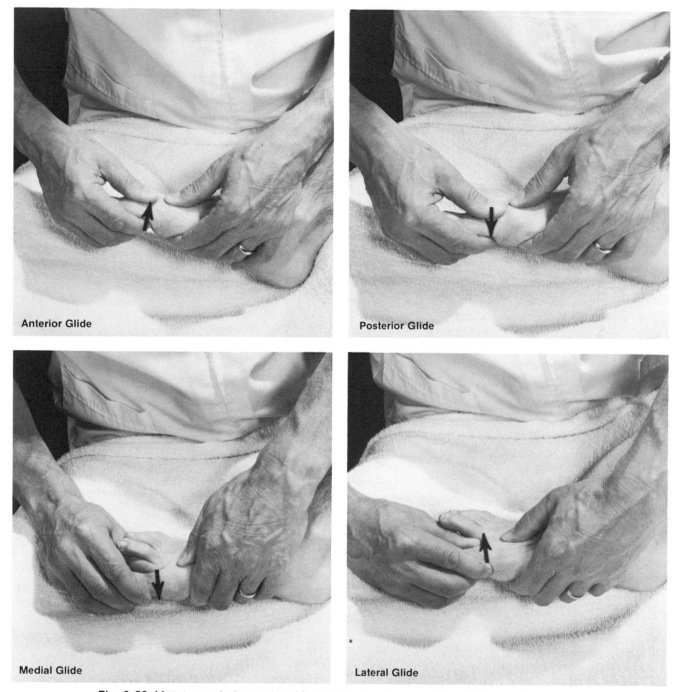

Anterior Glide

Posterior Glide

Medial Glide

Lateral Glide

Fig. 8-53. Metatarsophalangeal and interphalangeal joints. (Fig. 8-53 is continued on next page.)

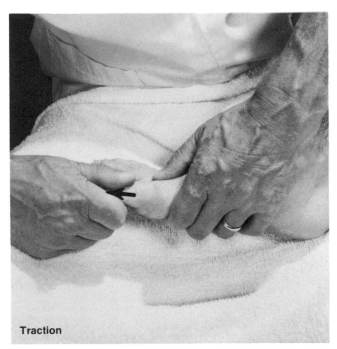

Traction

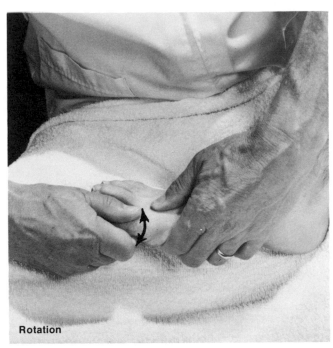

Rotation

Fig. 8-53. Metatarsophalangeal and intermeteatarsal joints. (Continued)

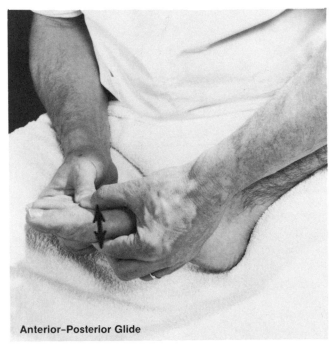

Anterior–Posterior Glide

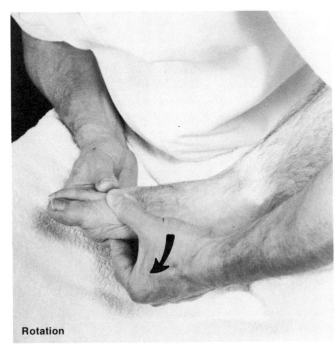

Rotation

Fig. 8-54. Distal intermetatarsals.

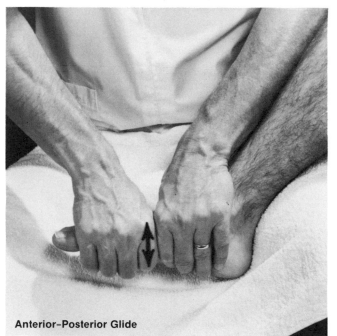

Anterior–Posterior Glide

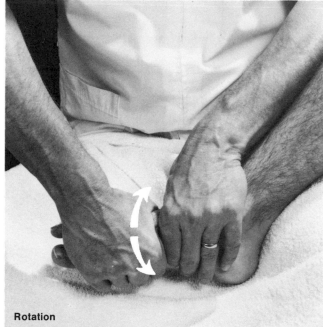

Rotation

Fig. 8-55. Tarsometatarsal joints.

joint for mobilization and joint play testing. The three cuneiforms and the cuboid make up the proximal portion of this joint and the bases of the metatarsals make up the distal portion. The therapist grasps and stabilizes the proximal side of the joint near the joint line with the web space of the hand across the dorsum of the foot and the fingers wrapping around onto the longitudinal arch. The other hand grasps the bases of the metatarsals in a similar fashion. Anterior-posterior glide and rotation can be performed at this joint. It is possible to concentrate more force laterally or medially with any of the mobilization techniques when desired.

Cuneionavicular Joint (Fig. 8-56)

The articulation between the first cuneiform and navicular allows the joint play movement of anterior-posterior glide. The technique is performed in exactly the same position as described for the TMT joints. The stabilizing hand grasps the navicular bone (prominent on the medial side of the foot) as the mobilizing hand grasps the cuneiforms. Since this joint is located on the medial side of the foot, the force is directed accordingly.

Midtarsal Joint (Fig. 8-57)

The midtarsal joint is made of the navicular and cuboid distally and the talus and calcaneus proxi-

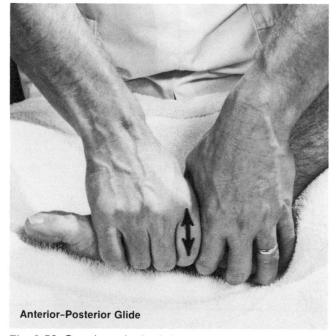

Anterior–Posterior Glide

Fig. 8-56. Cuneionavicular joint.

mally. The therapist and patient may be in the same position as described for the tarsometatarsal joints for this technique. If this position is used, the therapist may grasp the talus and calcaneus with one hand for stabilization and grasp the cuboid and navicular to mobilize. If, however, the talus and calcaneus are too large to hold with one hand, stabilization may be made easier by holding the calcaneus against the therapist's thigh or the patient may be positioned supine on a treatment table and the talus and calcaneus stabilized by holding the calcaneus against the treatment table as the therapist stands beside the table to perform the technique. Anterior-posterior glide is the only mobilization and joint play movement performed at this joint.

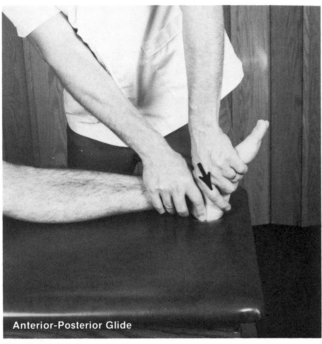

Fig. 8-57. Midtarsal joint.

Talocalcaneal Joint
(Subtalar Joint) (Fig. 8-59)

Inversion and eversion are the primary movements at the talocalcaneal joint. Mobilization and joint play movements performed at this joint are traction, medial tilt and lateral tilt. The techniques are performed with the patient supine and the therapist sitting between the patient's legs with his back toward the patient. The patient's knee is flexed to 90° with the lower leg in front of the therapist. The posterior aspect of the thigh is braced against the therapist's hip for stabilization. The therapist grasps the patient's foot with the web space of one hand over the dorsum of the foot next to the mortise of the ankle. The web space of the other hand is placed around the posterior aspect of the calcaneus. Both of the therapist's thumbs are now located on the medial aspect of the patient's foot and the fingers are lateral. A traction force is applied as the therapist flexes the patient's knee around his hip and simultaneouly pushes both hands distally. Medial tilt is applied with traction by pressing with the thumbs against the medial side. Lateral tilt is also applied with traction and is done by pressing with the index fingers against the lateral aspect of the calcaneus to open the joint on that side. These maneuvers can also be used to test for medial and lateral ligamentous stability.

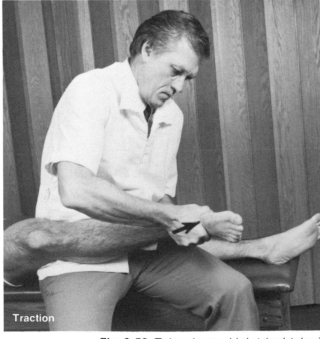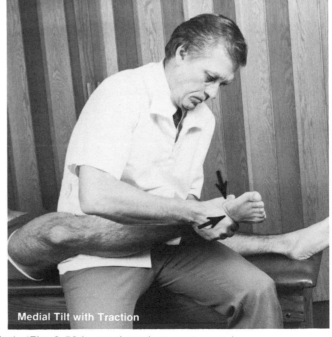

Fig. 8-58. Talocalcaneal joint (subtalar joint). (Fig. 8-58 is continued on next page.)

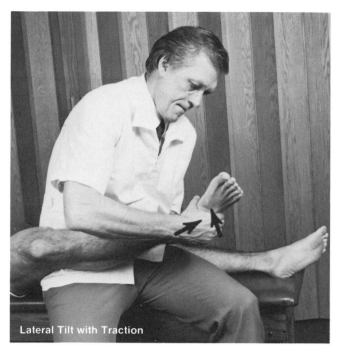

Fig. 8-58. Talocalcaneal joint (Subtalar joint).(Continued)

Tibiotalar Joint (Fig. 8-59)

Dorsiflexion and plantar flexion are the primary movements at this joint. The traction technique described for the talocalcaneal joint also effects a mobilization force and joint play movement across the tibiotalar joint and can, therefore, be considered as one of the techniques for this joint as

well. The traction technique may be modified so that the patient lies supine with the foot extended over the end of the treatment table. The therapist sits facing the plantar surface of the foot, grasping it with his fingers interlocked over the dorsum of the foot. The ulnar borders of the small fingers are at the joint line and the thumbs are on the plantar surface. While distracting the joint with a straight-line pull, the therapist passively dorsiflexes the foot through pressure with the thumbs. The mobilization is

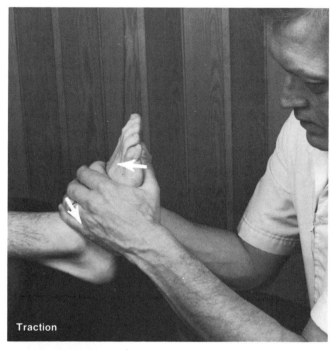

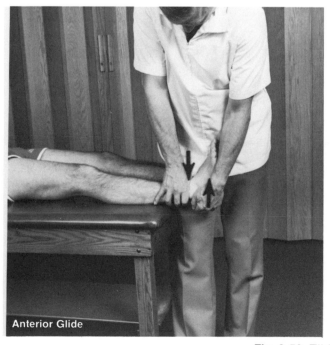

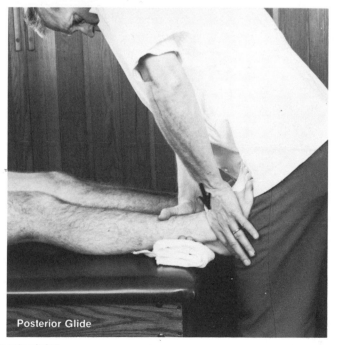

Fig. 8-59. Tibiotalar joint.

carried out with a quick downward tug on the talus through the ulnar aspect of the interlocked fingers.

Anterior-posterior glides are also performed at this joint and each should be done separately. Since the articulating surface of the talus glides posteriorly as the foot is dorsiflexed, posterior glide of the talus on the stabilized tibia is an important technique to use when dorsiflexion is restricted. Posterior glide is done with the patient lying supine and the foot hanging over the edge of a padded table. The talus is moved posteriorly with the web space of the therapist's hand contacting the dome of the talus just distal to the mortise. The distal tibia and fibula are stabilized against the table. For maximal mobilization force, the joint should be carried into as much dorsiflexion as possible before the technique is performed. Anterior glide is necessary for full range in plantar flexion. While it is seldom necessary to perform this technique for mobilization, it is very helpful in assessing the integrity of the joint following a sprain. The patient is supine with the foot extending off of the end of the treatment table. The therapist stabilizes by applying a posterior force with the web space of his hand against the anterior surface of the distal tibia. The therapist grasps the calcaneus with the other hand and directs an anterior force perpendicular to the distal tibia. The joint is held in a mid-range position to test joint play and for mild mobilization, but may be carried into plantar flexion for more vigorous mobilization. An alternate method may be done with the knee flexed and the calcaneus stabilized against the treatment table. With one hand, the therapist holds the foot in a neutral position. With the other hand, the therapist directs a posterior force perpendicular to the distal tibia. This posterior movement of the tibia on the talus is the same as an anterior movement of the talus on the tibia.

Inferior Tibiofibular Joint (Fig. 8-60)

The box-like mortise of the ankle is formed by the articulation of the distal tibia and fibula, otherwise known as the inferior tibiofibular joint. During dorsiflexion, the mortise must spread in order to accommodate the widening articular surface of the talus. This is an important component motion of dorsiflexion and should be checked in those patients experiencing difficulty in dorsiflexion. Anteroposterior glide of the fibula on the tibia can be effected by the therapist stabilizing the tibia with one hand as he grasps the lateral malleolus with the thumb and

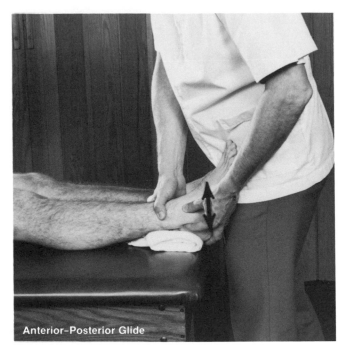

Fig. 8-60. Inferior tibiofibular joint.

index and middle fingers of the other hand and imparts an anterior-posterior force. A stronger grip may be accomplished by using the thenar eminence instead of the thumb to grasp the lateral malleolus.

JOINTS OF THE KNEE

Superior Tibiofibular Joint (Fig. 8-62)

The superior tibiofibular joint is mobilized and tested for anterior-posterior joint play with the patient supine, the knee and hip flexed and the foot

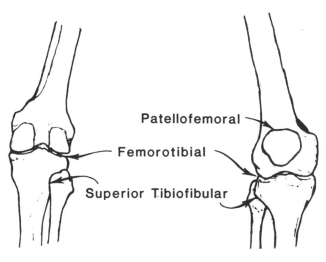

Fig. 8-61. Joints of the knee.

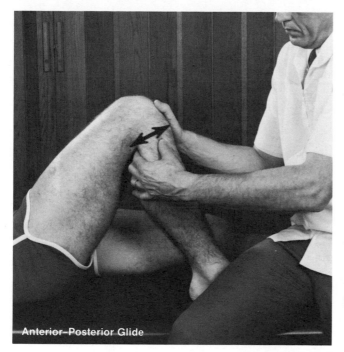
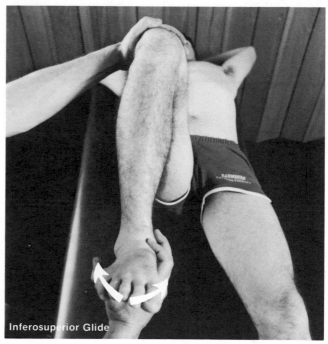

Anterior-Posterior Glide

Inferosuperior Glide

Fig. 8-62. Superior tibiofibular joint.

fixed on the table. The therapist stabilizes the knee with one hand and grasps the head of the fibula with the thumb, index and middle finger of the other hand to mobilize in an anteroposterior direction. Care must be taken when grasping the fibular head so that the common peroneal nerve is not pinched.

The fibula has a slight inferosuperior glide along the long axis of the tibia during certain ankle movements. These glides can be appreciated by palpating the head of the fibula and passively inverting or everting the ankle through the calcaneus.

Patellofemoral Joint (Fig. 8-63)

The movement of the patella on the femur is examined and mobilized with the patient lying supine with the knee slightly flexed and supported with pillows.

a. Cephalad movement is performed by placing the web space of the hand against the inferior pole of the patella and directing a proximal force. This movement tests the relative mobility of the patella and the patellotibial tendon in the direction of knee extension.

b. Caudal movement is performed by placing the web space of the hand against the superior border of the patella and directing a force distally. This movement tests the rela-

tive mobility of the patella and quadriceps muscle in the direction of knee flexion.

c. Medial movement is performed by placing both thumbs against the lateral surface of the patella and directing a force medially.

d. Lateral movement is performed by placing the index and middle fingers against the medial surface and directing a force laterally. Both medial and lateral movements test the relative mobility of the patella. Since mobility of the patella is necessary for full range of motion of the knee, assessment of these movements is very important when examining the knee and should not be neglected when trying to gain range of motion in the knee.

Femorotibial Joint (Fig. 8-64)

Although joint play testing and mobilization often play an important role when treating the knee, one must exercise additional caution when mobilizing this joint. Restrictions of range of motion at the knee are often due to the patellofemoral joint and/or adaptive shortening or contracture of the muscles. **If these restrictions are mistaken for femorotibial restriction, one may overmobilize the joint structures while attempting to gain full range of motion.**

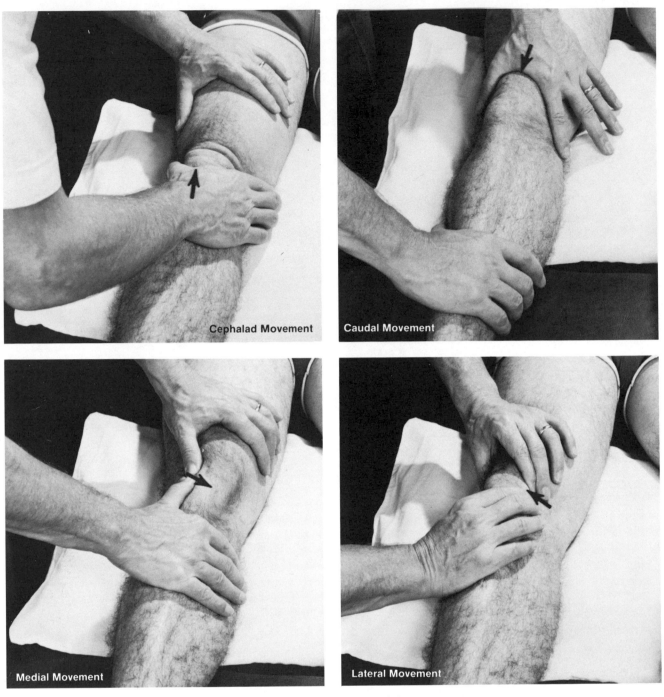

Fig. 8-63. Patellofemoral joint.

a. Medial and lateral rotatory mobilizations are applied with the patient supine. The knee is brought to its limit of flexion or to 90°. The therapist imparts a medial or lateral rotatory movement to the tibia along its long axis through the ankle or distal tibia-fibula. This technique may also be done in the prone position with the knee flexed.

b. Medial tilting (valgus stress) and lateral tilt-ing (varus stress) are done in two positions to test the integrity of the collateral liga-ments. When done with the knee in exten-sion, not only are the collaterals tested, but the posterior cruciate, posterior capsule and arcuate complex as well. Increased laxity in this position is indicative of serious knee pathology. The same tests are also applied to the knee in 30° of flexion. Laxity in this

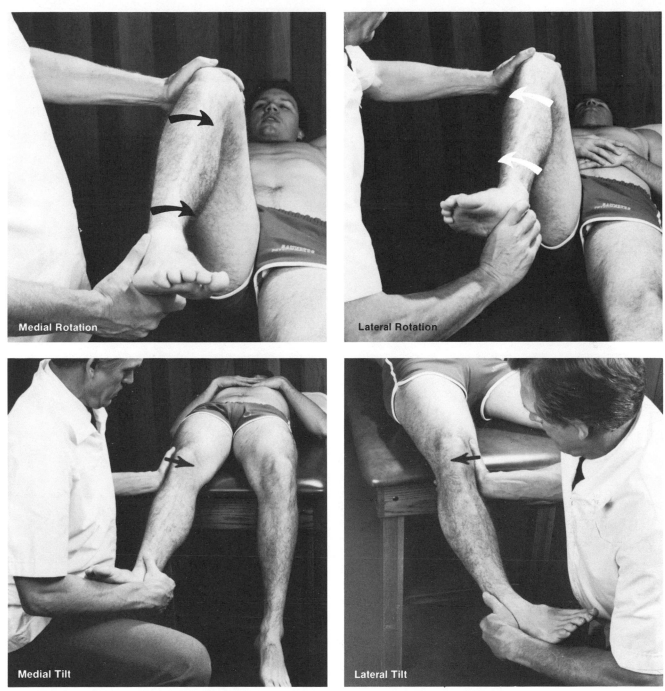

Fig. 8-64. Femorotibial joint. (Fig. 8-64 is continued on next page.)

position is more indicative of pathology localized to the collaterals. The tests and mobilizations are performed with the therapist stabilizing the leg at the ankle and applying the appropriate force either medially or laterally proximal to the knee joint.

c. Anteroposterior glides are performed with the knee and hip flexed and the foot stabilized on the treatment table. It is helpful for the therapist to sit on the dorsum of the foot to anchor it to the table. These gliding techniques are commonly called the "drawer" tests and can be used to detect laxity of the cruciate ligaments or restriction in joint play. The therapist interlocks his fingers behind the knee at the proximal tibia. Using the radial borders of his index fingers and web space, he can detect relaxation or

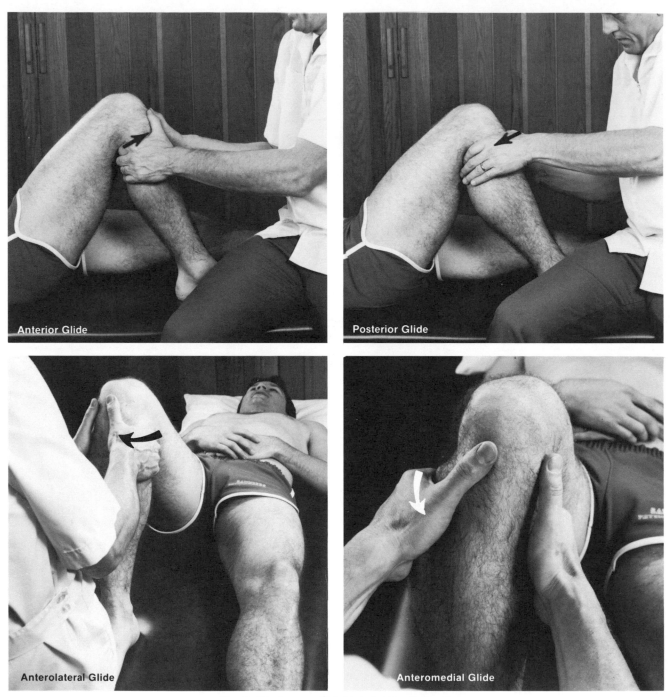

Fig. 8-84. Femorotibial joint. (Continued)

guarding of the hamstrings. The hamstrings must be relaxed in order to do this maneuver. The therapist then either pulls forward or pushes backward with a force perpendicular to the tibia. Pulling forward tests the anterior cruciate and joint play for extension, and pushing backward tests the posterior cruciate and joint play for flexion.

A somewhat more sensitive test of the anterior cruciate and a more gentle mobilization can be done with the knee in slight flexion with the heel resting on the treatment table. The therapist simply grasps the knee on either side of the joint line. The proximal hand stabilizes and the distal hand performs an anterior glide. This test is also known as the Lachman test.

d. The various portions of the anterior cruciate

and the presence of rotatory instability can be tested using slight variations of the technique described above. The tibia is either internally or externally rotated on the femur, and these rotated positions are held by the therapist sitting on the foot. The therapist then applies an anterior force in a lateral direction to the medial side of the tibia (foot externally rotated) in a wringing or circular fashion. Conversely, he can apply an anterior force in a medial direction to the lateral tibia and fibula (foot internally rotated).

HIP JOINT (FIG. 8-65)

The hip, due to its inherent stability, relative inaccessability and weight of the lower limb, is sometimes difficult to test and mobilize. Traction must be used in almost any technique in order to adequately assess the joint capsule. It is helpful to remember that the hip, like the shoulder, has redundant folds in the anterior-inferior capsule to allow range of motion into abduction and other extremes of motion. In arthritis and capsulitis, the hip tends to assume a posture of flexion, adduction and external rotation with loss of motion into extension, abduction and internal rotation.

Joint play may be best tested by taking the hip into its maximal loose-packed position (approximately 15° abduction, 15° flexion and 15° external rotation) and applying a distractive force through the long axis of the leg at the ankle. It is necessary to have an assistant stabilize the pelvis by a strap through the groin area or by applying a superiorly directed force against the ASIS while such distractive techniques are applied. This technique may become a manipulative thrust as the therapist applies maximal distraction to take up the slack and then gives a quick, sharp tug. The therapist and patient will both feel the joint distract and the head of the femur impact against the acetabulum upon cessation of the tug.

Joint play may also be tested with the patient supine and the hip and knee flexed to 90°. The therapist rests the patient's lower leg over his shoulder and interlocks his hands around the proximal thigh at the groin. He can then apply an inferolateral distraction to the hip joint.

The best mobilization techniques for the hip employ the use of a 2-inch strap. When using the strap, the therapist can mobilize the posterior, lateral and inferior portions of the joint and capsule. Standing at the side of the patient, the therapist loops the strap around the medial side of the patient's thigh and around his own waist. The strap is at the level of the patient's groin (a towel for padding eliminates undue pressure from the strap) and the level of the therapist's buttocks. The hip can be brought into any amount of flexion while the therapist stabilizes with his hands on the lateral aspect of the knee. The mobilizing force is applied to the hip as the therapist uses his body against the

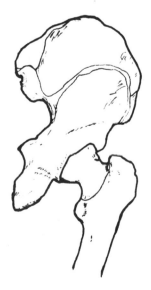 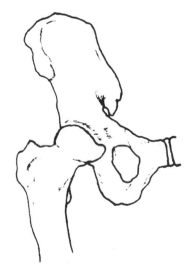

Fig. 8-65. Hip joint.

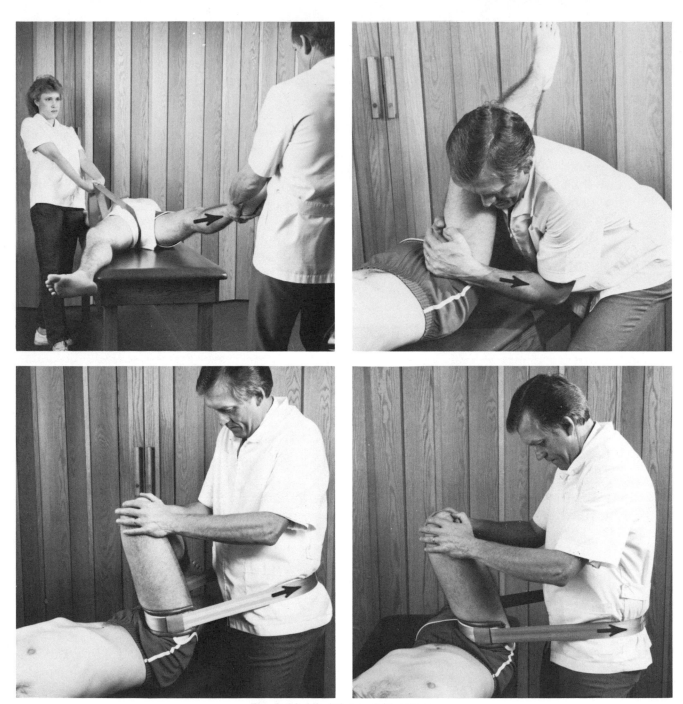

Fig. 8-66. Hip joint mobilizations.

strap. Oscillations and articulations can be performed without difficulty. For example, if the posterolateral capsule needs to be stretched, the therapist flexes the hip, stabilizes it into adduction by pushing medially and distracts the capsule by moving his hips laterally.

The anterior portion of the capsule is best mobilized with the patient lying prone with the knee in flexion. The therapist reaches around the knee,

grasping the distal femur on the medial side and cradling the lower leg against his arm and trunk. The other hand stabilizes the pelvis at the level of the PSIS. The leg is then brought out into some abduction and the slack is taken up as the leg is brought into extension at the hip. Stretch articulations are most effective with this technique.

See Fig. 8-66 for mobilization techniques of the hip joint.

MUSCLE ENERGY TECHNIQUES

Muscle Energy Techniques (MET) for joint mobilization are becoming quite popular among certain physical therapists who have advanced skills in mobilization. MET's have been developed primarily by osteopathic physicians, most notably Drs. Fred Mitchell Sr. and Jr. For sake of completeness, a brief description of the principles on which these techniques are based follows. As these techniques can be quite complicated without first-hand instruction, they are considered to be beyond the scope of this basic text and are introduced to stimulate the reader into pursuing higher level skills.

The mobilization techniques discussed up to this point are primarily passive in nature; they require specific positioning of the patient and his relaxation. The forces imparted by the therapist may then be directed either into the restriction or away from it in order to gain joint mobility and/or stretch soft tissue. Thrust and oscillation techniques are passive in nature.

Muscle Energy Techniques, on the other hand, are active in nature. MET's may be likened to PNF contract-relax techniques except that they employ submaximal rather than maximal contractions. In fact, these techniques may be **isotonic** (where the counterforce is less than the force of the patient's muscular contraction, producing motion into or toward the motion barrier); **isometric** (where the counterforce meets the force of the patient's muscular contraction, producing no joint motion); and **isokinetic** (where the counterforce increases during contraction to meet changing contraction forces as the muscle shortens and its force increases[14].) Generally, MET's for joint mobilization are gentle, isometric contractions as opposed to maximal isometric contractions which tend to tighten and compress the joints. MET's which employ hard maximal contractions are useful for loosening tight muscles and fascia, however. The concept for the employment of MET's may be summarized as follows:

After a positional and motion assessment of the spinal segments in question has been done, the patient is placed in a position which corresponds to and which facilitates the impartation of motion. The patient is then stabilized and the slack at the particular spinal segment is taken up in all three planes. The patient is then asked to perform a submaximal isometric contraction against a counterforce in a direction which will produce the desired

effect. These techniques are particularly safe and gentle, especially in the upper cervical spine where risk of vertebral artery compromise is present with thrust and rotatory techniques. Thus, the patient moves the joint himself by his own muscle power.

Manual therapy techniques for the spine are usually taught to the beginner via assessment through the spinous processes because they are easily palpated. Problems sometimes arise using this method when one is trying to determine whether a joint dysfunction is on the left or right side. For example, palpating the T5 spinous process to be offset to the left of T6 determines only that the vertebral body is rotated to the right. By palpating between the spinous processes, one might detect that two adjacent spinous processes are closer together than the spinous processes of two other adjacent segments. Does this mean that the superior element is backward bent or that the inferior element is forward bent? To clarify this problem, osteopaths indirectly palpate the transverse processes through fascial planes to determine the exact position of the facets as well as their ability to move in all three planes of motion. Thus, the lesion can be precisely defined and a treatment maneuver prescribed which exactly corresponds to the dysfunction. The basic principles which govern the use of MET's are outlined as follows:

1. **Motion Barriers** — Normal joints all have physiological barriers to motion at opposite ends of their ranges of motion. These barriers are produced by the protective resiliency and elasticity of the soft tissues. Any other factor which impedes the free motion of the joint between these range limits is considered to be pathological. In the normal spine, both in backward and forward bending, the facets at each segment should glide symmetrically in superior and inferior directions (open and close.) This means that in flexion, the facets on each side should fully open and in extension the facets should fully close (Fig. 8-67)

Vertebral Motion by Facet Function	
1. Forward Bending	Facets Open
2. Backward Bending	Facets Close
3. Sidebending Right	Right Facet Closes Left Facet Opens
4. Sidebending Left	Right Facet Opens Left Facet Closes

Fig. 8-67

2. **Positioning** — Motion takes place in all three planes simultaneously. Positioning of patients for both active and passive techniques should account for motion in all planes. Fryette's Third Law of Spinal Motion applies here in that if motion is introduced into a segment in any plane, motion in the other planes is reduced. This means, for example, that if a spinal segment is in extension, the available range for sidebending and rotation is reduced. If the segment is both extended and sidebent, the available range for rotation is even further reduced.[14]

3. **Diagnosis and Treatment** — Diagnosis and treatment by MET is based on the position of the segment and the motion restriction. The nomenclature of spinal lesions is based on the palpation and visual inspection (using the transverse processes) with the spine in neutral, flexed and extended positions.

Example:

Level	Position	Motion Restriction
T3 on T4	Flexed,	Extension,
	Left Rotated,	Right Rotation,
	Left Sidebent	Right Sidebending

The suffix of the descriptive word used is the key to precisely indicating both the position of the joint and its restriction of movement:

-ion	motion term
-ed	position term

Example:

Position	*Motion Restriction*
Flex**ed**	Extens**ion**
Extend**ed**	Flex**ion**
Right Rotat**ed**	Left Rotat**ion**
Left Sidebe**nt**	Right Sidebend**ing**

Figure 8-68 shows two figures which appear to represent identical lumbar facet lesions. However, functionally and from a treatment aspect, they are nearly opposite lesions. In Figure 8-68A, the left facet will not **close**. This has been determined because during backward bending, the transverse process on the right becomes more prominent and during forward bending, the transverse processes become more equal. Positionally, the lesion is described as *flexed, right sidebent,* and *right rotated.* Its motion restriction will be in *extension, left sidebending* and *left rotation.*

Conceptually, by having the patient perform the motions of backward bending and forward bending in the above example and by palpating the change in position of the transverse processes, the following deductive thought process might occur: Since the **left** facet will not close, this means that the **right** facet is in an already extended (closed) position. Having the patient actively recruit extension of the entire spine will force the transverse process on the right to become more prominent (it will come from an extended position into more extension.) In forward bending, the left facet is already in an open position. Since the right facet is free to move, the transverse processes tend to become more symmetrically placed. This does not mean that the left facet

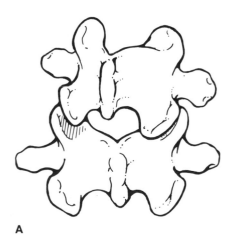
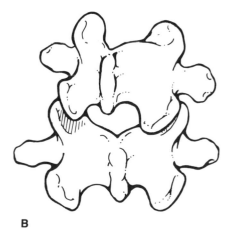

A   B

Fig. 8-68. A) Lumbar facet lesion in which the left facet will not close (approximate); B) Lumbar facet lesion in which the right facet will not open (distract).

has moved into closure, only that the right facet has moved into opening.

In Figure 8-68B, the right facet will not open. In this example, a similar line of reasoning will apply. When the patient forward bends, the right transverse process becomes more prominent. When he backward bends, the transverse processes become more equal. Positionally, this lesion is described as *extended, right sidebent,* and *right rotated.* Its motion restriction will be in *flexion, left sidebending* and *left rotation.*

Since the position and motion restrictions of these two lesions are different, it stands to reason that they should be approached differently from a treatment aspect in order to restore motion. To illustrate this, the following brief descriptions of MET's for the two examples are given so that the reader may appreciate the differences:

Lesion A - The left facet will not close. It is diagnosed by the posterior prominence of the right transverse process when the spine is in a hyperextended position.

Lateral Recumbent Technique:

1. The patient is sidelying on a table on the side of the more posterior transverse process. The operator stands at the side of the table facing the patient. The patient is close to the edge of the table.
2. The patient's head is supported by a pillow and the lower leg is straight with the upper leg flexed at the hip and knee.
3. The operator's left hand palpates the interspinous space of the involved segment while the right hand reaches under the knee of the patient's uppermost leg to extend the patient's lower leg at the hip joint until the extension movement is localized to the lesioned segment.
4. The operator repositions his hands, placing the right hand in a position to palpate movement of the spine while the left hand introduces rotation down to the segment by moving the patient's upper shoulder backward toward the table surface. The patient is instructed to inhale, and as he exhales the rotation is produced, localizing movement to the segment.
5. The patient is then instructed to grip the edge of the table behind him.
6. The operator repositions the hands again.

The hand that rotated the shoulder palpates the segment. The opposite hand grasps the patient's uppermost leg at the ankle.

7. The operator lifts upward on the upper leg of the patient to sidebend to the level, then presses downward with his elbow on the patient's knee to rotate to the level. Finally, the operator extends the upper leg to localize extension to the segment.
8. The patient is instructed to pull the upper foot down toward the table. After a 5-10 second contraction, the patient relaxes.
9. The operator relocalizes movement to the segment, then sidebends, rotates and extends again.
10. Steps 8 and 9 are repeated three times. The patient is retested and treatment is repeated if necessary.

Lesion B - The right facet will not open. It is diagnosed by the posterior prominence of the right transverse process when the spine is in a hyperflexed position.

Lateral Recumbent Technique:

1. The patient lies on his side, but with the chest down toward the table surface. The patient lies with the prominent transverse process on the top side. Thus, in this example, he will be on his left side.
2. The operator stands at the side of the table facing the patient. The operator's left hand palpates the interspinous space below the vertebra to be treated, while the right hand flexes the hips so that flexion is localized to the involved segment.
3. While supporting the knees against the body, the operator lowers the patient's feet until sidebending to the left is localized to the segment.
4. The patient is then asked to reach toward the floor until rotation to the left is localized to the segment (at times, this step can be omitted since rotation may be localized simultaneously with sidebending.)
5. The operator instructs the patient to lift his feet up toward the ceiling against unyielding resistance (isometric right sidebending — hold/relax.) The patient maintains the contraction for 5-10 seconds then relaxes. The force required is approximately five pounds.
6. The segment is relocalized by sidebending

(dropping patient's feet further), flexing and rotating if needed.

7. Steps 5 and 6 are repeated three times.
8. The patient is retested and the treatment is repeated if necessary.

While a beginner may not be able to perform either of the two techniques described, the purpose of the above examples has been to show the nearly opposite approaches that are employed for two different types of dysfunctions. The unskilled practitioner may apply the same treatment to two very different joint dysfunctions just because they may appear similar. Obviously, a specific technique employed to a specific segment for a specific dysfunction is a preferable approach to treatment.

The range of possibilities for MET's in application to the spine (and, to a lesser degree, the extremities) is almost unlimited. These techniques are gentle, safe and neurophysiologically based. As the physical therapist grows in his knowledge and skill in mobilization, MET's should become a part of his regular treatment regimen, balancing active versus passive and specific versus non-specific techniques.

References:

1. Nwuga, V: Manipulation of the Spine. Williams and Wilkins, Baltimore 1976.
2. Freeman, M and Wyke, B: The Innervation of the Knee Joint: An Anatomical and Histological Study in the Cat. Joul Anat 101:505-532, 1967.
3. Polacek, P: Receptors of the Joints: Their Structure, Variability and Classification. Acta Fac Med Univ Brunensis 23:1-107, 1966.
4. Halata, Z: The Ultrastructure of the Sensory Nerve Endings in the Articular Capsule of the Knee Joint of the Domestic Cat (Ruffini Corpuscles and Pacinian Corpuscles). Joul Anat 124:717-729, 1977.
5. Newton, R: Joint Receptor Contributions to Reflexive and Kinesthetic Responses. Phys Ther 62:22-29, 1982.
6. Kaltenborn, F: Manual Therapy of the Extremity Joints. Olaf Norlis Bokhandel, Oslo 1976.
7. Mennell, J: Joint Pain. Little-Brown, Boston 1964.
8. Paris, S: Course Notes — The Spine. Atlanta Back Clinic, Atlanta, GA 1975.
9. MacConaill, M and Basmajian, J: Muscles and Movements. Williams and Wilkins, Baltimore 1969.
10. Burkart, S: Personal Communication. Physical Therapy Department, University of West Virginia, Morgantown, VW 1980.
11. Cyriax, J: Textbook of Orthopaedic Medicine; Diagnosis of Soft Tissue Lesions. Vol 1, 8th ed. Bailliere-Tindall, London 1982.
12. Maitland, G: Vertebral Manipulation, 2nd ed. Butterworth, London 1968.
13. Mennell, J: Back Pain. Little-Brown, Boston 1964.
14. Mitchell, F, Moran, P, and Pruzzo, N: An Evaluation and Treatment Manual of Osteopathic Muscle Energy Procedures, Mitchell, Moran and Pruzzo Associates, Valley Park, MI, 1979.

CHAPTER 9

SPINAL TRACTION

The purpose of this chapter is to present and discuss the types of spinal traction, the effects of spinal traction, the indications and contraindications for spinal traction and effective spinal traction techniques. The chapter contains a review of important points on traction found in earlier literature, as well as the introduction of new ideas and concepts. A portion of this chapter deals with the rationale of using spinal traction for the treatment of the herniated disc and other spinal nerve root syndromes. Detailed descriptions of proper positioning and considerable discussion of the forces necessary to achieve therapeutic results with spinal traction are included. The importance of the use of proper equipment for mechanical spinal traction is stressed. The chapter emphasizes the beneficial aspects of spinal traction as an effective treatment for certain musculoskeletal disorders, but points out that its administration is not as easy as it may seem.

Use of tractive forces for the treatment of back problems probably can be found in antiquity. Certainly, Hippocrates and other early medical authors have described the use of traction in their writings. However, even into the first half of this century, the literature has been sketchy as to certain aspects of the techniques used, such as body type and weight of subjects, amounts of forces used, duration of treatments, etc . . . Opinion varied as to indications, contraindications, weights and techniques.

Many physicians, therapists and patients recall the poor results of the continuous, or "bed", traction that was used for many years. These poor results caused many physicians and therapists to become disinterested in using spinal traction. However, when used appropriately and correctly, traction is claimed to be an effective and beneficial method of treatment by numerous authors [1-16]. Some controlled studies, however, have shown either poor results of treatment or that positive effects of traction were of limited or marginal significance [17-21]. One noted exception is the study of Lind [22] in which exceptionally good results were obtained in a controlled trial using autotraction.

The word traction is a derivative of the Latin "tractico", which means a process of drawing or pulling. In order to achieve separation between two objects or surfaces, two opposing forces are required — traction and countertraction. Various authors have suggested the word "distraction" as being more descriptive. If the term "distraction" is used, the reference relates to the joint surfaces and suggests that these surfaces move perpendicular to one another. This is not always the case, as one can see in the spinal segment. As traction is applied, the movement produced at the segment is a combination of distraction and gliding.

EFFECTS OF SPINAL TRACTION

Correctly performed, spinal traction can cause many effects. Among these are distraction or separation of the vertebral bodies, a combination of distraction and gliding of the facet joints, tensing of the ligamentous structures of the spinal segment, widening of the intervertebral foramen, straightening of spinal curves and stretching of the spinal musculature.

The relative degree of flexion or extension of the spine during the traction treatment determines which of these effects are most pronounced. For example, greater separation of the intervertebral foramen is accomplished with the spine in a flexed position during the traction treatment, whereas greater separation of the disc space is achieved with the spine in a neutral position.

TYPES OF SPINAL TRACTION

CONTINUOUS TRACTION

Continuous spinal traction is applied for as long as several hours at a time. This long duration requires that only small amounts of weight can be used as the patient's skin cannot tolerate prolonged traction at high poundages. Thus, it is generally accepted that this form of traction, when applied to the lumbar spine, is ineffective in achieving separation of the vertebrae [10].

SUSTAINED (STATIC) TRACTION

Sustained traction involves application of a constant amount of traction for periods of a few minutes up to one-half hour. The shorter duration is usually coupled with heavier weight. Sustained lumbar traction is most effective if a split table is used to reduce friction. The traction source can be either hanging weights or a mechanical device specially made to produce the traction force. Mechanical devices must maintain constant tension. In other words, any slack developed as the patient relaxes during the treatment must be automatically taken up and the desired amount of traction maintained. This method is most widely used in Europe, and much of the European literature describes various applications of sustained traction[23].

INTERMITTENT MECHANICAL TRACTION

This form of traction involves a mechanical device that alternately applies and releases traction every few seconds. When applied to the lumbar area, a split table is utilized to reduce friction[7-10]. This is probably the most popular form of traction currently used in the United States.

MANUAL TRACTION

To apply manual traction the therapist grasps the patient and manually applies a traction force. Manual traction is usually applied for a few seconds, but it can be applied as a sudden, quick thrust. It allows the therapist to feel the patient's reaction[24-26]. It is sometimes more difficult for the patient to relax with manual traction than with mechanical traction because the exact amount of force that will be applied cannot be anticipated.

POSITIONAL TRACTION

The patient is placed in various positions using pillows, blocks or sandbags to effect a longitudinal pull on the spinal structures. This form of traction usually incorporates lateral bending and only one side of the spinal segment is affected[26].

AUTOTRACTION (LUMBAR)

A special traction bench composed of two sections that can be individually angulated and rotated is used with autotraction. Patients apply the traction by pulling with their own arms and can alter the direction of the traction as the treatment progresses. Treatment sessions can last one hour or longer and are supervised by a clinician[18, 22, 27].

GRAVITY LUMBAR TRACTION

With gravity lumbar traction, the lower border and circumference of the rib cage are grasped by a specially made vest which is secured to the top of the bed. The patient is tilted on a circular bed or specially made table into a vertical or nearly vertical position. In this position the free weight of the legs and hips (about 40% of the body weight) exerts, by gravity, a traction force on the lumbar spine[28].

Two other types of gravity traction have become very popular recently through commercialization efforts. One technique utilizes specialized boots which attach to the subject's ankles. The individual is then able to suspend himself from a frame into a fully inverted position. The other technique involves a device in which the individual is supported on the anterior thighs and is able to hang inverted in a hip and knee flexed position. Both techniques will achieve a traction force of approximately 50% of the total body weight on the lumbar spine[29]. An excellent study by Kane showed significant separation of both the anterior and posterior margins of the lumbar vertebral bodies at all levels as well as increased dimension of the intervertebral foramina using the inversion boot method. These techniques are not without some risks which will be discussed later[30].

INDICATIONS FOR SPINAL TRACTION

HERNIATED NUCLEUS PULPOSUS WITH DISC PROTRUSION

Spinal traction is indicated for the treatment of herniated nucleus pulposus with disc protrusion[1, 2, 4-11, 13, 20-22, 31, 32]. There is evidence that a disc protrusion can indeed be reduced and spinal nerve root compression symptoms relieved with the application of spinal traction. Mathews[31], using epidurography, studied patients thought to have lumbar disc protrusion. Applying sustained traction forces of 120 pounds for 20 minutes, he showed that the protrusions were flattened and that the contrast material was drawn into the disc spaces. He also found recurrence of the bulging defects later (Fig. 9-1). Also using epidurography, Gupta and Ramarao[4] demonstrated reductions of lumbar disc protrusions in 11 of 14 patients treated with 60-80 pounds of weight. The weight was applied for intermittent periods every three to four hours for ten to 15 days. They also found definite clinical improvement in the patients in whom defects were reduced (Fig. 9-2). Such studies as these show that traction can indeed separate lumbar vertebrae and lead to decreased pressure at the disc space with a resulting suction force. In addition, material can be drawn from the epidural space into the disc space. Similarly, it may be concluded that any anatomical correction produced is unstable. Thus, if patients are not carefully treated with a total management regimen, traction alone is likely to be unsuccessful (Fig. 9-3).

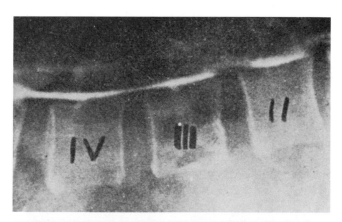

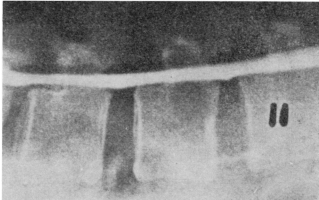

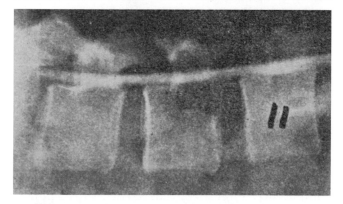

Fig. 9-1. A disc protrusion before traction is shown in the top view. It is being reduced with traction in the middle view and the bottom view shows a partial return of the protrusion after release of traction (copied with permission from Mathews[31].)

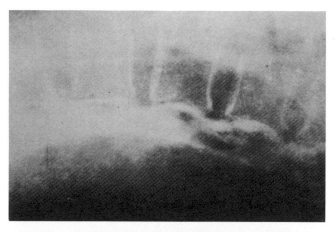

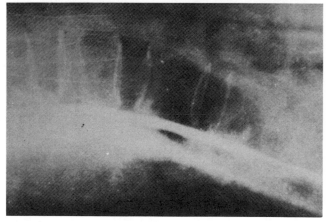

Fig. 9-2. A disc protrusion being reduced by traction. The top view is before traction and the bottom view is during traction (copied with permission from Gupta and Ramarao[4].)

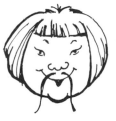

Fig. 9-3. Confusion say: "Man with herniated disc cannot get well on traction alone — Must have total management."

As with all conservative treatment approaches for disc protrusion, patient education and a gradual, cautious return to activities are necessary if the traction is to be successful. Once disc protrusion is reduced and spinal nerve root symptoms have been relieved, patients may need the support of a lumbosacral corset or a modified Taylor or chairback brace. These supports remind patients to limit their activities, especially forward bending, and they also promote proper posture and relieve some of the compressive forces on the disc when the patients are standing or sitting[33-36]. It is important that muscle guarding and spasm be reduced throughout the treatment period, because they add an additional compressive force on the disc. Also, extension principles often are important in helping to reduce herniation and to maintain the correction once it has been reduced. These principles follow the rationale that forward bending moves the nuclear gel posteriorly, backward bending moves the nuclear gel anteriorly and an exaggerated spinal extension posture will keep the gel in the correct position once it has been reduced[33,35,37]. It is often necessary to use spinal traction to achieve the initial reduction,

following which the extension principles can be used to maintain the correction until healing occurs[2,4,13]. Positions and activities that increase intradiscal pressure (e.g., forward bending and sitting in lumbar flexion) should be avoided[38]. Obviously, flexion exercises, such as knee-to-chest exercises and partial sit-ups, should be avoided (Fig. 9-4). Generally, activities that decrease pain and other symptoms are permissible, while those that increase pain and symptoms are to be avoided. An exception to this rule involves the supine or side lying flexed position that is often used for patients with disc protrusion because it seems to provide relief of symptoms. Relief is accomplished because flexion draws the bulging annulus taut, thus moving it away from the nerve root. However, this flexion also causes anterior narrowing of the disc space and a posterior force on the nuclear gel[33,37]. Therefore, the supine or side lying flexed position does not appear to be of lasting benefit in patients with herniated disc, although it does afford patients comfort while they are in the position (Fig. 9-5). Additionally, activities which cause the pain and other symptoms to move away from the central area of the spine toward the

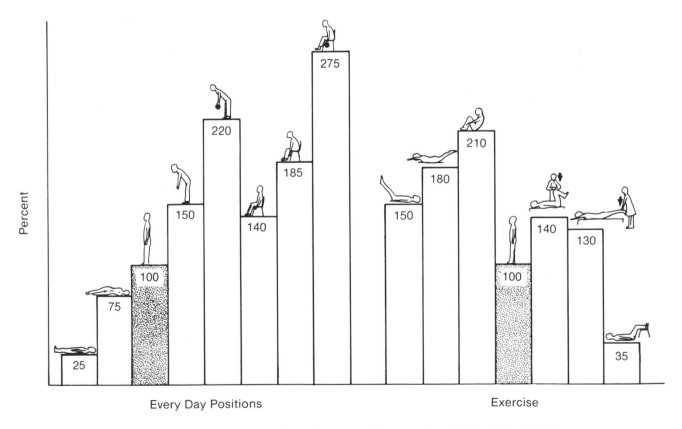

Fig. 9-4. Intradiscal pressure in various positions and activities (adopted from Nachemson[38].)

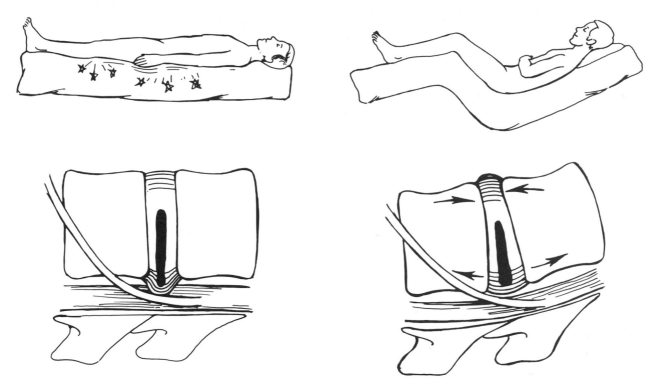

Fig. 9-5. The supine, flexed position draws the posterior annulus taut and may draw the bulge away from the spinal nerve root. However, the flexion also causes anterior compression and the net result may not be beneficial in the long run, even though the patient may feel relief in this position. Therefore, this position is only recommended in the early stages of treatment of the very acute patient.

periphery are to be avoided, while activities that may cause some increased central pain but a decrease in peripheral symptoms are beneficial. This rule of central pain and symptoms versus peripheral pain and symptoms is an extremely important concept and should govern all activities, including the application of spinal traction, spinal mobilization and exercises.

DEGENERATIVE DISC/JOINT DISEASE

The argument is often raised that although traction can cause separation and widening of the intervertebral foramen and intervertebral disc space, the effect will only be temporary. It is true that the separation shown on x-rays will at least partially disappear soon after traction has been discontinued. If traction is applied to a patient with a narrowed intervertebral foramen or one who has osteophyte or ligamentous encroachment, the disc space and intervertebral foramen will not be restored to their original size and structure. The relief experienced by these patients after the traction treatment must be explained from another basis. Many people have

narrowing of the disc space and intervertebral foramen without signs and symptoms of spinal nerve root impingement. Often, patients in whom the degenerative changes have obviously been present for some time will have a sudden onset of symptoms related to a certain activity or position. The same can be said of osteophytes that do not cause symptoms. A very fine line must exist between cases in which encroachment on the spinal nerve root occurs and does not occur. The traction treatment must, in some manner, move, separate or realign the segment in such a way as to relieve the impingement.

JOINT DYSFUNCTION

Traction may be regarded as a form of mobilization since it involves the passive movement of joints by mechanical or manual means. Any condition of joint dysfunction (joint hypomobility) may respond favorably to traction. One argument against using traction for mobilization is that it is nonspecific and simultaneously affects several joints. However, when traction is applied to a series of spinal segments, each segment in that series receives an equal amount of traction; if that amount is sufficient to mobilize the segment, it is irrelevant that other segments are also receiving the same amount of traction unless, of course, traction is contraindicated at those other segments. If this is the case, a more specific technique of joint mobilization should be selected[14, 26].

CONTRAINDICATIONS

Traction is contraindicated in structural disease secondary to tumor or infection, in patients with vascular compromise and in any condition for which movement is contraindicated[16].

Relative contraindications include acute strains, sprains and inflammation that would be aggravated by traction. Traction applied to patients with joint instability of the spine may cause further strain. Other relative contraindications may include pregnancy, osteoporosis, hiatal hernia and claustrophobia.

LUMBAR TRACTION TECHNIQUE

Many physicians and physical therapists routinely use cervical traction and appear reasonably satisfied with the beneficial results in patients with joint dysfunction, degenerative joint/disc disease and nerve root symptoms. Yet many do not use traction for treatment of similar conditions in the lumbar spine. The author attributes this general attitude to inadequacies of equipment and basic techniques. With proper equipment and technique, however, the same satisfactory results that have been experienced with cervical traction can also be accomplished with lumbar traction.

As previously mentioned, disappointment with the use of continuous traction has caused many physicians and physical therapists to lose interest in any form of lumbar traction. Some patients are reluctant to have traction treatments, recalling the continuous traction they may have received earlier. Any benefit accredited to this technique was probably the result of the rest and immobilization experienced by the patient while undergoing treatment.

The coefficient of friction of the human body lying on a couch or mattress is 0.5. In other words, a force equal to one-half of the patient's body weight is required to move the body horizontally (Fig. 9-6). It is necessary to move the lower one-half of the body horizontally before any force is effected to the lumbar spine (Fig. 9-7). As one-half of the body weight lies beneath L3, a force equal to $\frac{1}{2} \times 0.5 = \frac{1}{4}$ of the body weight is all that can effectively cause a traction force if conventional bed traction techniques are applied[10]. Any force less than one-fourth of the patient's body weight will not be enough to overcome friction and any more than one-half will cause the patient to slide to the foot of the bed. Nowhere in the literature was this author able to find any evidence that traction forces of one-fourth of the patient's body weight or less could effect any change in the structures of the lumbar spine.

The following points are essential to the administration of therapeutically effective lumbar traction:

1) The traction force must be great enough to effect a structural change (movement) at the spinal segment. Cyriax[2] reported a visible separation with sustained traction of 120 pounds for 15 minutes. Other studies have reported measurable separation in the lumbar spine at forces ranging from 80 to 200 pounds [6, 32, 39]. Judovich[10] advocated a force equal to one-half of the patient's body weight on a friction-free surface as a minimum to cause therapeutic

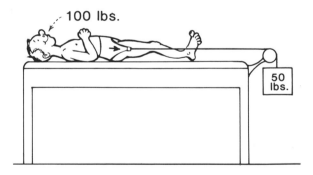

Fig. 9-6. A pull of 50 pounds is necessary to slide a 100 pound person horizontally on a couch or mattress.

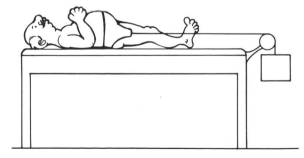

Fig. 9-7. It is necessary to move the lower one-half of the body horizontally before any traction force is effected to the lumbar spine.

effects in the lumbar spine. It is not necessary that the first treatment be administered at that weight, and it must be remembered that the minimum weight necessary to cause a measurable separation will not always be enough to produce satisfactory results. It is important in every case that the patient's reaction and results of the treatment be assessed; adjustments can then be made until satisfactory results are achieved.

The weights required to effect damage to the vertebral structures have also been studied. Most often cited is the study by Ranier in which fresh cadavers were used. According to DeSeze and Levernieux, Ranier found that a force of 400 pounds was necessary to produce a rupture of the dorso-lumbar spine (T11, T12[40].) Harris[6] indicated that enormous traction forces were necessary to cause damage to the lumbar spine with the breaking load possibly being as high as 880 pounds.

2) A split table is necessary to eliminate friction. As mentioned previously, it is the effective traction force on the spine that is important, and any friction involved must be considered. A split table, on frictionless guides, essentially eliminates this factor (Fig. 9-8).

3) Patients must be able to relax. The amount of force alone does not determine the effectiveness of the traction treatment. Patient comfort is of utmost importance. If patients are unable to relax during

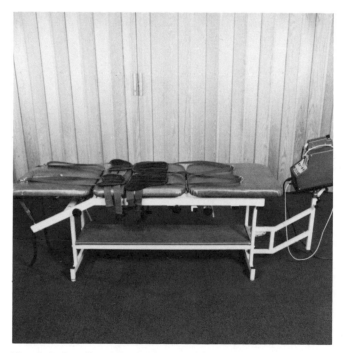

Fig. 9-8. A split table used for lumbar traction.

treatment, the treatment will probably be ineffective. Evidence shows that *narrowing* of the intervertebral spaces can actually occur during the traction treatment in patients who are unable to relax[41]. The treatment must not aggravate the condition and patients must feel secure and well supported. It may be beneficial to administer modality treatments before the application of traction. Such agents as ice, heat, ultrasound and massage are often effective.

4) The use of a heavy duty, non-slip traction harness is essential [14, 42]. If patients do not feel secure, they will almost certainly remain tense during treatment. An effective, one-size-fits-all heavy duty lumbar traction harness is seen in Fig. 9-9. This harness is lined with a vinyl material that causes it to adhere to the patient's skin, thus eliminating the slipping that is common with cotton lined belts. Both the pelvic and thoracic pads should be placed next to the patient's skin (Fig. 9-10). If clothing is left under the harness, it will be more likely to allow slippage. Clothing can also take some of the traction force if it is bound tightly under both belts. Even something as simple as a velcro strap around the patient's thighs will add support and help relaxation (Fig. 9-11). The pelvic harness should be secured to the patient first. It is properly positioned when the top web belt crosses at approximately the umbilical line (Fig. 9-12). The thoracic pads should be positioned so that they lie on the lateral-inferior chest wall. The thoracic pads are in proper position when both web belts are below the xiphoid process and are actually positioned and held on the inferior rim of the eighth, ninth and tenth ribs. The patient's arms should be placed through the thoracic harness. The anterior strap should always lie over the anterior aspect of the shoulder joint when the thoracic pads are in correct position. When properly positioned, the pelvic and thoracic belts will overlap slightly (Fig. 9-13).

5) All of the slack in the harnesses must be taken up before the split table is released. It is a good idea to begin the treatment with progressively stronger pulls with the split table locked. After two or three progressions the split table is released during a rest phase if one is using intermittent traction. If using sustained traction, the table is released with care being taken to avoid a sudden jerk. This may be accomplished by holding or blocking the movement of the table top as the mechanism is released, then gradually letting the table apart manually.

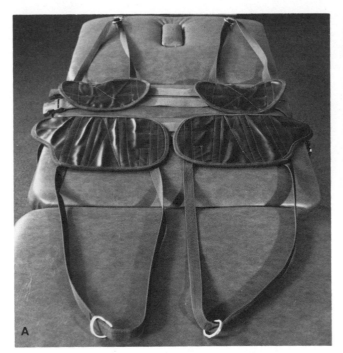
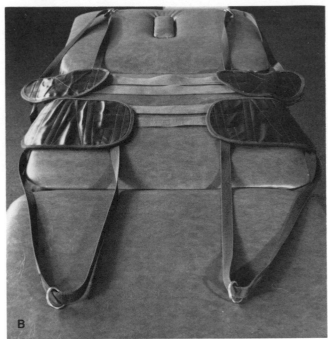

Fig. 9-9. A heavy duty lumbar traction harness A) adjusted for a small patient and B) adjusted for a large patient.

6) The patient position (prone or supine) and the amount of flexion or extension used will depend upon the disorder being treated and the comfort of the patient [2, 42]. In this author's experience, disc herniation with protrusion is effectively treated with the patient lying prone with a slightly flattened to normal lordosis. Joint hypomobility and degenerative disc disease are usually more effectively treated with the patient lying supine and the lumbar spine in a straight (flattened) position. However, patient comfort and the ability of the patient to remain relaxed during the treatment are also important

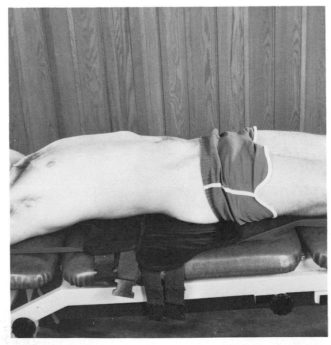

Fig. 9-10. Both the pelvic and thoracic pads should be placed next to the patient's skin to eliminate slipping.

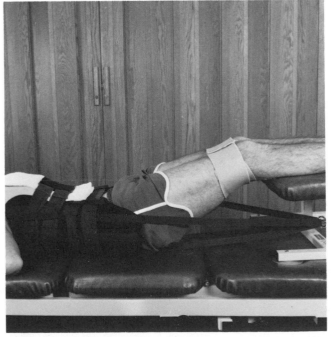

Fig. 9-11. A velcro strap is used to stabilize the patient's thighs.

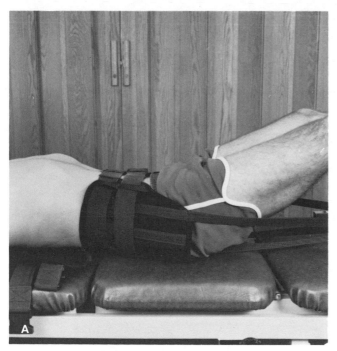

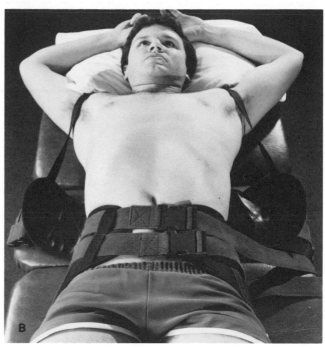

Fig.9-12. The pelvic harness is properly positioned when A) the top web belt is above the crest of the ilium and B) the top edge of the top web belt crosses at the umbilical line.

considerations when choosing which position to use and no absolute rule applies. Variations of flexion, extension and lateral bending should be tried to find the most beneficial position for each individual patient.

There is often a postural component involved with disorders of the lumbar spine. Initially, traction treatments may have to be administered in positions which accommodate the patient's postural position, but as progress is achieved, the treatment should be given in positions which encourage the return to normal posture. For example, most patients with disc herniation with protrusion will have a flattened lumbar lordosis and will be limited in spinal

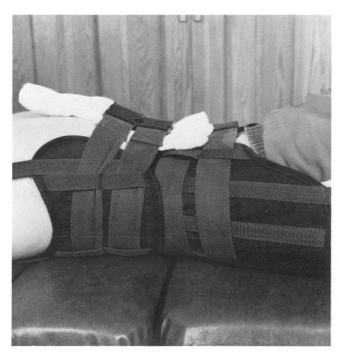

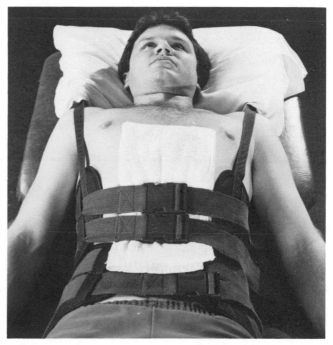

Fig. 9-13. When properly positioned, the pelvic and thoracic pads will overlap slightly.

extension. One of the treatment goals will be to return this patient to normal posture. Although it may be impossible to place the patient in a position of normal lordosis initially, one will want to work in that direction as treatment progresses. Thus, it may be necessary to give the traction treatment in a position involving some flexion (supine with a posterolateral pull or prone with a posterolateral pull with pillows under the lumbar spine.) However, as progress is noted and the patient is able to achieve a position of normal lordosis, the traction treatments should be given in a position that helps achieve the normal lordosis (prone with an antero-lateral pull.)

When applying lumbar traction in the supine position one should remember that it is not necessarily the position of the legs or the rope angle to the table which control the amount of lumbar flexion. The position of the legs controls hip flexion and has only a slight effect on lumbar lordosis. Likewise, the rope angle to the table does not always effectively control the amount of spinal flexion. The choice of pelvic harness is probably the most important determinant of the amount of spinal flexion achieved. If the pelvic harness pulls from the sides only, it is possible to maintain considerable lumbar lordosis. For this reason a pelvic harness that pulls from the posterior is essential. The knees and hips can be flexed moderately for comfort, while the rope angle to the table should remain relatively in line. This is especially true if heavier poundages are used. It should be noted that certain commercial traction tables are not recommended for heavy poundages unless a straight or zero degree rope angle to the table is maintained (Fig. 9-14).

Lumbar traction can be effectively administered in the prone position as well as supine. Patient comfort and the ability of the patient to remain relaxed during the treatment are considered when choosing which position to use. When using prone traction, the amount of lumbar flexion can be controlled with pillows under the pelvis and, as mentioned above, by using the correct pelvic harness. If one desires to apply lumbar traction with the spine in a normal amount of lordosis or in extension, the prone position is probably best. The harness should be positioned with an anterolateral pull. The patient lies flat on the table and the rope angle to the table is varied to control the exact amount of lordosis (Fig. 9-15).

Prone traction can be especially effective with the patient who has moderate to severe pain and/or

muscle guarding. The patient can be positioned prone for modality treatments and the traction can follow without moving the patient. Another advantage of prone traction is that the therapist can palpate the interspinous spaces to ascertain the

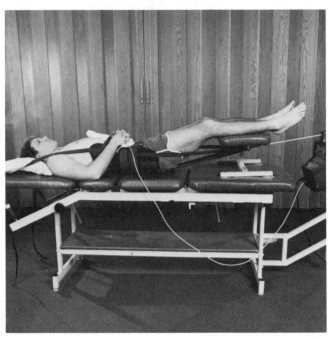

Fig. 9-14. Supine lumbar traction with the lumbar spine in a neutral (non-lordotic) position.

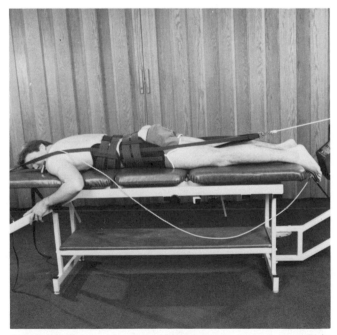

Fig. 9-15. Prone traction with an anterolateral pull. This technique enables the treatment to be given with the lumbar spine in some lordosis. The exact amount is controlled by the rope angle and adjustment of the table into extension.

amount of movement that is taking place during the treatment (Fig. 9-16).

7) The traction mode (sustained or intermittent) selected will depend on the disorder being treated and the comfort of the patient. Disc protrusions are usually treated more effectively with sustained traction or with longer hold-rest periods (60 second hold, 20 second rest) of intermittent traction, whereas joint dysfunction and degenerative disc disease usually respond to shorter hold-rest periods of intermittent traction. Some mechanical traction devices are relatively ineffective in administering sustained tration due to their inability to take up slack during the treatment. To be effective it is essential that a mechanical traction device continue to take up slack as the patient relaxes[43].

8) When disc protrusion is treated with spinal traction, the treatment time should be short. As the disc space is widened the intradiscal pressure is decreased[44]. This is a beneficial effect and, at least in the opinion of this author, explains the demonstration by Mathews of movement of contrast medium into the disc space. It seems that this decrease in pressure will only be maintained for a short time, as osmotic forces will soon equalize pressure to that of the surrounding tissue. If equalization does occur, the suction effective on the protrusion would be lost. Theoretically, an increase in intradiscal pressure with respect to the surrounding tissue might result when the traction is released. Consequently, the patient may experience a sharp increase in pain after treatment. The author has not observed this adverse reaction in intermittent treatments of less than ten minutes and sustained treatments of less than eight minutes. Often, the first treatment is only three to five minutes long.

9) Recently, mechanical traction devices have been introduced that have the ability to gradually increase the traction force at the beginning of the treatment and to regressively step down the force at the end of the treatment. Progressive-regressive application of traction is actually like a "warm up-cool down" period known to all trainers, therapists and physicians. The gradual application and removal of traction forces made possible with the progressive-regressive traction modes may enhance the potential effectiveness of traction in certain patients[45].

OTHER CONSIDERATIONS FOR LUMBAR TRACTION

MANUAL TRACTION

Paris uses manual lumbar traction for treatment of herniated disc. These techniques are sometimes used with a sudden thrust and can be directed unilaterally[26]. Kaltenborn also describes various

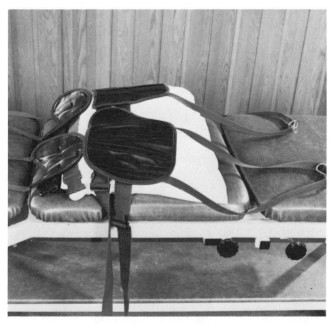
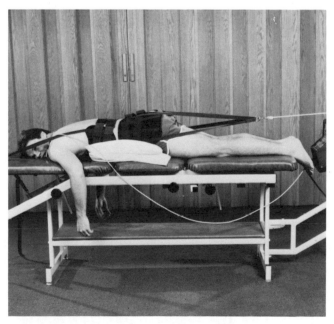

Fig. 9-16. Prone traction with a posterolateral pull and a pillow under the hips. This technique allows for more flattening of the lumbar lordosis.

manual traction techniques that can be used for the purpose of spinal mobilization[25]. Manual traction can be helpful in testing the patient's tolerance to traction or to find the most comfortable direction in which to administer the treatment (Fig. 9-17). Manual lumbar traction is of questionable value in most cases because of the physical difficulty encountered in applying and sustaining forces great enough to be effective.

POSITIONAL TRACTION

Positional traction is applied by placing the patient in a side lying position over a rolled pillow or blanket. The roll should be approximately six to eight inches in diameter and should be placed at the level of the spine where the traction or separation is to occur. The effect is a unilateral stretch of the soft tissue structures and gapping of the facet joints on the side opposite to the roll. The technique can involve only side bending or can also incorporate rotation (Fig. 9-18). This technique may also be used (side bending only) to correct a lateral scoliosis sometimes seen in patients who have a herniated nucleus pulposus — protrusion.

GRAVITY LUMBAR TRACTION

Although gravity lumbar traction with the patient in an upright position has been claimed to be

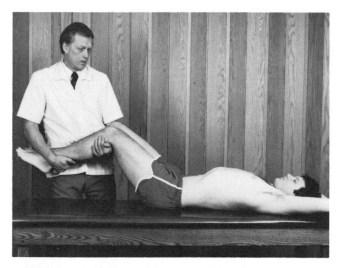
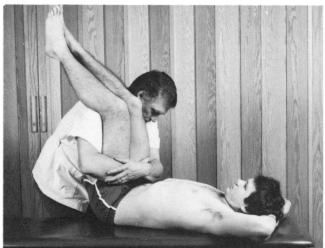
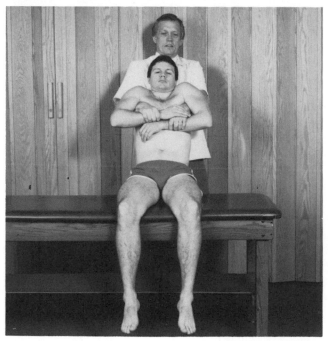
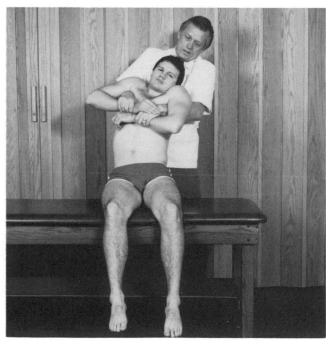

Fig. 9-17. Manual lumbar traction techniques.

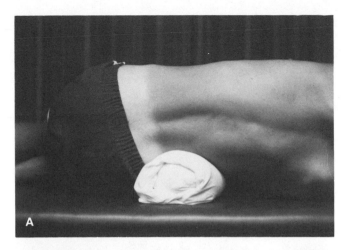

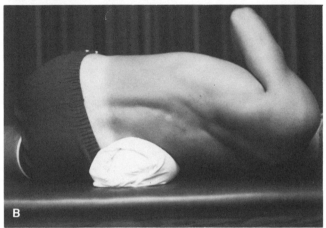

Fig. 9-18. A) Positional traction with side bend only; B) Positional traction with side bend and rotation.

effective in the treatment of disc protrusion, the amount of force that can be applied is limited (approximately 40% of body weight[28].) A moderate amount of physical effort is also required on the part of patients. This form of traction is recommended only for medically screened, well motivated patients whose body size and shape allows this form of treatment[12]. The program usually consists of one hour of traction twice daily. This treatment time is not consistent with the previously mentioned theory that an initial suction force caused by the vertebral bodies separating is soon lost due to osmotic movement of body fluids into the disc.

Gravity traction with the individual inverted has been shown to be effective in separating the intervertebral disc and foramenal spaces and therefore, may be an effective method of administering lumbar traction in certain cases[30]. This method is not without some risks, however. Recent investigation has shown that the inverted position can produce marked changes in heart rate and blood pressure in young adults. There is also evidence of increased ocular pressure and the potential for retinal damage in the inverted position[46]. Inversion traction may be dangerous for hypertensive individuals and those with cardiac anomalies or cerebral vascular disease. In any case, blood pressure, heart rate and patient comfort should be closely monitored during inversion and the patient should be acclimated to the inversion position on a gradual basis[30]. Other disadvantages of gravity traction include the difficulty in controlling the direction (flexion — extension — lateral bending) and the force (poundages).

It is this author's opinion that inversion devices can be effective as a treatment to improve joint mobility and general flexibility, but that they do not offer the control of direction and, in some cases, the amount of force that is necessary when treating patients with herniated nucleus pulposus or degenerative disc/joint disease with nerve root involvement.

UNILATERAL LUMBAR TRACTION

In some cases, lumbar traction involving a pull at a lateral angle to the midline of the body has been demonstrated to be more comfortable and more efficacious for unilateral disorders (including protective scoliosis) than is bilateral lumbar traction[6, 15, 27, 47, 48]. Although the technique seems sound, very little unilateral lumbar traction has been used clinically because of problems with patient positioning and with availability and adaptability of equipment. Lumbar traction involving a pull at a lateral angle to the midline of the body involves two problems: First, most commercially available traction equipment does not adapt to this technique. Also, when using equipment that does adapt to a lateral pull, the patient's body simply slides to the side of the table and aligns itself with the traction force and the pull on the lumbar spine remains straight (Fig. 9-19). When attempts are made to stabilize the spine to prevent this realignment, the exact area of lateral bending is difficult, if not impossible, to control. For instance, when attempts are made to stabilize the patient with a belt across the torso, most side bending occurs at the segment just inferior to the belt and the exact segment can only be determined by x-ray.

The technique preferred by this author to produce unilateral lumbar traction utilizes the con-

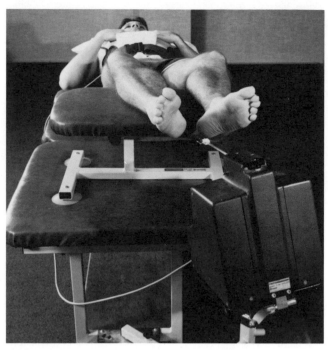

Fig. 9-19. When using a traction technique that involves a lateral pull, the patient's body slides to the side of the table and aligns itself with the traction force.

ventional heavy duty traction harness described earlier. By hooking only one side of the harness to the traction source, or by varying the length of the harness straps between sides, effective unilateral lumbar traction can be administered. With this method, the lateral bending and separation of the vertebrae is uniform throughout the lumbar spine. The technique can be applied in either the prone or the supine position (Fig. 9-20).

This author investigated the effects of unilateral traction to determine if vertebral separation occurs and, if so, where it occurs and whether a lumbar scoliosis occurs when the unilateral pull is applied. The information obtained is based on comparison of x-ray findings in one 200 pound man with no apparent lumbar disorder. This investigation was done with the subject in the supine position with a 100 pound pull from the right side only (Fig. 9-20a). Measurements were taken from the lateral aspect of the inferior edge of the T12 vertebral body to the superior surface of the sacrum at a point adjacent to the lateral aspect of the L5 vertebral body. The unilateral traction produced a separation of ten millimeters on the side of the pull and a separation of two millimeters on the side opposite the pull. Lumbar lateral bending of 12 degrees was also observed with the curve being convex on the side of the pull. The separation and curve occurred uni-

formly throughout the lumbar part of the spine (Fig. 9-21). These findings were then compared to supine side bending at the same degree without the traction force, which showed a separation of seven millimeters on the convex side and a narrowing of eleven millimeters on the concave side (Fig. 9-22). Investigation of a patient with a lumbar disorder has revealed similar findings (see section on unilateral facet joint hypomobility.)

The general indications and contraindications for applying conventional lumbar traction are also applicable to unilateral traction techniques. A complete and thorough evaluation and assessment is necessary before a patient receives lumbar traction. A part of that assessment should involve consideration of the factors which favor the unilateral as opposed to the bilateral technique.

Whenever there are general indications for lumbar traction, a unilateral pull may be considered, especially if the disorder is unilateral. Often, the determining factor is the patient's comfort and his ability to relax with the treatment. Daugherty and Erhard recommend a trial of manual traction and compression tests to ascertain if the patient is a suitable candidate for traction[49]. They theorize that if manual traction causes no pain or offers relief, the patient may be a suitable candidate for mechanical traction. Likewise, if manual traction aggravates the patient's condition, he is unlikely to be a suitable candidate. The series of manual tractions should be given at various degrees of flexion, extension and lateral bending in order to find the most comfortable and beneficial positioning of the patient[15]. When the disorder is unilateral, the most comfortable position will often be one that does involve some lateral bending of the spine along with traction. It is wise to take advantage of this more comfortable position in these cases[15].

Three specific instances when unilateral traction may be preferred to the conventional bilateral technique are for unilateral facet joint hypomobility, protective lumbar scoliosis and lumbar scoliosis caused by unilateral lumbar muscle spasm[15].

UNILATERAL FACET JOINT(S) HYPOMOBILITY

Conventional lumbar traction has been suggested as a mobilization technique[15, 42]. When the hypomobility involves the facet joint(s) on one side

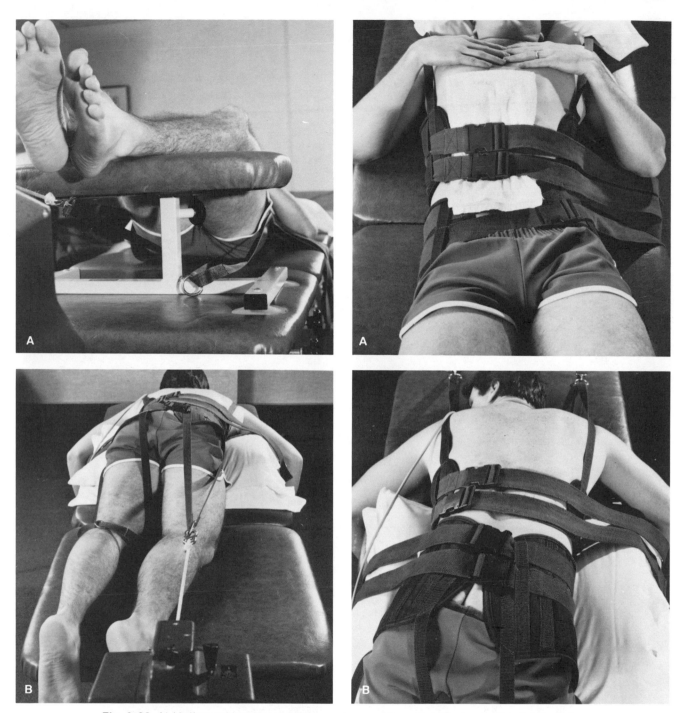

Fig. 9-20. A) Unilateral lumbar traction-supine position. Note that only the right pelvic pad is hooked to the traction force. B) Unilateral lumbar traction-prone position. Note that only the right pelvic pad is hooked to the traction force. This technique can be done with a posterolateral pull as shown, or with an anterolateral pull.

only, unilateral technique should be considered. The following is a case study of unilateral facet joint hypomobility involving the use of unilateral lumbar traction[15].

The patient reported that the onset of symptoms had occurred three months previously, after a compression type of fall with the spine extended.

The pain was only minor at first but had stiffened his spine. He had not sought medical help. His chief complaint, when seen three months after injury, was that it hurt in the area just lateral to the L5-S1 interspace on the right when he ran. He was otherwise doing the full activities of daily living for a 17 year old, 155 pound athlete/student[15].

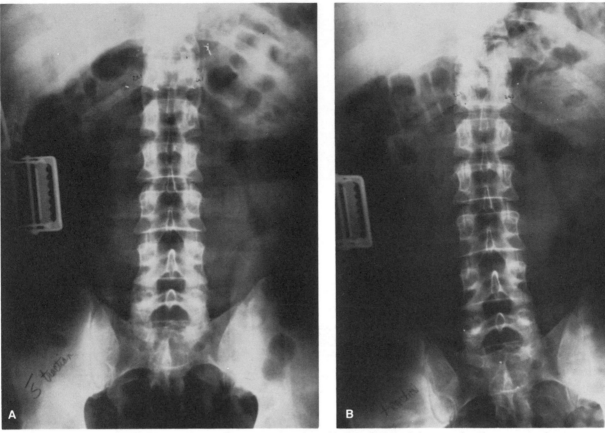

Fig. 9-21. Comparison of x-rays showing A) the patient lying supine in an anterior-posterior view with no traction and B) the patient lying supine in an anterior-posterior view with 100 pounds of traction pulling from the right side only.

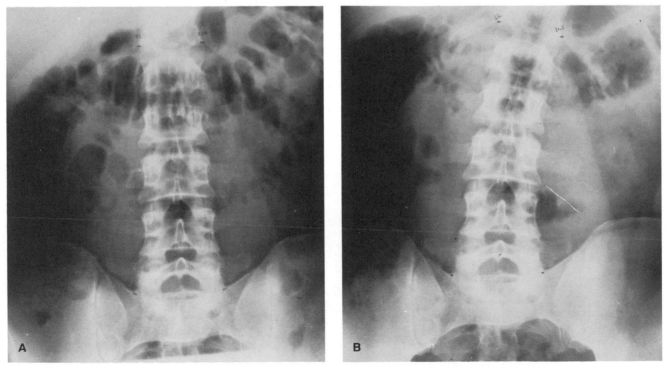

Fig. 9-22. Comparison of x-rays showing A) the patient lying supine in an anterior-posterior view with the spine straight and no traction and B) the patient lying supine in an anterior-posterior view with the spine side bent to the left and no traction.

The x-ray revealed apparent narrowing of the right facet joint (Fig. 9-23). Mobility tests revealed hypomobility at the L5-S1 level with the greatest restriction in right rotation and left side bending. Other clinical signs and symptoms supported the presence of facet joint hypomobility at that level. There were no positive neurological findings[15].

The patient was given continuous ultrasound for six minutes at 20 watts, followed by intermittent unilateral lumbar traction with a right sided pull of 100 pounds for 10 minutes. An x-ray was taken while the traction was being applied, showing visible separation (mobilization) of the right L5-S1 facet (Fig. 9-24). The patient was nearly symptom free after two treatments, and received a total of four treatments. He has returned to full activities of daily living, including varsity cross-country running, and has remained symptom free for several months[15].

PROTECTIVE SCOLIOSIS

If a patient has a herniated nucleus pulposus and the protrusion is encroaching upon a spinal nerve root, lateral bending of the spine often offers relief. This is referred to as a "protective scoliosis." Many musculoskeletal problems involve lateral bending of the spine, and the protective scoliosis is only one of several possibilities. Most patients with protective scoliosis lean away from the side of the symptoms. However, when the disorder involves a herniated disc with a protrusion medial to the nerve root, the patient may bend toward the side of the symptoms. If the herniation is lateral to the nerve root (most common), the patient will bend away from the painful side (Fig. 9-25). In all cases, the patient assumes the position that offers symptomatic relief [50, 51].

When the patient with a protective scoliosis is placed in conventional bilateral traction, the scoliosis straightens which may result in increased pain. The traction does not appear to be beneficial. On the other hand, if the scoliosis can be maintained while the traction is applied, the treatment may be given without increasing the patient's discomfort. Such a technique enhances the chances of achieving the desired results of the treatment.

A protective scoliosis differs from the condition McKenzie describes as a lateral shift[35]. With a

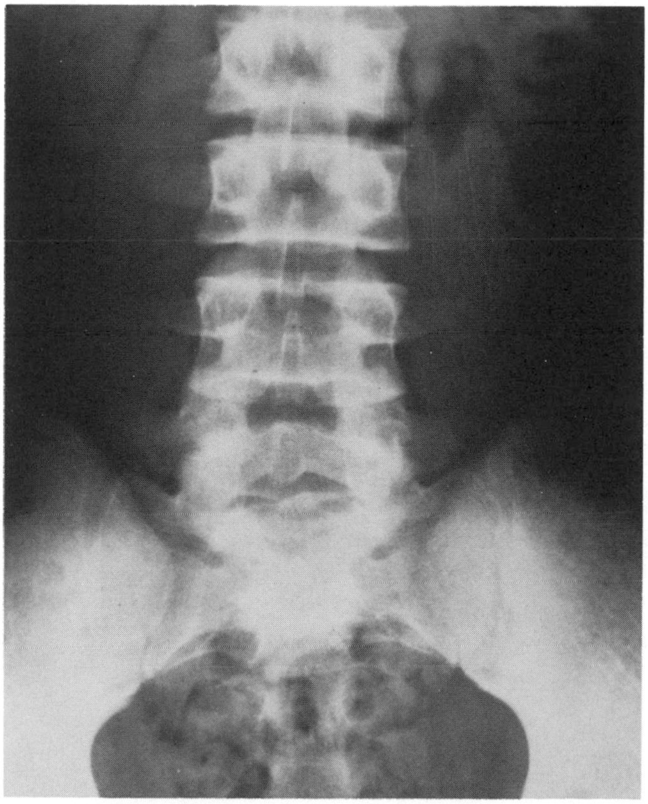

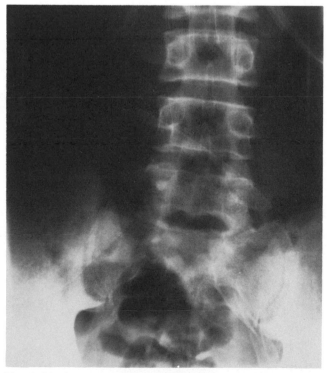

Fig. 9-23. An x-ray showing a narrowed right facet joint and a position change of right rotation at interspace L5-S1 (posterior-anterior view) (Reprinted with permission from Saunders[15].)

Fig. 9-24. An x-ray showing the amount of movement (separation) occurring in a right facet joint of the L5-S1 interspace with 100 pounds of intermittent unilateral lumbar traction (same patient and view as in Fig. 9-23) (Reprinted with permission from Saunders[15].)

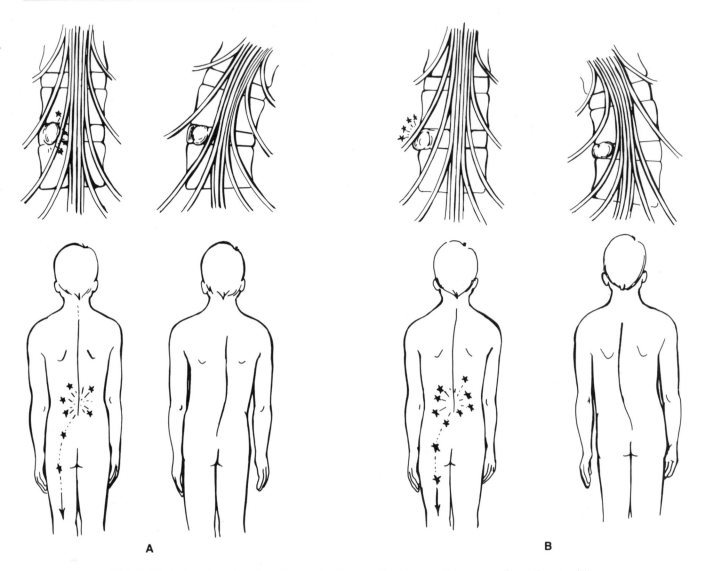

A   B

Fig. 9-25. A drawing showing the protective scoliosis sometimes seen in patients with herniated disc syndrome (Adopted from Finneson[50].)

protective scoliosis, the patient places himself in the most comfortable position. A lateral shift is a mechanical phenomenon that occurs when the nuclear gel moves laterally. It is difficult to distinguish between these conditions clinically unless manual correction is attempted. When manual correction causes increased peripheral symptoms, one may be dealing with a protective scoliosis and lumbar traction will be more effective if the scoliosis is not disturbed.

To maintain the protective scoliosis for the patient who leans away from the side of the symptoms, the pull should be from the same side as the symptoms. For the patient who leans toward the affected side, the traction pull should be from the side opposite that of the symptoms (Fig. 9-26).

LUMBAR SCOLIOSIS CAUSED BY MUSCLE SPASM

Unilateral lumbar traction can also be effective in reducing a lumbar scoliosis caused by unilateral paravertebral muscle spasm in the lumbar area. To do this the unilateral pull should be from the concave side of the scoliosis[15] (Fig. 9-27).

THREE-DIMENSIONAL LUMBAR TRACTION

Postural changes accompany many of the spinal disorders treated by physical therapists. It is sometimes difficult to determine if the abnormal

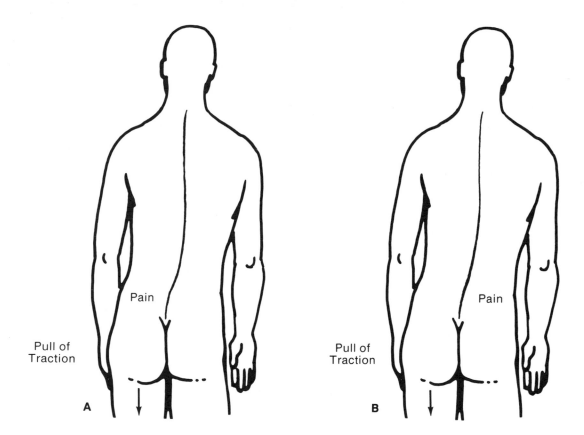

Fig. 9-26. A drawing showing A) a patient with a protective scoliosis away from the side of the symptoms and B) a patient with a protective scoliosis toward the side of the symptoms. In order to maintain the scoliosis in both cases, the unilateral pull should be from the convex side of the scoliosis (Adopted from Saunders[15].)

posture is the result of the pathological disorder, or if the postural change is the cause of the disorder. However, regardless of this relationship, return to normal posture is always one of the treatment goals. For example, the patient with herniated nucleus pulposus-protrusion is often seen with a flattened lumbar spine and a lateral scoliosis. One of the goals of treatment should be to return this patient to normal posture. However, this is not always possible initially in the course of treatment and attempts to straighten the lateral scoliosis and/or restore the lordosis often cause an increase in the peripheral signs and symptoms and a general worsening of the condition. When this is the case, traction is often the treatment of choice if it can be administered in such a way that the patient's flexed and laterally shifted posture is not disturbed. As previously discussed, the initial treatment is often given in the prone position with pillows under the lumbar spine to maintain flexion. The harness strap from the convex side of the scoliosis is hooked to the traction source.

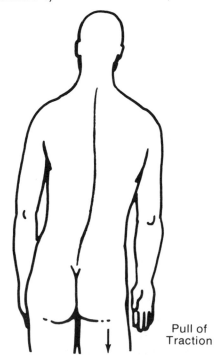

Fig. 9-27. A drawing showing a patient with a unilateral muscle spasm causing a lumbar scoliosis. To stretch this condition, the unilateral pull should be from the concave side of the scoliosis (Adopted from Saunders[15].)

Thus the traction treatment is given without disturbing the patient's postural position. On subsequent treatments, the amount of flexion and the amount of unilateral pull is lessened as the patient is gradually worked back into a normal postural position.

A three-dimensional traction table may offer an advantage to this method of treatment in that the table can be positioned initially to accommodate to the patient's abnormal posture; as the traction force is being given, the table can be adjusted gradually to return the patient toward the normal posture. Since three-dimensional traction tables have only been commercially available for a very short time, clinical experience with them is limited. This author, however, believes that they may offer considerable advantage, especially in the ease and convenience of administering treatment (Fig. 9-28).

CERVICAL TRACTION TECHNIQUE

Many of the comments concerning lumbar traction technique are equally appropriate for cervical traction. In addition, the following points are essential:

1) The first question that should be resolved concerning cervical traction technique is seated versus supine positioning. Although both positions are commonly used, research reveals that the supine position is superior [5, 41, 52].

2) Colachis and Strohm have demonstrated a relationship between separation of the vertebral bodies and the angle of pull. They studied angles of pull at 6, 20 and 24 degrees and found that as the angle was increased, the posterior separation of the cervical vertebrae also increased[52]. One must not forget, however, that the space available for the spinal nerve in the intervertebral foramen decreases as flexion beyond the neutral or straight position of the spine occurs[53]. Therefore, if opening of the intervertebral foramen and/or mobilization of the posterior cervical structures is the desired effect, the most advantageous position for cervical traction is flexion of the cervical spine to 25 to 30 degrees. This position effectively straightens the normal lordosis but does not go beyond that point. However, if greater separation is desired at the intervertebral disc space or if one is using traction to mobilize to improve cervical extension and/or axial extension (the head back, chin in posture), any amount of flexion would render the treatment less effective. This concept does not apply to the atlanto-occipital and atlanto-axial joints. The optimum angle to

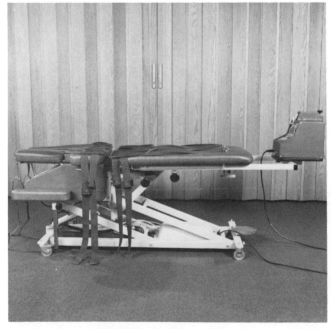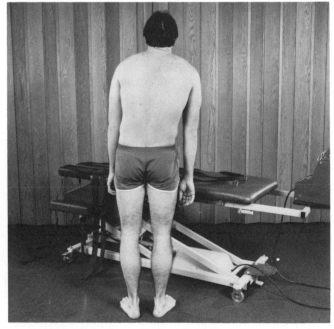

Fig. 9-28. Three-dimensional mechanical traction. The table is positioned initially to accommodate the patient's abnormal posture. As the traction force is being given, the table can then be adjusted to correct (or overcorrect) the patient's posture. (Fig. 9-28 is continued on next page.)

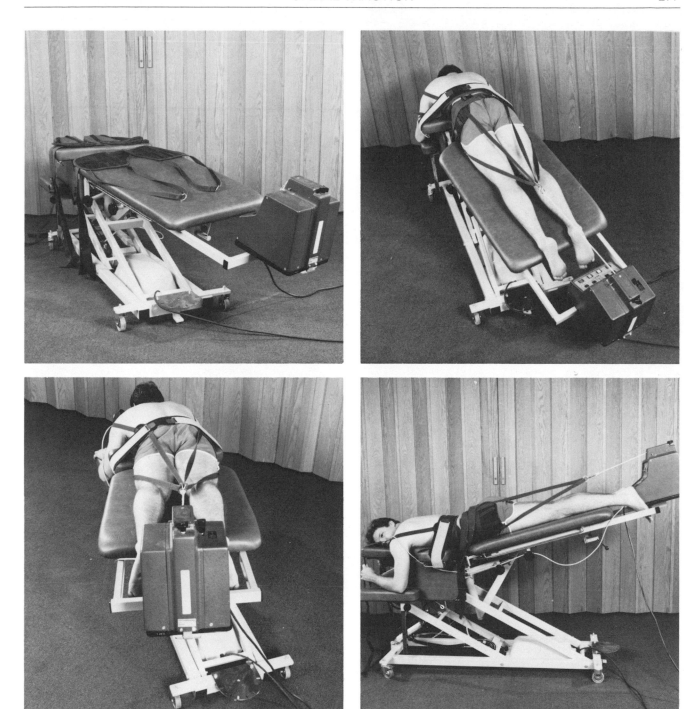

Fig. 9-28. Three-dimensional mechanical traction. (Continued)

achieve separation at these levels is a straight or zero degree angle which allows the normal cervical lordosis to remain[49].

DeLacerda measured the electromyographic activity of the upper trapezius muscle when a force of 30 pounds of intermittent cervical traction was applied at angles of 10, 25 and 35 degrees with the subjects positioned supine. He found that a positive relationship existed between an increase in the angle of pull and muscle activity[54].

3) The angle of the rope to the table is not the only factor influencing the correct amount of flexion or extension that must be considered. In fact, it is probably less important than the choice of head halters or cervical traction devices. If a poorly adjusted or constructed head halter is used, a different degree of flexion may be effected even if the angle of the rope to the table is within the recommended limits[15]. Many head halters are available. The most satisfactory seem to be those that position

the head in a neutral position, enabling the pull to be exerted more at the occiput than at the chin. This is more comfortable for the patient and also concentrates the force in line with the cervical spine (Fig. 9-29).

4) Judovich[9] found that forces of 25 to 45 pounds were necessary to demonstrate a measurable change in the posterior cervical spine structures. Jackson[8] confirmed this finding. In another comprehensive work, Colachis and Strohm[52] demon-

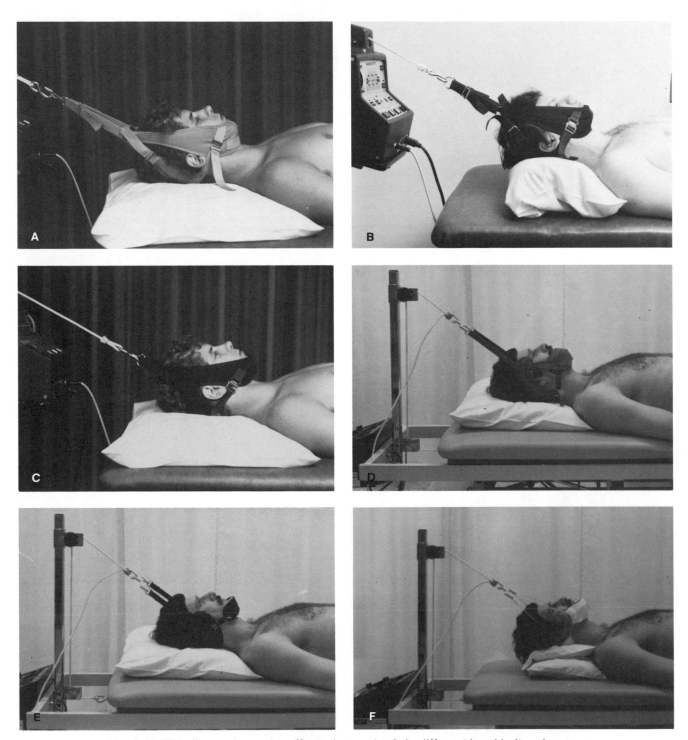

Fig. 9-29. This figure shows the effects that each of six different head halters have on head and neck positions. All are taken with the same rope angle to the table. Head halters shown are listed in order of the author's preference: A) Hill head halter, B) Chattanooga 1405 head halter, C) Chattanooga 1403 head halter, D) Repo Upper Seven head halter, E) Universal head halter, F) Disposable head halter.

strated that tractive forces of 30 pounds produce separation of the cervical spine. A search of the literature disclosed no evidence of separation occurring at lesser forces in the mid and lower cervical spine. Weights of 25 to 40 pounds, therefore, appear necessary to produce vertebral separation[14]. Daugherty and Erhard[49] demonstrated separation of the atlanto-occipital and atlanto-axial joints with 10 pounds of traction. Therefore, it appears that less force is necessary when treatment is directed to that area.

5) It is also of interest that some researchers have found compression or narrowing of the joint space with application of cervical traction. This narrowing is often attributed to muscle guarding and to the patient's inability to relax during traction. These findings are most common when patients are seated[41].

6) Research has been done concerning the forces necessary to cause damage to the cervical structures. Ranier[40] found that a tractive force of 120 pounds was necessary to cause a disc rupture at the C5-C6 level.

7) When receiving traction treatments, the patient must feel secure and be able to relax. The force of the traction must not cause pain to the extent that the patient cannot relax. The use of modalities preceding the traction treatment may be helpful in this regard. Patient comfort should be considered when making a choice between intermittent or sustained cervical traction, as either can be effective.

8) Treatment time should be relatively short (five to ten minutes) when treating herniated nucleus pulposus-protrusion. Times can be increased slightly for other conditions. Patient comfort should always be of primary consideration when determining duration of the treatment.

THE SAUNDERS' CERVICAL TRACTION DEVICE

Conventional cervical traction methods utilize head halters that fit under the chin anteriorly and on the occipital bone posteriorly. A common problem encountered in administering cervical traction is aggravation of the temporomandibular joints because of the force applied at the chin. The exact amount of force on the chin depends upon the design and adjustment of the head halter, the direction (flexion or extension) of the traction force and the amount of the traction force. Nevertheless, even when the utmost care is taken to minimize the force on the chin, there often exists enough force to cause an undesirable effect on the temporomandibular joints[55].

The cervical traction device shown in Fig. 9-30 does not contact the chin or place any force on the temporomandibular joints. The device consists of a shaft that connects to the traction source of a commercial traction table at one end as the other end rests near the head of the traction table. Mounted on this shaft is a friction-free carriage that holds an adjustable V-shaped device. The V-shaped device fits against the back of the patient's neck just below the occipital bone. There is also a small head rest on the carriage and a strap that fits over the patient's forehead to hold the patient's head in position as treatment is given. Treatment is given with the patient lying supine. This device allows complete control of head and neck positions both in flexion and in extension and is adjustable to allow a side bending (unilateral) pull.

Of particular interest is the literature concerning temporomandibular joint dysfunction associated with cervical traction. During the cervical traction treatment using one of the standard head halters, force is transmitted via the chin strap to the teeth and the temporomandibular joints become weight bearing structures. Crisp[56], and Shore, Frankel and Hoppenfeld[57], have drawn attention to the fact that during treatment some of the patients experience considerable discomfort in the temporomandibular joints. This is particularly true if an abnormal dental occlusion exists such as the absence of posterior teeth. In some cases, the discomfort is so great that the treatment has to be discontinued. With advancing age, the tissues become more susceptible to disruption and joint trauma which, in some cases, may be irreversible[56,57]. Franks suggests that cervical traction should be carried out with caution. He reports that, in the older patient particularly, excessive pressure on the jaw can give rise to intracapsular bleeding and hematoma in the temporomandibular joint[58].

The Saunders' Cervical Traction Device meets all of the general requirements for application of cervical traction. It can be utilized in the optimal range of head and neck positions with any amount of force and duration (intermittent or sustained.) The most favorable patient position (supine) is used and the chin and temporomandibular joints are not encroached upon.

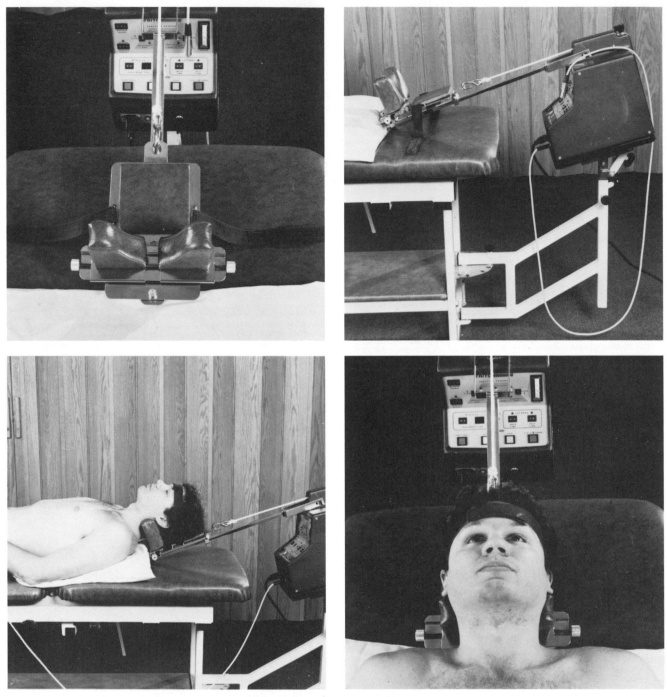

Fig. 9-30. Cervical traction device that does not contact the chin. This eliminates many of the problems associated with the conventional head halters now in use. This device is available from Chattanooga Corporation.

MANUAL CERVICAL TRACTION

Cyriax advocates manual cervical traction and estimates that he exerts forces as high as 200 pounds[24]. He often incorporates passive range of motion with the manual traction (Fig. 9-31). Inhibitive manual traction is a technique used by Paris

that has a beneficial relaxing effect as well as a tractive force[26] (Fig. 9-32).

UNILATERAL CERVICAL TRACTION

Unilateral cervical traction can be incorporated if the therapist wants to direct a stronger force to one

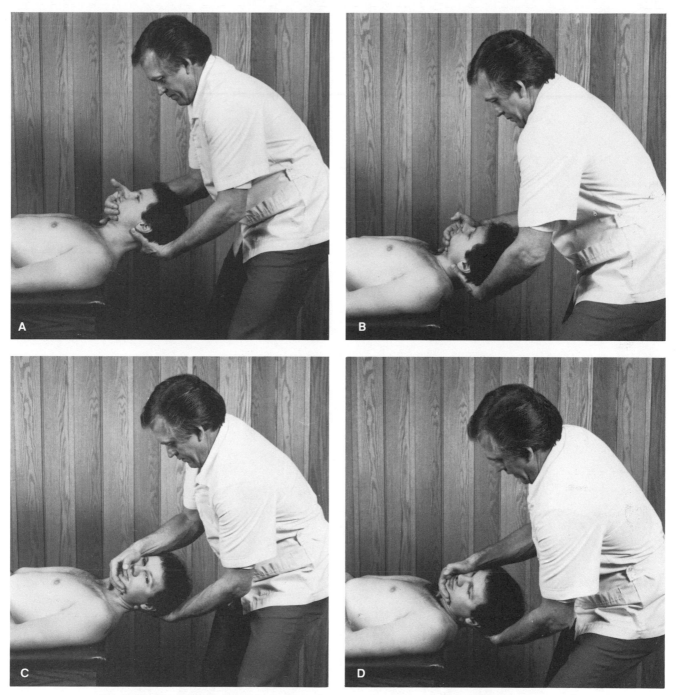

Fig. 9-31. Manual cervical traction may incorporate range of motion. The greatest pull should be from the occiput. A) Straight manual traction, B) Manual traction with side bending, C) Manual traction with rotation, D) Manual traction with rotation and side bending, E) Backward Bending and F) Axial Extension (head back, chin in). (Fig. 9-31 is continued on next page.)

side of the cervical spine, or to maintain a protective scoliosis (see discussion under "Unilateral Lumbar Traction".) When using the unilateral or three-dimensional cervical traction, a stabilization strap must be used over the patient's chest. Otherwise, the patient will align himself with the angle of the rope and the unilateral effect will be lost (Fig. 9-33). A unilateral effect may also be achieved by shortening only one of the two straps that attach the head halter to the traction source. As previously mentioned, the cervical traction device shown in Fig. 9-30 is also adjustable to allow a unilateral pull.

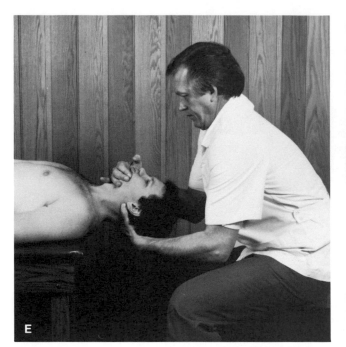
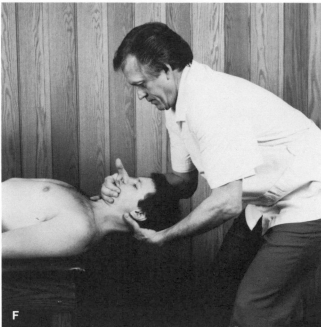

Fig. 9-31. Manual cervical traction. (Continued)

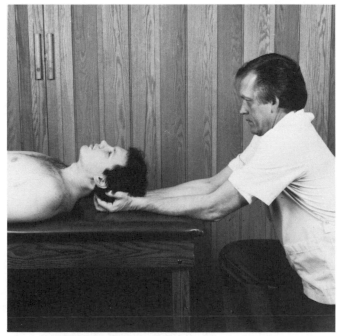

Fig. 9-32. Inhibitive manual traction.

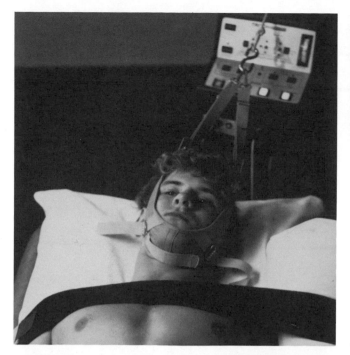
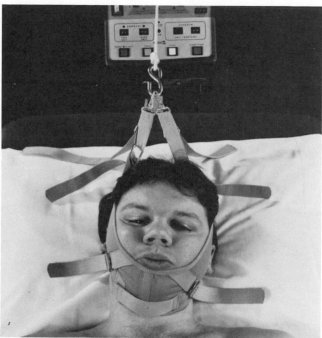
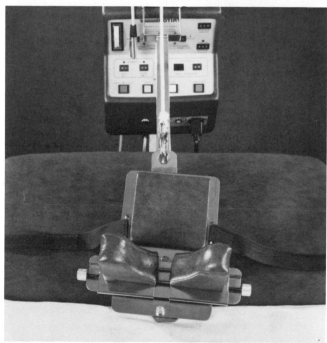
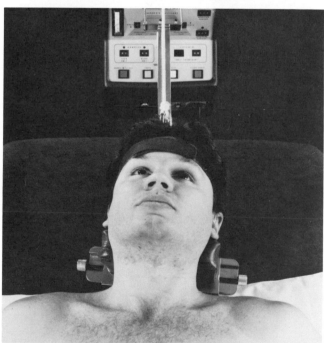

Fig. 9-33. Unilateral cervical traction. Note the rolled pillow and stabilization strap to prevent the patient's body from sliding to the side of the pull.

References:

1. Crisp, E: Discussion on the Treatment of Backache by Traction. Proc R Soc Med, 48:805, 1955.
2. Cyriax, J: The Treatment of Lumbar Disk Lesions. Br Med Joul 2:1434, 1950.
3. Frazer, E: The Use of Traction in Backache. Med J Aust, 2:694, 1954.
4. Gupta, R; Ramarao, S: Epidurography in Reduction of Lumbar Disc Prolapse by Traction. Arch Phys Med Rehabil, 59:322, 1978.
5. Harris, P: Cervical Traction: Review of Literature and Treatment Guidelines. Phys Ther, 57:910, 1977.
6. Harris, R: Massage, Manipulation and Traction. New Haven, E. Licht, 1960.
7. Hood, L, and Chrisman, D: Intermittent Pelvic Traction in the Treatment of the Ruptured Intervertebral Disc. J Am Phys Ther Assoc, 48:21, 1968.
8. Jackson, B: The Cervical Syndrome. Springfield, Charles C Thomas, 1958.

References: (Continued)

9. Judovich, B: Herviated Cervical Disc. Am J Surg 84:649, 1952.

10. Judovich, B: Lumbar Traction Therapy. JAMA 159:549, 1955.

11. Masturzo, A: Vertebral Traction for Sciatica. Rheumatism, 11:62, 1955.

12. Oudenhoven, T: Gravitational Lumbar Traction. Arch Phys Med, 59:510, 1978.

13. Parsons, W and Cummings, J: Mechanical Traction in the Lumbar Disc Syndrome. Can Med Assoc J, 77:7, 1957.

14. Saunders, H: Spinal Traction: A Continuing Education Module for Physical Therapists. University of Kansas, Independent Study, Division of Continuing Education, 1979

15. Saunders, H: Unilateral Lumbar Traction. Phys Ther 61:221, 1981.

16. Yates, D: Indications and Contraindications for Spinal Traction. Physiotherapy, 58:55, 1972.

17. Christy, B: Discussion on the Treatment of Backache by Traction. Proc R Soc Med, 48:811, 1955.

18. Larsson, V; Sholer, U; Lidstrom, A; Lind, G; Nachemson, A; Nilsson, B and Roslund, J: Auto-Traction for Treatment of Lumbago-Sciatica. Acta Orthop Scand, 51:791, 1980.

19. Lindstrom, A; Zachrisson, M: Physical Therapy on Low Back Pain and Sciatica: An Attempt at Evaluation. Scand J Rehabil Med 2:37, 1970.

20. Mathews, J and Heckling, H: Lumbar Traction: A Double Blind Controlled Study for Sciatica. Rheumatol Rehabil 14:222, 1975.

21. Weber, H: Traction Therapy in Sciatica Due to Disc Prolapse. J Oslo City Hosp, 23(10):167, 1973.

22. Lind, G: Auto-Traction: Treatment of Low Back Pain and Sciatica. Thesis, University of Linkoping, 1974.

23. Hickling, J: Spinal Traction Technique. Physiotherapy, 58:58, 1972.

24. Cyriax, J: Textbook of Orthopaedic Medicine; Treatment by Manipulation, Massage and Injection. Vol 2, 10th ed, Balliere-Tindall, London, 1980.

25. Kaltenborn, F: Proceedings, International Federation of Orthopaedic Manipulative Therapists. Kent, B (ed), Vail, Colorado, 1977.

26. Paris, S: Course Notes, The Spine. Atlanta Back Clinic, Atlanta, 1976.

27. Natchev, E: A Manual on Auto-Traction Treatment for Low Back Pain. Natchev, Stockholm, Sweden, 1984.

28. Burton, C: Low Back Pain. 2nd ed, Philadelphia, Lippincott, 1980.

29. Nosse, L: Inverted Spinal Traction. Arch Phys Med Rehabil, 59:367, 1978.

30. Kane, M: Effects of Gravity Facilitated Traction on Intervertebral Dimensions of the Lumbar Spine. Master's Thesis, U.S. Army-Baylor University Program in Physical Therapy, Academy of Health Sciences, Fort Sam Houston, Texas, 1983.

31. Mathews, J: Dynamic Discography: A Study of Lumbar Traction. Ann Phys Med, 9:275, 1968.

32. Mathews, J: The Effects of Spinal Traction. Physiotherapy, 58:64, 1972.

33. Kapandji, I: The Physiology of the Joints. Vol 3, 3rd ed, London, Churchill Livingstone, 1974.

34. Morris, J; Lucas, M and Bresler, M: Role of the Trunk in Stability of the Spine. J Bone Joint Surg, 43A:327, 1961.

35. McKenzie, R: The Lumbar Spine. Spinal Publications, Waikanae, New Zealand, 1981.

36. Nachemson, A and Morris, J: In Vivo Measurements of Intradiscal Pressure. J Bone Joint Surg, 46A:1077, 1964.

37. Shah, J: Shift of Nuclear Material With Flexion and Extension of the Spine. Structure, Morphology and Mechanics of the Lumbar Spine: The Lumbar Spine and Low Back Pain. Jayson, M (ed), London, Pitman Medical, 1980.

38. Nachemson, A: The Lumbar Spine: An Orthopaedic Challenge. Spine, 1:59, 1976.

39. Lawson, G and Godfrey, C: A Report on Studies of Spinal Traction. Med Serv J Can, 12:762, 1958.

40. DeSeze, S and Levernieux, J: Les Tractions Vertebrales. Sem Hop Paris, 27:2075, 1951.

41. Deets, D; Hands, K and Hopp, S: Cervical Traction: A Comparison of Sitting and Supine Positions. Phys Ther 57:255, 1977.

42. Saunders, H: Lumbar Traction. J Orthop Sports Phys Ther, 1:36, 1979.

43. Saunders, H: The Use of Spinal Traction in the Treatment of Neck and Back Conditions. Clinical Orthopaedics and Related Research, 179: 31-38, October, 1983.

44. Nachemson, A and Elfstom, G: Intravital Dynamic Pressure Measurements in the Lumbar Discs; Scand J Rehabil Med (Suppl 1): 1, 1970.

45. Petulla, L: Clinical Observations With Respect to Progressive-Regressive Traction (Unpublished), Los Gatos, California, 1983.

46. LeMarr, J; Golding, L and Crehan, K: Cardiorespiratory Responses to Inversion. Phys Sportsmed, 11:51-57, 1983.

47. Brodin, H: Manueli Medicine ooh Manipulation. Lakartidningen 63:1037-1038, 1966.

48. Brodin, H, et al: Manipulation av Ryggraden. Scandinavicen University Books, 1966.

49. Daugherty, R and Erhard, R: Segmentalized Cervical Traction. Proceedings, International Federation of Orthopaedic Manipulative Therapists; Kent, B (ed), Vail, Colorado, 1977, pp. 189-195.

50. Finneson, B: Low Back Pain. Philadelphia, J.B. Lippincott, 1973, pp. 149-155.

51. Waitz, E: The Lateral Bending Sign. Spine 6:388-397, 1981.

52. Colachis, S and Strohm, M: Cervical Traction. Arch Phys Med 46:815, 1965.

53. Maslow, G and Rothman, R: The Facet Joints, Another Look. Bul NY Acac Med 51:1294-1311, 1975.

54. De Lacerda, F: Effect of Angle of Traction Pull on Upper Trapezius Muscle Activity. J Orth Spts Phy Ther 1: 205-209, 1980.

55. Frankel, V; Shore, N and Hoppenfeld, S: Stress Distribution in Cervical Traction Prevention of Temporomandibular Joint Pain Syndrome. Clin Orth 32:114-115, 1964.

56. Crisp, E: Disc Lesions. Livingstone, Edinburgh, 1960.

57. Shore, N; Frankel, V and Hoppenfeld, S: Cervical Traction and Temporomandibular Joint Dysfunction. Joul Am Dental Assoc 68 (1):4-6, 1964.

58. Franks, A: Temporomandibular Joint Dysfunction Associated with Cervical Traction. Ann Phys Med 8:38-40, 1967.

CHAPTER 10

SPINAL ORTHOTICS

Support or bracing is an important adjunct in the management of many musculoskeletal disorders of the spine. Physical therapists play an important role in determining the need for and selection and fitting of spinal braces and supports. The purpose of this chapter is to: 1) Discuss the effects of spinal braces and supports commonly used for the treatment of musculoskeletal disorders; 2) Review the indications for spinal bracing; 3) Review the types of spinal braces; 4) Discuss fitting procedures and 5) Discuss total management of the patient using a spinal brace or support.

Spinal braces can be grouped into two major categories: corrective and supportive/immobilizing[1]. Corrective braces are used in the treatment of disorders such as scoliosis and kyphosis and will not be considered here. This chapter will instead direct attention to the spinal braces which provide support and/or immobilization for conditions commonly seen by the physical therapist. The types of spinal orthoses discussed are lumbosacral corsets, chairback braces, Knight spinal braces, Williams' braces, sacroiliac belts, dorsal-lumbar corsets, Taylor braces, Knight-Taylor braces, hyperextension braces, soft cervical collars, hard cervical collars, Philadelphia collars, two and four poster cervical braces and Somi braces.

EFFECTS OF SPINAL BRACING

A review of the literature reveals the following effects of spinal bracing: 1) Immobilization of the intervertebral joints; 2) Increased motion of intervertebral joints adjacent to those that are immobilized; 3) Transfer of part of the vertical load from the spine to other structures; 4) Increase in intra-abdominal pressure (lumbar supports); 5) Decrease in intradiscal pressure; 6) Decrease of venous return from the lower extremities (lumbar supports); 7) Control of lordosis or kyphosis; 8) Providing the user with an awareness of correct posture; 9) Providing the user with a placebo (psychological) effect; 10) Decrease of abdominal and/or spinal muscular activity and 11) Increase of spinal muscular activity.

Thoracolumbosacral Spine

The ability of spinal braces to immobilize thoracolumbosacral rotation, flexion and extension has been studied extensively. Norton and Brown[2] showed that lumbar flexion-extension was reduced but not eliminated by many of the braces that they studied. At the same time, in many cases they found increased motion toward the upper and lower margins of the braces tested. Long braces, such as the Taylor brace, provided considerable immobilization in the upper lumbar and lower to mid-thoracic spine, but considerable increase of lower lumbar movement resulted. Thus, it appears that bracing can be used effectively to restrict flexion-extension movements from the mid-lumbar to the mid-thoracic area. However, in the lower lumbar area, the effect of bracing on flexion-extension movements may be lost or even reversed. If bracing is effective in limiting flexion-extension in the lower lumbar spine, it is probably because the brace serves as a reminder to the patient that certain movements are to be restricted and teaches the patient the position of correct posture.

Lumsden and Morris[3] showed that immobilization of the lumbosacral joint with the use of a modified chairback brace was relatively effective in restricting rotation, but that the effects of a lumbosacral corset on immobilization were varied and unpredictable. Adequate fixation of the pelvis is essential to achieve restriction of motion in the lower lumbar region as opposed to the more obvious fixation that occurs at higher levels, according to Wasserman and McNamee[4]. They found a 50% reduction in rotation at regions in the center of the garments they tested.

If intra-abdominal pressure is increased, the vertical load on the spine (intradiscal pressure) is decreased. Morris and associates[5] found that an inflatable corset raised the resting abdominal pressure but did not change the maximum intra-abdominal pressure that was produced during exercise. This implies that the peak loading on the disc from bending is not reduced with the use of a lumbosacral brace or corset. However, Wasserman and McNamee suggest that lumbosacral orthoses can reduce axial and bending loading on the spine because of increased abdominal pressure[4]. Nachemson and Morris[6] found that in inflatable corset decreased the intradiscal pressure by 24%. This decrease was noted in both the standing and the sitting positions.

It should also be noted that as intra-abdominal pressure is increased, a corresponding decrease in venous return from the lower extremities may occur. Although this would not cause a problem in most cases, it should be kept in mind when prescribing lumbar braces and corsets for patients with vascular insufficiency in the lower extremities. Garments that surround the circumference of the thigh, such as the panty girdle, or garments with a crotch are especially restrictive of venous return.

Waters and Morris[1] found that with subjects at rest both the chairback brace and the lumbosacral corset either decreased or had no effect on the electrical activity of the back muscles or the internal and external oblique abdominal muscles. When subjects walked at a comfortable speed, neither support had a significant effect on muscular activity. When the subjects walked at a fast pace wearing the chairback brace, the activity of the spinal muscles was increased in the majority of subjects when compared with the activity of those muscles when no support was worn. They reasoned that because of the chairback brace's restrictive nature, the back muscles had to work harder to produce the transverse rotation of the trunk that is an inherent feature of ambulation. Since persons with lower back pain do not ordinarily walk fast, this finding is presumably of little clinical significance.

In summary, lumbosacral and thoracolumbosacral supports have been shown to have certain protective functions. The functions include an increase in intra-abdominal pressure and a decrease in intradiscal pressure, which thereby lessen the loading of the spine. These devices limit range of motion of the spine so that there is a reduction in the amount of flexion-extension and rotation for the regions in which the supports are applied. The supports also provide the user with an awareness of correct posture and the fact that certain motions should be restricted. This provides protection against the rapid kinds of dynamic motions which occur during the normal day.

These functions suggest that such devices should be used in the role of adjunct therapy since no other means has been shown to reduce stresses to a level that is sometimes required. The limitations do not, however, rule out the application of such supports as they can provide a protective role, especially in the acute stages of certain conditions.

The effect of the hyperextension brace is one of preventing flexion or forward bending of the upper lumbar and lower and mid-thoracic spine. It is an effective brace for this function, but does not have any of the other effects described for other thoracolumbosacral braces.

Sacroiliac Joints

Sacroiliac belts or supports serve to immobilize the sacroiliac joints by circumferential pressure around the pelvis. Most sacroiliac supports have a sacral pad which presses against the sacrum to add further immobilization. The only effect of a sacroiliac support is that of immobilization.

Cervical Spine

There have been relatively few quantitative evaluations of the effects of cervical orthoses. Colachis and associates[7] found that the soft collar did little to limit cervical motion and that the more rigid plastic collars were only somewhat more effective. Johnson and associates[8] found that, in general, increasing the length and rigidity of a cervical orthosis improved its ability to restrict motion. However, lateral bending and rotation throughout the entire cervical spine, as well as flexion-extension at the upper levels, were not well controlled by any of the conventional orthoses.

The goals of cervical bracing vary according to the patient's problem. Minor cervical muscle and joint injuries may only require gentle support which reminds the patient to restrict his own neck motion. A flexible collar should satisfy these goals. A more rigid orthosis may be necessary to actually limit cervical motion. No orthosis, including the halo with skeletal fixation, restricts all motion.

Another function of cervical collars and braces is to transfer the weight of the head to the shoulders, thus unloading the cervical spine. Although no scientific study supports such an effect, clinical experience indicates that collars and braces that lift under the mandible and occiput do accomplish this task.

INDICATIONS FOR SPINAL BRACING

In general, any patient with a musculoskeletal disorder who might benefit from immobilization, unloading of compressing forces on the spine and/or postural correction may be a suitable candidate for a spinal brace.

Perry[9] found that opinion among orthopaedic surgeons was divided concerning indications for braces, but that the majority of orthopaedists did prescribe a support for treatment of post-operative fusions, spondylolisthesis and pseudoarthrosis. The chairback brace was the most commonly prescribed device for these conditions. Interestingly, less than 25% of the orthopaedists surveyed prescribed supports for acute strain, post-operative discs, disc syndromes and chronic situations, with the lumbosacral corset being the device most often prescribed by this group.

Acute Sprains and Strains

It seems reasonable that acute muscle strains and joint sprains need rest and immobilization in order for healing to take place. Any movement and activity allowed should be painfree. If the injury is moderate or severe, bedrest may be required for a few days. However, a support may lend enough protection in the way of immobilization and may serve as a reminder to the patient to move carefully. This will permit greater activity without risk of aggravation. The use of supports with acute strains and sprains should be of short duration. Usually a week or so is sufficient; certainly six to eight weeks is the longest treatment time, even in the most severe cases.

Post-Surgical Fusion, Laminectomy and Discectomy

Most orthopaedic surgeons prescribe a support such as a lumbosacral corset or chairback brace for lumbar fusions and laminectomies, and a cervical support such as a soft collar, Philadelphia collar or four poster brace for cervical fusions and laminectomies. It is less common to use them following discectomies. The goal with such supports is to immobilize the area, thus relieving pain, and to remind the patient to restrict movement while allowing early ambulation and activities. Such supports are usually used for short periods of a few days to a few weeks.

Congenital or Traumatic Joint Instability

Congenital defects and severe injuries which result in spinal joint instability may be a source of constant aggravation for the patient who attempts to lead an active life. In such cases, bracing may allow the patient to participate in a vocation or in activities that otherwise would result in chronic pain and discomfort. The patient should be advised to use his support only when he needs the protection that the brace provides. It is also wise for these patients to exercise regularly to maintain adequate strength of the spinal and abdominal muscles. One should also remember that it is not always possible to cause an immobilizing effect on the spine when the patient is doing full, normal activities. This is especially true in the lower lumbar and upper cervical spine[2, 8].

If a spondylolisthesis is unstable, it can be a constant source of aggravation. In such cases, a chairback spinal brace may be effective in immobilizing the involved segments or at least may serve as a reminder to the patient that forward bending and rotation should be limited.

Spondylolisthesis is frequently associated with hyperlordosis of the lumbar spine. In such a hyperlordotic state, the shear forces between the two segments that are slipping apart is greatly magnified. Reduction of the hyperlordosis can reduce the shear forces. These cases can often be effectively managed in a brace designed to flatten the lumbar spine[10].

Children in their preteen years participating in sports requiring excessive lumbar lordosis (e.g., gymnastics) and teenagers indulging in sports of violence are more frequently found to have spondylolysis. The assumption is made that the break in the pars interarticularis represents a stress fracture. If a bone scan demonstrates an increase in activity over the pars interarticularis, this assumption is justified. Such patients can be treated with a brace that maintains the spine in lumbar flexion in an attempt to heal the stress fracture. There are not sufficient data to confirm that such healing takes place, although pain can readily be eliminated. In patients whose scans are not "hot", the assumption is made that nonunion has resulted. If pain is a problem in these cases, a lumbar brace often provides relief[10].

Herniated Nucleus Pulposus-Protrusion

Herniated nucleus pulposus-protrusion is characterized by a bulging defect caused as the nuclear gel pushes against the outer rings of the annulus. Treatment is directed toward reducing those factors that increase the compression load on the disc. Spinal bracing has been shown to reduce the intradiscal pressure in the lumbar disc by 25-35% in both the sitting and the standing positions[5, 6]. Rotation and forward bending also increase intradiscal pressure and spinal bracing can aid in restricting these movements. A brace can at least serve as a reminder to the patient to avoid these movements as well as remind the patient to maintain correct posture (lumbar extension) during recovery.

Cervical supports may also unload the disc by transferring the weight of the head onto the shoulders, but scientific research is unavailable to substantiate such claims. Such supports are sometimes helpful in maintaining the proper head and neck posture required during recovery of herniated disc syndrome.

Postural Backache (Lumbar Extension)

Postural backache caused by weak abdominal muscles and excessive lumbar lordosis is probably most effectively treated with postural correction and abdominal strengthening exercises. Extreme cases may require bracing with a lumbosacral corset, chairback brace or a Williams' brace. Since evidence shows that lumbar bracing can decrease the activity of abdominal muscles, one should be reluctant to prescribe a support or brace for treatment of postural backache. When one is prescribed, it should be accompanied with an exercise program.

Muscle Guarding and Spasm

Since spinal braces have been shown to decrease the lumbar spinal muscle activity in certain cases, it is feasible that such supports may be effective in alleviating muscle guarding and spasm.

Fractures

Various types of fractures of the spine are often treated with braces or supports. In any case requiring immobilization and/or unloading of the spine, bracing may be considered. It must be remembered that conventional lumbar and cervical orthoses do not completely immobilize the spine. Even the halo with a plastic body vest does not totally restrict movement[8]. In general, the upper cervical and lower lumbar spine are the most difficult to immobilize and fractures in these areas will be the most difficult to support with bracing. It is common to use bracing for support of fractures after some healing has taken place and restricted movement is allowed. The fact that the brace reminds the patient that he should restrict movement and maintain correct posture is often beneficial.

Compression fractures which occur in the upper lumbar and lower and mid-thoracic spine are often treated with braces. The goals of a bracing program for compression fractures are to keep the injured part of the spine in extension and to prevent flexion. This keeps the vertebral body space as wide as possible and allows the body to heal with as much height as possible. The braces are effective both because they prevent flexion and because they serve as a reminder to the patient that forward bending must be avoided. The Jewett[11] and Cash hyperextension braces are probably the most commonly used braces for treatment of compression fractures. Their sole function is to prevent flexion of the upper lumbar, lower and mid-thoracic spine and to remind the patient to maintain an extended posture.

While the hyperextension braces are effective in treating compression fractures, it has been this author's experience that some patients (especially geriatric) cannot tolerate the rigid nature of this support. In such cases, a Taylor brace or dorsal-lumbar corset may be a reasonable alternative. They offer less rigid support, but at least they offer some support and serve as a reminder to the patient to avoid flexion. An added benefit of either of these supports is that they decrease the vertical weight bearing force on the spine by increasing the intra-abdominal pressure. The hyperextension braces do not provide this effect.

Since the majority of compression fractures occur in geriatric females and are associated with severe osteoporosis, these supports may be utilized as a part of a preventive program, too. When this is done, active hyperextension exercises should be considered because in this and any other case that involves long-term wearing of a spinal support, there is the risk of muscle atrophy. Muscle atrophy occurs because the brace or support takes over the function of the muscles. Waters and Morris[1] have shown that certain braces cause a decrease in spinal and abdominal muscle activity. This phenomenon does occur if the patient assumes a passive role in the bracing program. However, muscle strengthening and improved posture can result if the patient assumes an active role in the bracing program. If the patient is instructed to avoid slumping into the brace and to hold himself in the correct posture that the brace is reminding him of, the patient will actually increase the use of the muscles needed for correct posture. For example, the shoulder straps of a Taylor or dorsal-lumbar corset are reminders to the patient to hold himself in correct posture. Their function is not to pull his shoulders back and hold him straighter. Likewise, the lordotic curve in a chairback brace is a reminder for the patient to stand and sit while actively maintaining the lordosis. Actually, this concept of active bracing is what the Milwaukee brace utilizes in the treatment of scoliosis.

Degenerative Joint/Disc Disease

Degenerative joint and/or disc disease is usually associated with joint hypomobility and treatment should be directed toward mobilizing the restricted joints and tight muscles. In severe cases, however, any mobilizing activity may tend to aggravate rather than relieve the pain and discomfort. The patient will report that any attempt to increase activities is accompanied by another flare up. In such cases, support with a spinal orthosis may at least allow the patient to participate in activities that would otherwise be too strenuous.

TYPES OF SPINAL ORTHOSES

Lumbar

Lumbosacral Corset (Fig. 10-1)

Perry[9] surveyed 5,215 orthopaedic surgeons and found that the most commonly used lumbar support was the lumbosacral corset and the second most commonly used lumbar support was the chairback. Other lumbar braces (prescribed by less than 10% of those responding to the survey) were the Williams' brace, the body cast, the flexion cast, the Goldthwait, the Bennett, the Norton-Brown and others not identified.

The lumbosacral corset is the most popular and most widely used of all spinal orthoses. Lumbosacral corsets are usually sized according to hip measurement and have a taller back than front. Most manufacturers feature styles with several different heights and developments. Development is the difference between waist size and hip size. In other words, a size 36" (hip size) with a 6" development will have a 30" waist. The most common lumbosacral corsets are made of a dacron or cotton material, have a snap front, have four to six inches of size adjustment in the side panels and are washable. Some are made out of elastic material and have velcro front closures. Most lumbosacral corsets have removable metal stays that fit in pockets along the length of the spine. The womens' lumbosacral corset has a larger development and is usually supplied with garter straps. The mens' corset is supplied with groin straps that are rarely needed if the garment is fitted correctly.

When fitting a woman's lumbosacral corset, it is important to choose a garment that does not crowd the breasts in front when the patient is sitting. The corset should come down onto the buttocks as far as possible if the lower lumbar spine is to be supported. The bottom front of the corset should

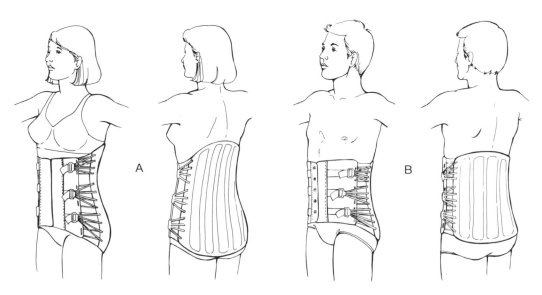

Fig. 10-1. Lumbosacral corset A) Womens' B) Mens'.

just touch the angle of the hip when the patient is sitting. The front is always closed from the bottom up. The corset should be put on the patient and adjusted to the proper size and position before the metal stays are shaped and put into place. If possible, the stays should be shaped to the normal standing lordosis of the patient. It is usually difficult to alter the lumbar lordosis with this type of support, but the corset serves as a reminder of correct posture and the patient alters the lordosis actively.

The lumbosacral corset is a flexible support and is relatively ineffective in restricting movement, especially lower lumbar movement, yet it can be effective as a reminder to the patient to avoid movement and to maintain correct posture. It is effective in increasing intra-abdominal pressure, thus reducing intradiscal pressure in the treatment of HNP-protrusion.

If the patient is in acute discomfort, he should put the corset on and take it off while lying down. Generally, the support is worn at all times when the patient is out of bed if the condition is severe. In other cases, the patient may only wear the support while doing activities that would cause possible aggravation. The support is seldom worn while lying down and resting.

Chairback brace (Fig. 10-2)

The chairback brace is a popular rigid lumbo-sacral brace that provides greater immobilization than the lumbosacral corset. It consists of two uprights, pelvic and thoracic bands posteriorly and a piepan abdominal support anteriorly. The brace effectively restricts lumbar and lumbosacral rotation and lumbar flexion. It is less effective in restricting flexion in the lumbosacral area. In addition, it has all of the support capabilities of the lumbosacral corset. Chairback braces are fitted according to hip size and length from the mid-sacral to the lower thoracic spine. The brace is made of metal covered with leather and is somewhat cooler to wear than the lumbosacral corset. The same fitting procedures outlined for the lumbosacral corset should be followed.

Knight Spinal Brace (Fig. 10-3)

The Knight spinal brace is similar to the chairback with the addition of lateral uprights and a full corset-like front. It is somewhat more rigid and restricts lateral bending better than the chairback. It is sized the same as the chairback brace.

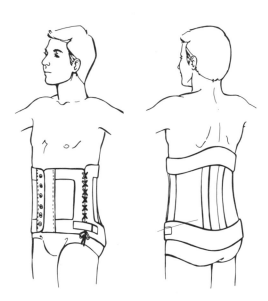

Fig. 10-3. Knight spinal brace.

Williams' Brace (Fig. 10-4)

The Williams' brace provides a three-point pressure system consisting of a posteriorly directed force from the pelvic adjustment strap and anteriorly directed forces from the pelvic and thoracic bands. This pressure system tends to limit lumbar extension and reduce lordosis. The brace also tends to limit lateral bending. The brace is made of metal covered with leather and has a corset front.

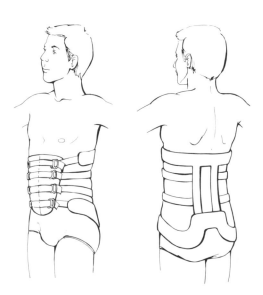

Fig. 10-2. Chairback brace.

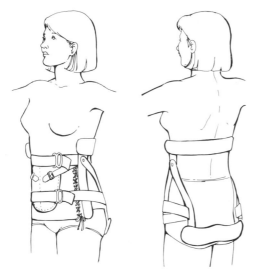

Fig. 10-4. Williams' brace.

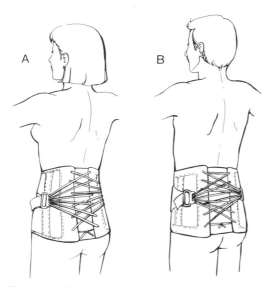

Fig. 10-5. Sacroiliac belt A) Womens' B) Mens'.

Sacroiliac

Sacroiliac Belt (Fig. 10-5)

The sacroiliac belt partially stabilizes the sacro-iliac joints and symphysis pubis. It is fitted by hip size. It must fit relatively tight to accomplish any degree of immobilization and must fit low around the pelvis to be effective. It is used post-partum, post-traumatic injury and for hypermobility of the sacroiliac joints[12]. The mens' sacroiliac belt is four to six inches wide and the womens' sacroiliac belt is six to nine inches wide with a larger development. A removable sacral pad is included.

Thoracolumbosacral

Dorsal-lumbar Corset (Fig. 10-6)

The dorsal-lumbar corset is sized according to hip measurement and is available in several lengths and developments. It is similar to the lumbosacral corset with additional height in the back and straps that loop around the shoulders. It provides the same function in the lumbosacral spine as the lumbosacral corset. It also provides immobilization and support to the lower and mid-thoracic spine. The shoulder loops serve as a reminder to the patient to stand and sit up straight. They are not effective in holding the patient straighter and, if they fit too tightly, they will irritate the underarms.

The dorsal-lumbar corset is used for treatment of compression fracture and osteoporosis for patients who do not require the more rigid support

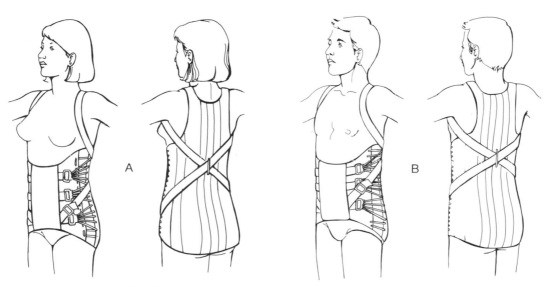

Fig. 10-6. Dorsal-lumber corset A) Womens' B) Mens'.

of a Taylor or hyperextension brace, or for those patients who are too feeble to wear one of the more rigid supports. Dorsal-lumbar corsets are also used for other conditions of the lower and mid-thoracic spine, such as sprains, strains and degenerative joint/disc disease.

Taylor Brace (Fig. 10-7)

The Taylor brace is similar to the chairback brace, except that the posterior uprights extend into the mid-thoracic region and there are straps that loop around the shoulders. The thoracic band may be absent. It is sized similarly and serves the same function as the dorsal-lumbar corset, except that it provides a more rigid immobilization support.

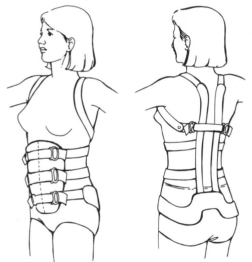

Fig. 10-7. Taylor brace.

Knight-Taylor Brace (Fig. 10-8)

The Knight-Taylor brace is similar to the Taylor with the addition of lateral uprights and a full corset-like front. It is somewhat more rigid and restricts lateral bending better than the Taylor.

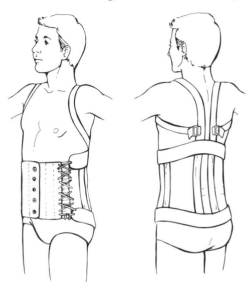

Fig. 10-8. Knight-Taylor brace.

Hyperextension Brace (Fig. 10-9)

The hyperextension brace provides a three-point fixation system consisting of posteriorly directed forces from the sternal and suprapubic pads and an anteriorly directed force from the thoracolumbar pad. This fixation system causes hyperextension and restricts flexion in the thoracolumbar

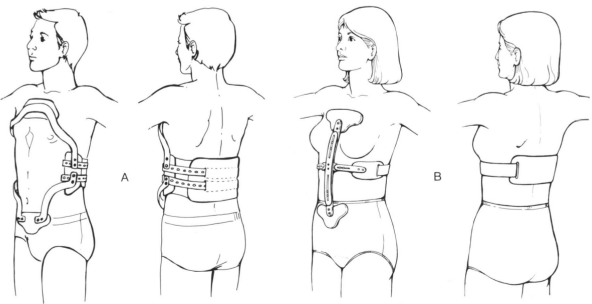

Fig. 10-9. A) Jewett brace B) Cash brace.

spine. Control of flexion is achieved by the pads only; the frame should not contact the patient. With the patient seated in the prescribed posture and the orthosis properly adjusted and aligned, the sternal pad will have its superior border 1/2 inch inferior to the sternal notch and the suprapubic pad will have its inferior border 1/2 inch superior to the symphysis pubis. Hyperextension braces are normally sized by height, hip circumference and chest circumference.

Cervical

Soft (Foam) Collars (Fig. 10-10)

Soft collars have very little, if any, immobilizing effect. They do, through sensory feedback, serve as a reminder to limit head and neck motion, especially flexion. They do not provide forces to position the head in certain postures. However, if they are properly positioned under the mandible and occipital line, they partially unload the cervical spine by supporting a portion of the weight of the head. They are sized according to neck circumference and height. Exact measurements will depend upon the desired head and neck position and expected function.

Hard (Plastic) Collars (Fig. 10-11)

Hard collars serve basically the same function as soft collars, but do so with greater immobilizing and supporting effect. Most collars are adjustable and are sized according to neck circumference and height. A chin support (plastic cup) may be added to the hard collar for additional support and control.

Philadelphia Collar (Fig. 10-12)

The Philadelphia collar is a molded plastic, semi-rigid orthosis designed to provide support effects similar to the other cervical supports described in this chapter. The Philadelphia collar is lightweight and may be more comfortable than other cervical orthoses. This collar may also serve as a foundation for cervical casting. This support is significantly more effective than the soft collar and is almost as effective as the more rigid cervical braces (four poster and Somi) in controlling flexion-extension between the occiput and third cervical vertebrae. It is less effective than other rigid braces at the middle and lower cervical levels.

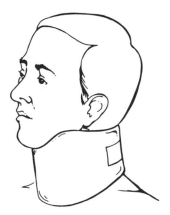

Fig. 10-10. Soft cervical collar.

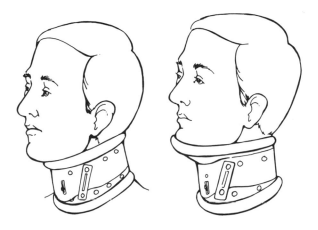

Fig. 10-11. Hard cervical collars.

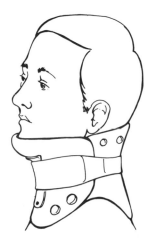

Fig. 10-12. Philadelphia collar.

Two and Four Poster Braces (Fig. 10-13)

The two or four poster brace applies forces under the chin and occiput to restrict flexion and extension of the head and cervical spine. These orthoses include an anterior section consisting of a sternal plate, one or two uprights and a chin support, and a posterior section consisting of a thoracic plate, one or two uprights and an occipital support. The two sections are connected by flexible straps between the chin and occipital supports and by over-the-shoulder straps between the thoracic and sternal plates. The uprights are adjustable for height and position of the chin and occipital supports. They are made of aluminum with leather or plastic padding of the parts that touch the body. A thoracic extension may be added to provide increased support and rotatory control. However, this may impart undesired thoracic movement to the cervical spine. The advantage of this support is that fine adjustments can be made and that it is more rigid than the soft or hard collars. This orthosis is effective in restricting flexion in the mid-cervical spine. If the thoracic extension is applied, it is also effective in restricting flexion in the lower cervical spine. It is only partially effective in restricting lateral bending and upper cervical flexion-extension. This brace is sized small, medium and large.

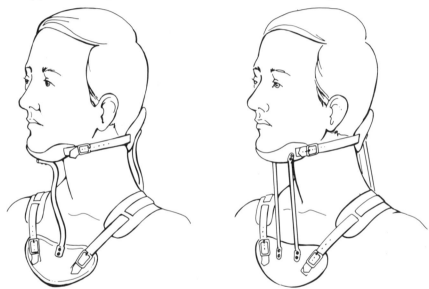

Fig. 10-13. Two and four poster cervical braces.

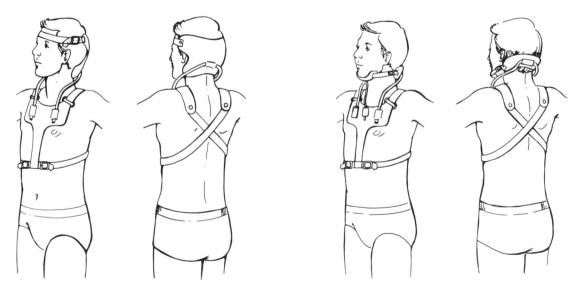

Fig. 10-14. Somi brace.

Somi Brace (Fig. 10-14)

The Somi brace is a prefabricated cervico-thoracic orthosis consisting of a rigid metal frame which rests on the front of the chest, two padded metal strips that pass posteriorly over the shoulders and adjustable uprights that extend up to the mandibular and occipital supports. Two straps connect to the shoulder extension, cross over the back and are secured to the lower portion of the frame in front. This brace is relatively easy to adjust and can be applied with the patient lying supine. Many patients find it more comfortable than the four poster cervical brace. Johnson[8] found that the Somi was the most effective conventional orthosis in controlling flexion in the upper cervical spine, but that it was less effective in controlling extension and lateral bending and flexion in the lower cervical spine than the four poster braces. This brace is sized small, medium and large.

Fitting Procedures

In addition to the sizing information mentioned for each type of spinal orthosis, the following tips for using a spinal orthosis are offered:

1. A spinal orthosis is seldom effective in mechanically correcting posture. Its effectiveness in correcting posture comes from reminding the patient to actively maintain the desired posture. For this reason, small corrections are often possible but one should not expect a brace to hold a patient in a posture that he cannot actively assume with some degree of ease. The therapist should have the patient assume his optimum posture, then the brace should be fitted to conform to that posture.

2. It is often desirable to explain to the patient the effects of the various braces and supports being considered for his condition, then fit each of them to the patient and let the patient make the final selection. In other words, a brace hanging in the closet that the patient will not wear is not going to help.

3. When the patient's condition is acute, he may need to wear a support at all times except when recumbent. If this is the case, the support must be put on and taken off while the patient is lying down. The best method of doing this is to roll to the side, place the support against the posterior spine, roll back onto the support and fasten the support in the front.

4. Most of the braces and supports described in this chapter are more comfortable with a cotton undershirt or T-shirt worn underneath. This also helps absorb perspiration and keeps the support clean longer.

MANAGEMENT OF PATIENTS WITH SPINAL ORTHOSES

In most cases, spinal bracing is an adjunct to other physical therapy treatment. The importance of exercises has already been mentioned. The value of using spinal supports as a reminder to the patient to maintain correct posture and restrict certain movements is often an important adjunct to other treatments. The unloading effect on the intervertebral disc is an important adjunct to the rest, traction and exercise programs that are often required for these patients.

Perry[9] found that many of the orthopaedic surgeons she surveyed indicated that spinal bracing is only one facet in the management of a spinal disorder. The value of exercise as either a preferable substitute for bracing or as an adjunct to bracing was emphasized. The use of braces as a short-term treatment rather than a long-term management was often mentioned. "Never prescribe a support without a plan to eliminate it" summarized the feelings of many.

MEASURING INSTRUCTIONS FOR BRACES AND CORSETS

These measurements are approximate only. Each garment must be fitted individually to the patient.

Lumbosacral Corset
Hip circumference
Waist circumference (to determine development)
Height in back from sacrococcygeal joint to lower thoracic area (approximately T10)
Height in front from angle of hip to comfortable clearance below breasts with patient seated

Chairback Brace-Knight Brace-Williams' Brace
Hip circumference
Height in back to patient's comfort (from ap-

proximately mid-sacral to lower thoracic spine)

Sacroiliac Belt

Hip circumference

Dorsal-Lumbar Corset

Hip circumference

Waist circumference (to determine development)

Height in back from sacrococcygeal joint to one inch below superior angle of scapula

Height in front from angle of hip to comfortable clearance below breasts with patient seated

Taylor Brace-Knight-Taylor Brace

Hip circumference

Height in back from mid-sacral spine to one inch below superior angle of scapula

Hyperextension Brace

Height in front from pubic symphysis to sternal notch, less one inch

Circumference of hips

Circumference of chest

Cervical Soft Collar-Hard Collar-Philadelphia Collar

Circumference of neck

Height to position and support head as desired

Two and Four Poster Braces-Somi Brace

Sized small, medium and large according to height and body build of patient

---

References:

1. Waters, R and Morris, J: Effect of Spinal Supports on the Electrical Activity of Muscles of the Trunk. Joul of Bone and Jt Surg, 52A:51-60, 1970.
2. Norton, P and Brown, T: The Immobilizing Efficiency of Back Braces. Joul of Bone and Jt Surg, 39A:111-139, 1957.
3. Lumsden, R and Morris, J: An In Vivo Study of Axial Rotation and Immobilization at the Lumbosacral Joint. Joul of Bone and Jt Surg, 50A:1591-1602, 1968.
4. Wasserman, J and McNamee, M: Engineering Evaluation of Lumbosacral Orthoses Using In Vivo Noninvasive Testing. Proceedings of the 10th Southeast Conference of Theoretical and Applied Mechanics, 1980.
5. Morris, J; Lucas, M and Bresler, M: Role of the Trunk in Stability of the Spine. Joul of Bone and Jt Surg, 43A:327-351, April 1961.
6. Nachemson, A and Morris, J: In Vivo Measurements of Intradiscal Pressure. Joul of Bone and Jt Surg, 46A:1077-1092, July 1964.
7. Colachis, S; Strohm, B and Ganter, E: Cervical Spine Motion in Normal Women: Radiographic Study of Effect of Cervical Collars. Arch of Phy Med Rehabil, 54:161-169, 1973.
8. Johnson, R: Hart, D; Simmons, E; Ramshy, G and Southwick, W: Cervical Orthosis. Joul of Bone and Jt Surg, 59A:332-339, 1977.
9. Perry, J: The Use of External Support in the Treatment of Low Back Pain. Joul of Bone and Jt Surg, 52A:1440-1442, 1970.
10. Watts, H: Bracing in Spinal Deformities. Orthopedic Clinics of North America, 10:769-785, 1979.
11. Jewett, E: Fracture of the Spine: New Treatment Without Plaster Casts. Joul of the International College of Surgeons, 13: 1950.
12. Atlas of Orthotics. American Academy of Orthopaedic Surgeons, CV Mosby, St. Louis, 1975.

CHAPTER 11

EDUCATIONAL BACK CARE PROGRAMS

Educational back care programs are most effective when designed to primarily teach people without back injuries. They may have had previous problems but at present they are working in industry, business or the professions. Educational back care programs can also be adapted as general education programs for people currently experiencing back problems. However, these people will also need individualized instructions specifically designed for them.

While most of this chapter deals with the educational aspects of back care, the principles that are presented can be incorporated into a total back care program. When a company or institution becomes involved in all phases of back care a truly comprehensive program develops. This enhances the overall effectiveness of each individual phase.

PHASES OF A COMPREHENSIVE BACK CARE PROGRAM

1) **Work Site Evaluation and Modification** — Many things can be done to make the work place safer. If the principles that an effective educational program teaches are applied to design or modify the work place, many back injuries can be avoided[1]. Special attention should be directed toward jobs that require forward bending and lifting and standing or sitting for prolonged periods of time in a slumped or forward bent posture.

According to Snook, the most effective control for low back injuries is the ergonomic approach of designing the job to fit the worker. This approach is only partially effective, however. His study shows that manual handling tasks (i.e., lifting, lowering, pushing, pulling and carrying) were implicated as the specific act or movement associated with back pain in 70% of the reported injuries from over 6,000 industrial clients of Liberty Mutual Insurance Company. Lifting tasks were implicated in almost one-half of those back injuries[1].

Manual handling tasks are often evaluated according to the weight of the material being handled. However, since strength varies greatly among individuals, there is no one maximum weight that applies to everyone. Snook feels that a better way to evaluate a manual handling task is in terms of the percentage of the working population that can be expected to perform the task without overexertion. He has analyzed various tasks and movements and has divided them into two categories: 1) Manual handling tasks which 75% or more of the working population can handle without overexertion, plus all acts or movements other than lifting, lowering, pushing, pulling and carrying; and 2) Manual handling tasks which less than 75% of the working population can handle without overexertion. His analysis includes object weights, horizontal and vertical distances from the lumbosacral joint, the number of repetitions per unit of time, the initial force, the sustained force, and the pushing, pulling or carrying distance[1-3]. The goal of ergonomic job analysis is thus to determine if a job or task can be done by 75% or more of the working population without overexertion and, if it cannot, to redesign the job so that it can be done.

2) **Preplacement Screening** — Pre-employment and preplacement examinations which use a variety of selection techniques such as medical histories, medical examinations and low back x-rays have not been shown to be effective methods of screening workers who are potential back injury risks[1]. Evaluations of physical fitness levels and spinal flexibilities have been shown to be effective ways of predicting incidence and severity of low back injuries[4-8]. Therefore, individuals who lack spinal flexibility and strength or who are in generally poor physical condition probably should not be placed on certain jobs. Although it is difficult to discriminate against these individuals unless it can be proven that they will be unable to perform a certain job or task, a preplacement screening program may demonstrate to an individual that he needs to improve his level of physical fitness and spinal strength and flexibility. This, then, is the beginning of the back care educational process.

3) **Medical Management of Acute Back Disorders** — Key management personnel in a company or institution should have knowledge and understanding of the medical management of acute back injuries. The injured worker can go to a variety of places for treatment of his disorder. Some of these treatments may be ineffective or may even cause

297

harm. Companies should be aware of this. They should also understand medical management well enough to direct the injured worker to medical practitioners who practice acute care management in a cost-effective, conservative and common sense manner which emphasizes education of the patient rather than expensive tests and passive treatment. Therefore, teaching the executive elements of companies and institutions how to manage back injuries when they do occur becomes a key part of a comprehensive educational program.

4) Back Fitness — Rehabilitation — Work Hardening Programs — The ultimate treatment for most back disorders involves exercises to restore strength, flexibility and physical fitness. Many times patients with back disorders are treated with medication, modalities and/or surgery during the acute phase. Nothing is actually done to rehabilitate the patient. Much more emphasis needs to be directed toward the rehabilitation phase to prevent the recurrence of the disorder. Companies can play an active role in this phase. Some actually have on-site exercise and fitness programs.

5) Educational Programs for Management and Supervisors — An effective educational back care program should contain material for teaching preventative back care to management and supervisory level personnel as well as instructions on managing back injuries when they do occur. As mentioned earlier, emphasis should be directed toward understanding of medical management as well as development of a proper attitude toward back injuries. Management and supervisors need to understand that most injured workers are not faking or exaggerating their problems and that management should work with the employee to get him back on the job rather than treating him with suspicion. This may involve assigning the worker to a light duty job to keep him in the habit of working.

6) Educational Programs for Workers — Back injury prevention training has been shown to be effective and is an important aspect of a comprehensive back care program[8-11]. A back care program should teach how the back works. It should help dispel misunderstandings about the various types of back disorders, what causes them and the value of various treatments. It should help the participant understand how to avoid a back injury, describe treatments for back disorders and explain what can be done if a back disorder is already present.

7) Chronic Pain Management — Although most back injuries can be prevented or managed effectively with treatment and education, there are occasions when severe, long-term disorders develop. In these cases, individuals must be treated with chronic pain management techniques and must be taught how to deal with their problems. Special clinics should be available to handle these cases.

8) Functional Capabilities Evaluation — A functional capabilities evaluation is devised to assess physical capabilities and limitations which relate to work, recreation or activities of daily living. This is a relatively new health care service arising from the needs of both the medical and vocational fields, primarily with regard to worker's compensation cases. Through objective testing, determinations are made of a person's safe level of lifting, carrying, pushing, pulling, sitting, standing and kneeling tolerances and other functional activities specifically relating to work demands[12, 13].

In addition to these objective findings, subjective information may be provided describing the observed levels of functioning, need for rest, usefulness of adaptations, pacing, cooperation, pain behavior and consistency[12].

As part of the assessment, the participant may be educated on movement and body mechanics. When performing heavy tasks, the client's body mechanics should be evaluated before and after the evaluation. Recommendations may then be made to assist the individual in performing tasks efficiently and safely to help prevent further injury and to increase on-the-job performance[12].

The functional capabilities evaluation program becomes a tool for the medical profession, providing data that are arrived at scientifically, with specific return-to-work recommendations[13].

9) Program Evaluation — Pretests and post-tests are not effective ways to evaluate a back care program. Such tests should be used to create interest and to summarize important points. The true test of a back care program is whether or not it effectively decreases the incidence and severity of back injuries. Companies should be encouraged to collect data and conduct longitudinal studies to determine the effectiveness of their programs.

10) Follow-up Review — Plans should be made to follow the initial educational effort with periodic review presentations. These can consist of a shorter stand-up presentation, a slide/tape program or a film. Time should be allowed to answer questions that have arisen since the previous presentation.

11) Ongoing Program and Consultation —

Because of constant change in both personnel and working conditions, a comprehensive back care program needs to be carried out as an ongoing process. New ideas should be incorporated into the existing program. As a company expands or changes the working environment, the "back care expert" should be consulted to make sure that the design and layout are as safe as possible.

12) **Promotion** — Educational back care programs can be promoted in many ways. The best way is to establish by documented results that the program is effective in reducing the incidence and severity of back injuries. Contacts with patients, physicians and occupational medicine departments are effective methods of promoting a back care program. Personnel managers and safety engineers are often the key people in companies who are concerned with development of a comprehensive back care program. Insurance companies, attorneys, labor unions and rehabilitation consultants are also valuable contacts. Brochures and informational letters can be sent to all of these prospective clients. Exhibits at health fairs, trade fairs and professional society meetings are also effective ways of promoting a back care program.

THE SCOPE

Educational back care programs are designed to help companies prevent and manage back injuries in industrial settings. They have emerged out of a need to control the epidemic rise of work-related back injuries.

Programs should be designed for supervisors and workers in areas where past experience has shown a significant incidence of back injuries. It is anticipated that this potentially includes all types of work settings, as statistics show that back injuries are not limited to heavy industry, but also occur in other groups such as office workers. There are considerable data available to indicate that a very serious problem exists, but there is only limited evidence to show that back injuries can be prevented by any means[1,8]. One of the long-range objectives of any back care program should be to determine if programs of this nature can be effective in reducing the number and severity of work-related back injuries.

Although the basic program should remain constant, the presentations will need to be varied to suit the individual needs of each participating company. Analysis of individual problems and specific work conditions should be made and incorporated into each program before it is actually presented.

The general objective of a total back care program should be to reduce the incidence and severity of work-related back injuries and to help the company manage back injuries when they do occur. This will result in cost savings to the company and reduce pain and suffering as well as avoid loss of income by the individual worker.

A brief introduction to the program should be presented to administrative and supervisory level personnel first so that they will be aware of and have input into the content of the final program. In this way, supervisors can support and reinforce the ideas and principles presented to their workers. This is important because one often encounters an atmosphere of suspicion between supervisor and worker. When a back injury occurs, it is essential that top and middle management be supportive of the principles that the program teaches.

THE NEED

Low back pain affects a large proportion of industrialized countries and causes an increasing number of lost work days each year. All working groups, social classes and both sexes are equally represented. Clerical workers suffer back pain as often as housewives and laborers. Although laborers may need longer periods of convalescence, the frequency of illness is the same. Recurrences are common. Adults of any age may be affected although the incidence of back pain does decline in people over 60. This is small comfort to people in their 20's who may lose many work days due to back problems and who statistically can expect several episodes of increasing pain during the following decades[14].

The number of cases of back pain has reached epidemic proportions in our society. It is estimated that 80% to 90% of the general population will experience back pain sometime in their lifetimes. Low back pain is the most expensive ailment in the 30 to 60 age group. In 1983, $17 billion dollars were spent in the treatment of industrial back injuries. The National Safety Council reports that 27% of all reported injuries were back injuries, accounting for 38% of workmen's compensation payments. The direct medical cost for a back injury presently averages $800 to $1000 per incident. This does not take into account the costs of replacement personnel, decreased production, retraining or down time[14].

With growing appreciation of what these and many more statistical surveys show, there is an obvious need for modification and progress in our efforts to control or limit the detrimental personal, societal and economic effects of back disorders. The short consultation time possible with the present medical organization does not allow the physician to analyze the patient's work situation in detail, inform him about his prognosis and raise his morale. Medical personnel have spent years working with patients who have back problems and have often become frustrated in trying to cure and rehabilitate this difficult disability. The logical solution thus becomes prevention in the form of educational programs.

THE PURPOSE

The general purposes of an educational back care program are: 1) To enable employees to play an active part in improving their working environment in order to reduce their back problems; 2) To provide increased knowledge and better understanding so as to reduce the risk of inappropriate therapy; 3) To reduce the demand on social, medical and economic resources resulting from avoidable back pain; and 4) To provide the participant with a positive, knowledgeable approach to exercises and activities.

Educational programs help to solve the back pain problem by approaching it in an organized, practical way, within the reach of often limited resources. It can certainly be seen that as research develops better treatment techniques and more definitive diagnostic procedures, the care of the back, both preventative and remedial, will improve.

The specific objectives of an educational back care program are: 1) To educate the participant in the basics of anatomy and mechanics of the spine; 2) To educate the participant in how to recognize and avoid potentially harmful situations, thus preventing the incidence and severity of back injuries; 3) To acquaint the participant with the common types of back disorders; 4) To create self-confidence so that the participant may effectively adjust to and manage a back disorder if it develops; 5) To inform the participant so that he may avoid excess or potentially harmful treatments; 6) To acquaint the participant with ways that he can change his lifestyle in order to avoid a back disorder; 7) To educate management and supervisory personnel in how to manage back injuries when they do occur; and 8) To decrease expenses and suffering.

THE METHOD

Although a program of this nature must be flexible in order to meet the individual needs of companies and institutions, a standard or model program should be developed. The basic program that this author uses consists of two 90-minute lessons conducted by a qualified and experienced physical therapist, physician or occupational nurse. A maximum of 30 participants should be included in each course. Instructions should be carried out by means of an audio-visual program, demonstration and active participation by the class members.

The first lesson should start with a summary of the contents of the whole course. The participants should be instructed in detail about the anatomy and function of the back and the results of research and studies on the back. It should be emphasized that almost all back problems are the result of months or even years of poor posture, faulty body mechanics, stressful living and working habits, loss of flexibility and a general decline in physical fitness, and not by the single event that may have started the pain.

The mechanical strain in different positions and during different movements should be discussed and the relationship between the center of gravity and strain on the back should also be explained. The function of the muscles and their influence on the back should be demonstrated.

Four common, unfavorable working postures should be analyzed in detail:

1) In the seated position, support should be provided behind (by means of a backrest) or in front of the body. The participants should be told, however, to avoid working for too long in the seated position if possible.

2) Working in the standing position and leaning forward is just as bad as the seated position unless the strain is lessened by using various aids and properly distributing the body weight.

3) Working in the standing position with the knees locked, stomach muscles relaxed and a sway back places the body weight on the ligaments and soon results in backache.

4) Bending forward and lifting is probably the most common position in which injury occurs.

The pathology of back injury (muscle, ligament, disc and joint) should also be discussed in relation to the above-mentioned stressful postures.

Different aspects of back disorders should be discussed. Various methods of treatment should be talked about and the body's natural capacity for healing should be emphasized. The fact that decreased strain on the back will help to relieve the pain and that increased strain on the tissues will lead to an increase in the symptoms should also be emphasized. From the outset of the program, participants should, as a matter of importance, be taught the most relaxing positions and postures for relief of discomfort.

In the second 90-minute lesson, the program should teach the individual what to do when a back injury occurs. Participants should be taught that what **they** do to manage their back injuries is almost always more important than what the doctor does.

Many workers recognize how to lift and carry, but they do not stop to think that the task which they are about to perform may threaten their backs. Instruction should be directed strongly toward attitudes, forcing one to recognize lifting, carrying, pushing and pulling tasks as potential problems, and toward helping one perform the tasks properly.

This lesson should encourage the participant to review his personal standards of fitness, nutrition and stress control. Participation in various types of physical activity and sports should be encouraged in order to improve psychological and physical tolerance to pain and stress. The participant should be informed that nutrition is often considered to be the foundation of health. Overweight people tend to have a vicious cycle going on within their bodies. Increased weight leads to greater wear and tear on joints, which can make them irritated and painful. This increased discomfort forces a person to become less and less active, thereby favoring further weight gain. It should be pointed out that stress has a direct effect on one's emotions and that stress affects the muscle tension. The participant should be told, if necessary, how relaxation exercises can be helpful in stress problems.

Special attention should be devoted to lifting and carrying methods and work positions. Advice on procedure during an acute attack of back pain should be given and some of the more common problems in activities of daily living, such as getting in and out of bed, should be addressed.

At the conclusion of the program the participants should actually participate in a flexibility and strength evaluation and should practice an exercise program that will help them maintain a healthy back. Participants should also practice proper body mechanics and posture techniques.

Considerable emphasis should be directed toward the company's role in management of back injuries when they do occur. Managers and supervisors play a key role in directing the injured worker to proper medical care. A company can do many things to influence the outcome of a back injury. A good educational program teaches managers and supervisors the things which can be done to effect a positive outcome.

Each participant should receive a booklet or pamphlet outlining the content of the course. The booklet should also contain a section of general flexibility and strengthening exercises for the spine. Each of the exercises should be demonstrated and discussed in the class.

THE PRESENTATION

In most cases, programs are more successful if presented by instructors who have had actual experience using the principles that the program teaches. Live, stand-up presentations are usually more effective than films or slide/tape presentations, although such audiovisuals can be used if time is allowed at their conclusion for live demonstrations, questions and active participation. Open discussion should be encouraged.

The following paragraphs outline the important points that should be included in an educational back care program.

Introduction — The instructor should begin by explaining that the program teaches how to avoid having a back injury, or if a back disorder already exists, the program will enable the participant to manage his back problem most effectively. The instructor should emphasize that the management, as the sponsor of the program, has invited him to present this program and that this is being done not just as a money saving venture, but also because the management is truly concerned about the welfare of its employees. If the participants do not know the instructor's background as an expert in the management of back problems, it would be appropriate at this point for the instructor to tell the participants what his education and experience background is and the reason for his interest in this subject.

Back pain is no joke (Fig. 11-1). Back disorders are real, even though some people do take advantage of workmen's compensation or insurance benefits. Back injuries that involve a worker who seems to be taking advantage of this system often involve a situation in which the supervisor was not supportive of the individual when the injury first occurred. Then, because the worker is treated as a faker, he becomes angry and turns what may be a minor back injury into a major back injury. This often happens because of frustration and anger toward the company and supervisor who treated him with suspicion in the beginning. If workers are given some attention, understanding and treatment or light duty immediately following the injury, most of them will be satisfied and will be able to return to work soon. When a worker does take advantage of the compensation system by exaggerating or faking a back injury, it tends to make a company or supervisor suspicious of all workers who have back disorders. We must all make an effort to be fair and honest when dealing with back injuries and must certainly recognize that most people are not faking or exaggerating their problems or pains. One of the major points that should be stressed throughout an educational program is that the doctor, therapist, company executives and supervisors must all have an understanding of back injuries and their management. They must work **with** the injured worker in order to get him back on the job rather than treat him with suspicion, possibly turning him into a "back cripple."

Back injuries are not new and throughout history there have been references to the suffering that has plagued man because of back disorders. The frequency and severity of back injuries is increasing, however, primarily due to two important factors: 1) Today people get very little physical exercise. Evidence shows that people in poor physical condition are much more likely to develop a back disorder. This idea should be developed throughout the presentation. 2) Back injuries are increasing because more time is being spent in flexed, forward bent postures. Sitting, standing in a forward bent posture, forward bending and lifting all involve flexion of the spine. It is believed that most back disorders are caused by the stress that this flexed position places on the spine.

It is important that the participants understand that back disorders are seldom caused by a single injury. Most people think that their back disorder occurred at a particular time and place. This is almost always not the case. A back injury is analogous to heart disease in that it takes months or even years for it to occur. Damage can be occurring long before pain is noticed. Then, a twist or fall causes pain. The twist or fall did not cause the injury but was like the "straw that broke the camel's back" and caused pain to become perceived. A healthy back is highly unlikely to be injured by a single twist, lift or fall.

We can cause considerable stress to our backs without injury. The instructor should point out that football players seldom have back injuries even though they are doing things that are quite stressful to their backs. The reason is that they maintain a

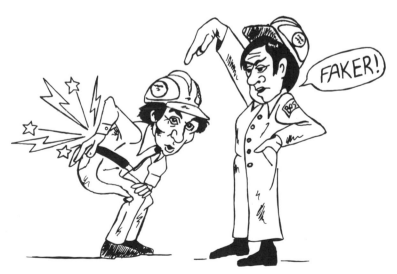

Fig. 11-1. Back pain is no joke. Back disorders are real, even though some people do take advantage of worker's compensation or insurance benefits.

high degree of general physical fitness, flexibility and strength. As long as these factors are operative, the back can withstand much stress without injury. The instructor also needs to emphasize that almost all back injuries are the result of poor posture, faulty body mechanics, stressful living and working habits, loss of flexibility and a general decline of physical fitness. These are the **real** causes of back disorders. Back disorders cannot be managed effectively unless these factors are recognized and dealt with.

Eight out of every ten people will have a significant back disorder in their lifetimes. Most back disorders occur in persons who are 30-50 years old with the incidence of back disorders actually declining after age 50. Once developed, a back disorder will typically recur on a fairly regular, intermittent basis. This is because treatment is seldom effectively directed toward correcting or eliminating the cause of the disorder. If we redirect our treatment efforts, the above statistics do not have to remain true. This idea is one of the major points of an educational back care program and should be stressed throughout the presentation.

Back injuries are incredibly costly. Ninety-three million work days are lost annually in industry and 17 billion dollars are spent annually (1983) in treatment, not to mention the individual pain and suffering that is also encountered. In many industries today, back injury claims account for over fifty percent of the total workmen's compensation benefits.

Generally speaking, medical treatment has failed because treatment has been directed toward symptoms such as pain and muscle spasm and has not addressed the real causes. Evidence shows that patients with back disorders are seldom helped by many of the costly treatments that are fostered upon them. American medical care is almost totally directed toward treatment rather than prevention. Ninety-seven percent of all medical expenses involve diagnosis and treatment of ailments and disorders **after** they occur. Only three percent is spent to help people learn how they can prevent problems and live healthy lives.

Although the problems associated with back disorders seem to be overwhelming, most back disorders are unnecessary and can be prevented. An effective back care program should teach how the back works. The program should help to dispel misunderstandings about back disorders, explaining the various types of back disorders and what causes them. It should help individuals understand how to avoid a back injury. It should also describe appropriate treatment for back disorders and tell what can be done if a back disorder is already present.

Anatomy — If an individual is going to have a healthy back, it is important that he understand how his back works. The spine must perform the dual, contrasting roles of *rigidity* to support the trunk and *flexibility* to allow mobility. It is recommended that the instructor have a flexible spine for demonstration and for examination by the participants. Using the spinal model, the instructor should demonstrate the flexibility of the spine, pointing out the normal physiological curves and explaining their role in strength and shock absorption. It should be pointed out that even if only one of the curves in the spine is lost, the shock absorbing capability of the spine is reduced considerably. The spine also provides protection for the spinal cord (Fig. 11-2). The four regions of the spine should be shown and explained in simple terms. The cervical or neck region is made up of seven vertebrae and is quite flexible. The thoracic or chest region is made up of twelve vertebrae. There is generally less mobility in this region because the ribs attach to these vertebrae. The lumbar or lower back region is made up of five vertebrae. The instructor should show how flexible the lumbar region is and emphasize that with forward bending, the lordosis tends to reverse, placing most of the weight on the anterior portion of the disc. With backward bending, the lordosis is increased and most of the weight is transferred to the posterior aspect of the disc and the facet joints. The sacrum is made up of the fusion of five vertebrae into a solid mass which supports the rest of the spine. The sacrum attaches the spine to the pelvis.

The fact that the spine is not straight but is actually made up of four continuous curves which allow for strength and flexibility, helping the spine in its role as a shock absorber, should be re-emphasized. One of the keys to having a healthy back is the maintenance of these curves in a balanced posture. If one of the curves becomes flattened or excessive, the balance and mobility of the spine will be altered and a disorder may eventually develop.

The differences between the cervical, thoracic and lumbar vertebrae should be noted, especially the size of the vertebral bodies and the orientation of the facet joints. The important parts of the vertebrae include the vertebral body, the disc, the intervertebral foramina, the spinal canal, the facet joints and the transverse and spinous processes. Most of

ANATOMY

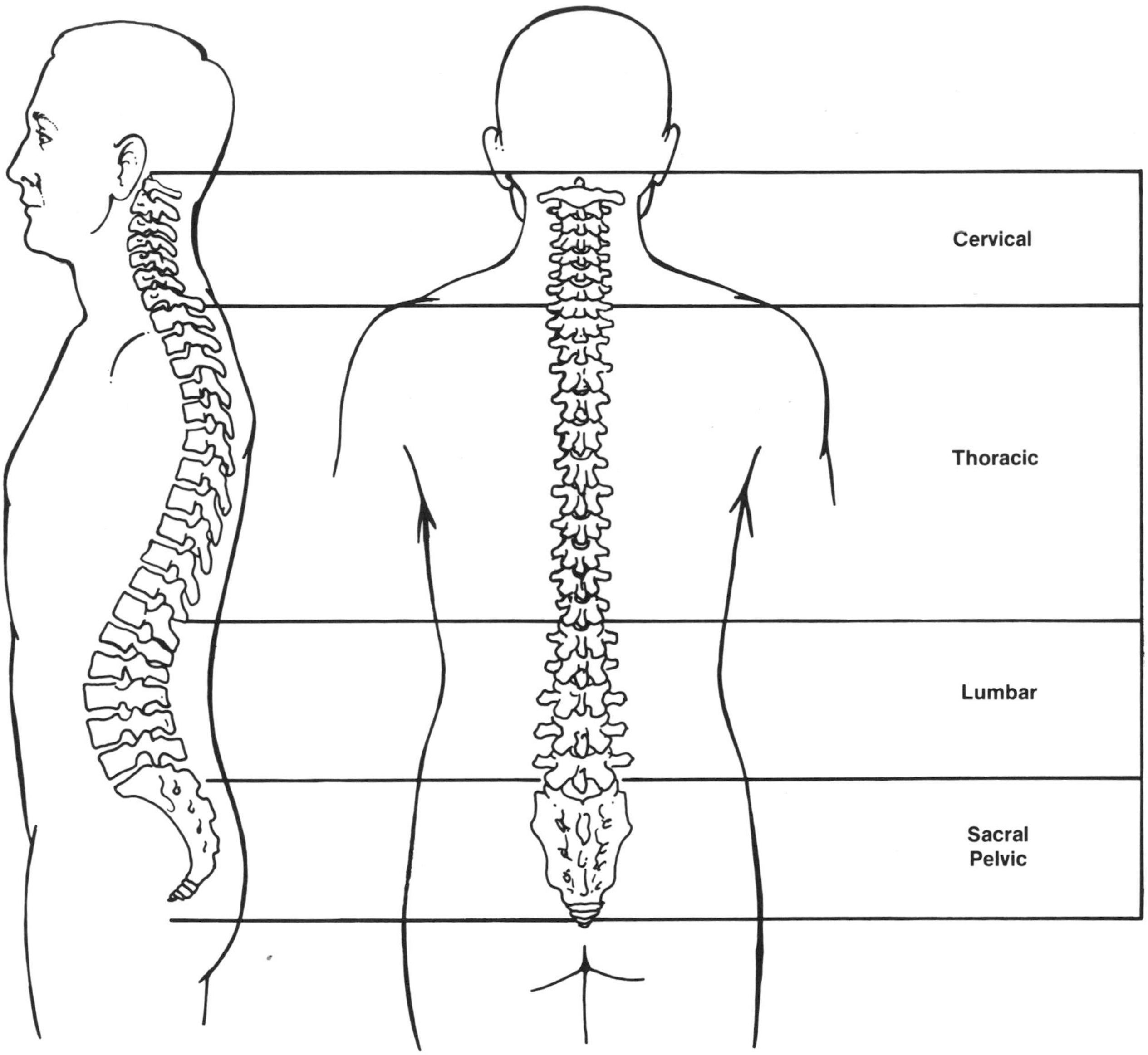

Fig. 11-2. The spine provides protection for the spinal cord, allows flexibility and acts as a shock absorber. The spine is not straight but is made up of four continuous curves. These curves allow for flexibility and help the spine in its role as a shock absorber.

the weight bearing is accomplished through the vertebral bodies and the discs. The facet joints control the amount and the direction of movement in the spine. The transverse and spinous processes are for ligament and muscle attachment. The spinal canal is the large opening just behind the vertebral bodies and the discs which contains the spinal cord. The intervertebral foramina are the openings on each side of the spinal canal. The spinal nerve roots exit through these openings.

Ligaments are strong, inelastic structures that support the spine and control motion. Ligaments "hold the bones together." They can be sprained by injury, such as a fall, or stressed because of poor posture.

Disc injuries are the most common and potentially the most serious of all back disorders. Therefore, a special effort should be made to teach the biomechanics of the disc in simple terms. The discs allow flexibility in the spine and act as shock absorbers. The center or nucleus of the disc is made up of a jellylike material that is similar in consistency to chewing gum. As one gets older, the consistency of this material gets somewhat stringy and less fluid. The nucleus is surrounded by fibrous rings which hold the jellylike material secure in the center of the disc. These fibrous rings are made up of the same material as ligaments and are somewhat like the nylon cords in the body of a car tire. The fibers run in an oblique direction and each layer of fibers runs in alternating directions. The fibers become stronger and thicker towards the outside of the disc. These fibrous rings are attached firmly to the vertebral bodies. There are no pain sensitive nerves within the disc itself and internal damage can be occurring without one having any sensation of pain whatsoever. Only the outer rings of the disc are supplied with pain sensitive nerves and it is not until damage spreads to the outer portion of the disc that one will begin to feel back pain.

When standing erect with the normal curve in the lower back, weight is distributed evenly on the discs with some weight being distributed to the facet joints. However, with forward bending, all of the weight bearing is on the disc, most of it to the front of the disc. This causes a backward pressure upon the nucleus. Backward bending has the opposite effect in that weight is distributed more to the back of the disc and to the facet joints. This causes a forward pressure on the nucleus. However, if the disc is healthy and the fibrous rings are strong, the nucleus does not actually move.

The nerves from the spinal cord pass through the intervertebral foramina at each segmental level. The nerves in the neck supply the arms and the nerves in the lower back supply the legs. There are two basic types of nerve fibers: motor and sensory. Motor nerve fibers carry impulses from the brain to the muscles. These impulses cause the muscles to contract and control movement of the body. Sensory nerve fibers send impulses from the body to the brain. Pain, touch, position, temperature and other senses are felt through the sensory fibers. The spinal nerves carry both sensory and motor nerve fibers. These nerves can sometimes become irritated by a bulging disc or another obstruction, either in the spinal canal or in the intervertebral foramina.

There are many muscles which control movement of the trunk. The shorter, deep muscles control rotation or twisting. The superficial muscles are longer and control forward, backward and side bending and hold the spine upright. The back muscles bring the spine into backward bending and the abdominal muscles aid in forward bending. The abdominal muscles also aid in compressing the abdominal cavity, which increases intra-abdominal pressure. This is important because if some intra-abdominal pressure is maintained when lifting, the abdominal cavity becomes a weight bearing structure.

Common Causes of Back Disorders — What are some of the causes of back problems? It has already been emphasized that most problems are related to poor posture, faulty body mechanics, stressful living and working conditions, loss of flexibility and a general decline of physical fitness. Course participants must realize that back disorders are usually not the result of a single injury. Now, the instructor should point out some of the specific causes.

Poor posture is thought to be one of the leading causes of neck and lower back disorders. Fig. 11-3 shows the common posture problems. With weak abdominal muscles, an increased lordosis may develop and cause a chronic strain on the facet joints and ligaments in the lower back. Sometimes the forward head, rounded shoulder posture is associated with hyperlordosis. This causes increased stress across the upper back and base of the neck. Many pregnant women develop this type of posture. Flat back posture places too much stress on the disc. This posture can develop because of bending and working in a stooped, forward bent position much of the time. The forward head posture often develops with this problem also. Slumped sitting is one of the leading causes of lower back disorders. Truck and bus drivers have a high incidence of lower back disorders. Studies have been done which measured the amount of pressure placed upon the disc in various positions. These studies have shown that there is nearly twice as much pressure on the disc in the sitting position as in the standing position.

Good posture involves a balance between forward bending and backward bending. It is this balanced posture in which the disc and facet joints are under the least amount of stress. The muscles and ligaments are also in balance and are not under stress. It is when we move out of this balanced posture that we tend to place stress on certain structures. The forward bent or slumped posture causes increased compression on the disc which can eventually cause a disc disorder. On the other hand, standing with hyperlordosis causes stress that can

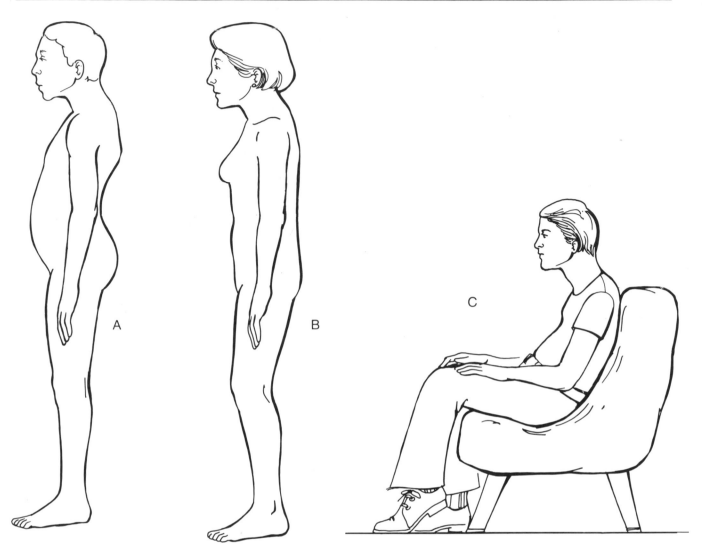

Fig. 11-3. Common posture problems: A) Hyperlordosis-hyperkyphosis B) Flat back and C) Slumped sitting. All may involve the forward head position which is stressful to the neck and upper back.

eventually cause a strain to the facet joints and ligaments (Fig. 11-4).

Faulty body mechanics and stressful living and working habits are closely related to poor posture and are contributing factors in most back disorders. Lifting with the back in a flexed posture, especially repetitive lifting, is one of the leading causes of back disorders even though one may not notice any problem at first. Injury to the disc occurs gradually as a result of perhaps hundreds of thousands of repeated forward bends and lifts. This forward bending and lifting is especially stressful on the lower back when done with the legs straight. If the legs are straight, as in Fig. 11-5, the trunk acts as a lever arm and increases the compressive load on the back by seven to ten times. For example, lifting a 20 pound box in this fashion can increase the load at the lower

back to as much as 200 pounds. Similarly, lifting objects at arm's length also significantly increases the compressive load on the back.

Many back injury prevention programs teach that one should squat and lift an object as shown in Fig. 11-6, but this person is still lifting incorrectly. The back is still flexed and the posterior disc is still being stressed in this position. This technique of lifting is better than the method shown in Fig. 11-5 because the weight is closer to the center of the body, but it is still incorrect. Later it will be shown that lifting should be accomplished with the back in an arched position with the head up and the feet spread out at a diagonal angle.

Standing and working in a forward bent position is similar to forward bending and lifting in that all weight bearing is on the anterior disc and the

Balance is the Key

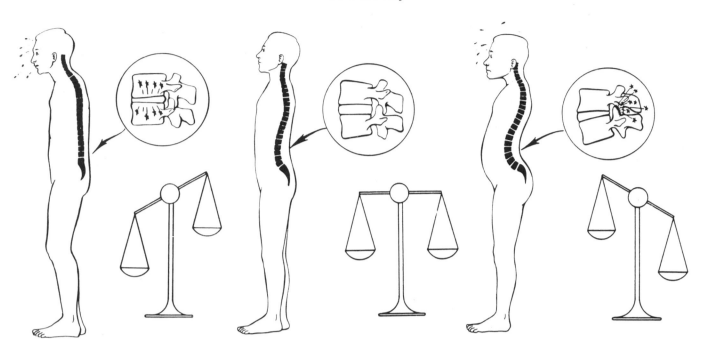

Fig. 11-4. Good posture involves a balance between forward bending and backward bending.

Lifting with Back Flexed

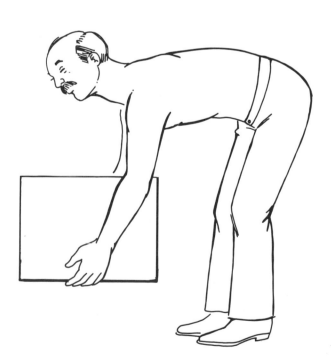

Fig. 11-5. Lifting with the back flexed causes stress to the back.

Lifting With Back Flexed

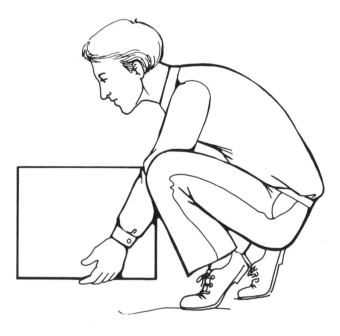

Fig. 11-6. Many back injury prevention programs teach that one should squat and lift as shown in this drawing, but this person is still lifting incorrectly. The back is still flexed and the disc is still being stressed in this position.

posterior ligaments are being stretched. This posture can lead to a disc disorder and/or chronic ligamentous strain (Fig. 11-7). Another common cause of disc injury is the slumped sitting posture. Having a working surface too low or a chair which is too high or does not support the lumbar arch and the entire back can produce the slumped posture. Correctly adjusting chairs and work surface heights are important factors in preventing fatigue and the resulting slumped posture. Working at arm's length serves only to increase the stress on the back.

Twisting the back, especially in a forward bent position, is perhaps the most stressful action on the back. The fibrous rings of the disc can be damaged by twisting. Just as in repetitive forward bending, in the early stages of injury, one would not notice if a back disorder was developing. Fig. 11-8 shows how the disc space is compressed by twisting and how one-half of the fibrous rings are drawn taut while the other one-half are slacked. This weakens the disc wall and makes it vulnerable to injury.

Reaching high over the head with a heavy load can produce a different type of stress on the lower back. This situation causes an increased arch in the lower back and, if repeated constantly throughout the day, irritation of the facet joints and ligaments can occur.

In any educational back program, the instructor should include slides throughout the presentation which show both good and bad examples of posture, working positions and body mechanics to illustrate his teaching points.

Sleeping postures are just as important as working and sitting postures. It should be emphasized throughout the presentation that the normal balanced position is best for the back. Either extreme of slumping into a flexed position or having an excessively arched back is harmful. It is at night when one sleeps that the disc absorbs fluids and regains its height. Therefore, balanced sleeping postures are essential for the maintenance of a healthy back. Mattresses which are either too soft or too hard are bad for the back. If too soft and saggy, the back will be unbalanced; if too hard, the back may be unsupported. Therefore, a mattress should be soft enough to conform to body contours, but firm enough to support the back in a balanced posture. Water beds are often recommended to meet these requirements.

Although most back injuries occur as a result of poor posture, faulty body mechanics and stressful living and working habits, we must also recognize

Work Too Low

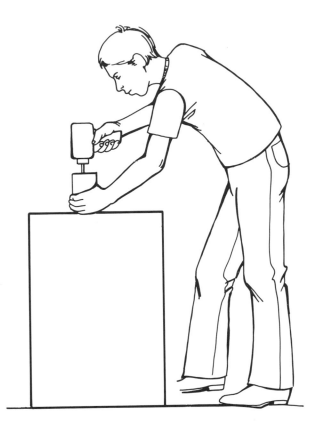

Fig. 11-7. Working in a forward bent position is one of the most stressful working positions.

that some back and neck injuries are caused by accidents. We must, therefore, practice the rules of safety at all times. Injuries caused by accidents will be much worse if the back is in generally poor condition. If a disorder has begun to develop, the effects of any accident will be much worse. A healthy back can endure most stresses and strains without being injured. Most traumatic neck and back injuries involve automobile accidents, falls or falling objects.

Loss of flexibility, not only of the ligaments, capsules and discs, but the muscles as well, contributes to back injury. The discs and facet joint surfaces do not have blood supplies. Nutrition is received through movement of body fluids into the disc and the movement of synovial fluid within the facet joints. Thus, if flexibility is lost the nutritional supply is decreased to these structures, which permits weakening and makes them vulnerable to injury. For example, tightness of the hamstring muscles will interfere with normal lumbo-pelvic movements, often producing loss of flexibility in the

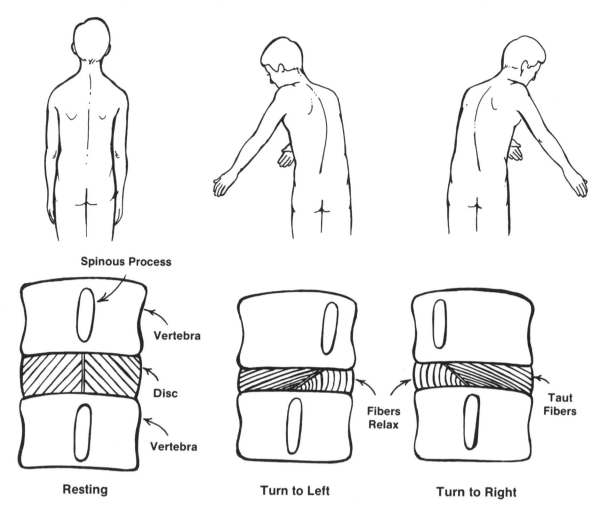

Fig. 11-8. Twisting the back, especially in the forward bent position, can cause stress to the back.

lumbar spine when one forward bends. Excessively tight hamstrings flatten the normal lordosis, thus when one forward bends strain occurs in the lower back and pain is often felt in the hamstrings.

It has been shown that people in poor physical condition are much more vulnerable to back injuries than those who maintain a high level of physical fitness (Fig. 11-9). A recent two-year study involving nearly 2,000 Los Angeles fire fighters showed a direct relationship between the level of physical fitness and the incidence of back injuries. The study divided fire fighters into three classifications of physical fitness. The physically fit group was found to have less than a 1% occurrence of back injuries, 3.5% of the moderately fit group had back injuries and over 8% of the unfit group had back injuries. This study would imply that most jobs can be done without back injury if one is willing to maintain a high level of physical fitness[4].

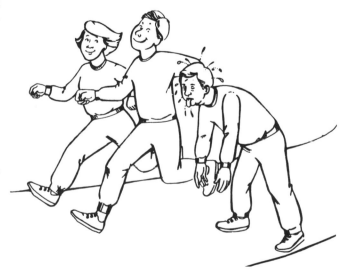

Fig. 11-9. It has been shown that people in poor physical condition are much more vulnerable to back injuries.

Other much less common causes of back disorders include congenital defects, psychosomatic problems, metabolic changes or problems, tumors and infections. These conditions should be mentioned as possible causes of back disorders, but it should be pointed out that they are quite uncommon.

At this point in the presentation, it is effective to emphasize that a lot of work situations are like athletic events in that they require a certain level of physical fitness, strength and flexibility. Many people attempt to work at jobs that require considerable physical labor and involve stressful positions, but they make no effort to keep their bodies in the physical condition required to do these jobs.

Companies can do many things to make the work place safer. A good program examines the principles of proper body mechanics. Many of these principles can and should be incorporated into the work place. However, a company cannot guarantee that all jobs will be totally free of stressful activities and positions that contribute to back injuries. Therefore, one must know how to maintain a healthy back. Certain jobs will require forward bending and lifting and standing and/or sitting in a forward bent position. Even when the work place is designed as safely as possible, these conditions will still exist. However, such stressful conditions need not lead to back injury if one maintains good flexibility and a high level of physical fitness and practices proper body mechanics and good posture whenever possible.

Common Types of Back Disorders — Muscle guarding and/or muscle spasm in the back and neck are common disorders which can be very painful. However, as previously pointed out, one does not have an attack of muscle guarding or muscle spasm unless there is some other disorder present. The muscle guarding results as the body attempts to protect itself from the pain caused by the underlying disorder. After muscle guarding has been present for a period of time, circulation is decreased. This decreased circulation restricts the metabolic processes within the cells. It also causes a restriction of movement which further decreases circulation. After a period of time, the muscle actually goes into spasm and becomes inflamed, due to the build-up of toxic metabolic waste products. This results in further pain and a vicious cycle is developed (Fig. 11-10). This cycle often needs to be interrupted by treatment such as pain and muscle relaxant medications or with physical therapy modalities such as heat, massage or electrical stimulation.

Disc strain or bulge is one of the most common back disorders. This disorder is actually an early stage of herniation which can eventually become a serious disorder. Forward bending increases weight bearing or pressure on the anterior portion of the disc and causes a backward force on the jellylike center of the disc. Disc injuries occur as a result of

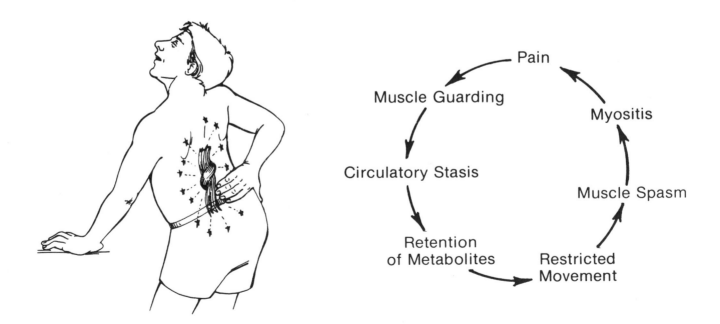

Fig. 11-10. A vicious cycle is developed with pain, muscle guarding and muscle spasm.

Disc Strain or Bulge

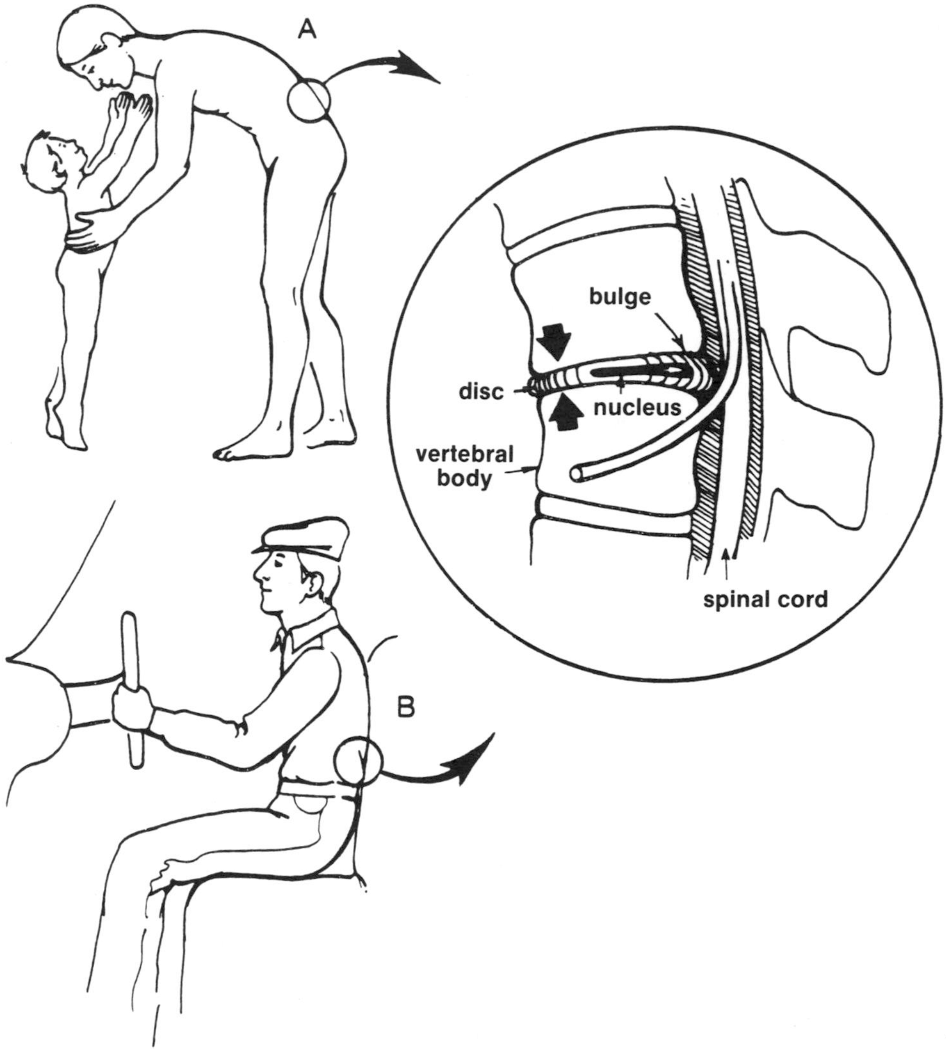

Fig. 11-11. Disc injuries occur as a result of months or years of forward bending and/or slumped sitting.

months or years of forward bending and/or slumped sitting (Fig. 11-11). Although one may experience a sudden onset of pain related to prolonged sitting or forward bending and lifting, the condition was progressing long before that single event occurred. Fig. 11-12 shows the progression of a disc strain or bulge. Drawing #1 shows a normal disc. Drawing #2 shows a very slight bulge. There are no sensory nerves supplying the inner portion of the disc, so at this stage no pain will be felt. Drawing #3 shows the continuation of the bulge. Pain will be felt when stress is placed on the outer wall of the disc. This pain is arising from the disc wall and the ligaments that surround the disc. The nerve is not being irritated or pinched at this stage. Note that the

bulge does not protrude straight back but that it usually protrudes posterolaterally to one side or the other. This condition is often not recognized as a disc disorder by many medical practitioners at this stage.

In the forward bent posture the disc is being squeezed. After a period of time, the disc begins to weaken and will eventually become irritated or start to bulge. The person with a disc problem will have more pain sitting and will tend to sit and stand with a flattened back. He will have difficulty standing up straight after prolonged sitting or lying. Walking will tend to make him feel better. Activities such as riding in an automobile or standing in a forward bent position will increase pain. The pain in the back

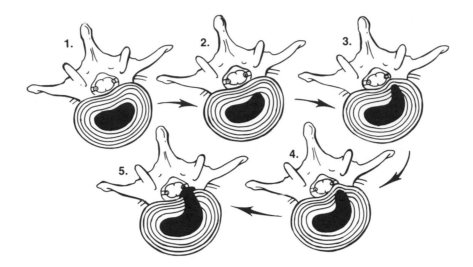

Fig. 11-12. Stages of a disc injury.

is usually on both sides although it may be worse on one side than the other. The pain may radiate into the buttock and thigh. Most individuals with this condition will have lost their lower back flexibility, especially the ability to backward bend.

This problem can be prevented by avoiding the stressful positions of forward bending and slumped sitting or by relieving or reversing these positions frequently when they are a necessary part of a working situation. If one has to sit a lot, stand in a forward bent position or do a lot of forward bending and lifting, one should stand and arch the back frequently to relieve this stress. This will also maintain good backward bending flexibility which is necessary to keep the disc healthy. By maintaining good flexibility, disc strain or bulge can be avoided. Even when a disc bulge is beginning to occur, backward bending as shown in Fig. 11-13 tends to correct it.

If the bulge is large, correction by backward bending may not be possible. If backward bending causes increased leg pain it should not be done, but if it causes some pain in the back but no increase in leg pain, it is permissible. Disc problems are the most common and potentially the most serious problem in the lower back. They can easily be prevented by maintaining good flexibility and interrupting the forward bent and slumped sitting posture frequently. If disc strain or bulge is allowed to worsen, the bulge may eventually touch the nerve root. At this point other signs and symptoms, such as numbness, weakness and reflex changes in the leg will begin to appear.

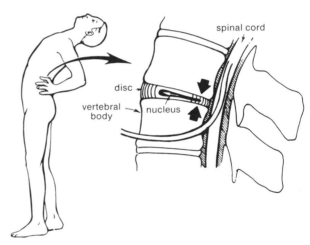

Fig. 11-13. In most cases, a small disc bulge can be prevented or corrected by backward bending and avoiding forward bending and slumped sitting for a while. However, if this backward bending exercise causes increased leg pain, one should stop. Some back pain with this exercise is okay.

Fig. 11-12 shows all stages of a disc injury. In stages two and three, the condition can be treated simply by avoiding forward bending and doing backward bending exercises occasionally. Stage four will require more extensive treatment such as traction, bedrest and a back support. Stage five shows how the nucleus can actually rupture through the wall of the disc. At this stage, most conservative treatment is ineffective, however, some do recover by simply maintaining good posture and avoiding aggravation. At other times, individuals with disc herniation as shown in stages four or five will require surgery. Fig. 11-14 shows the bulge in relationship to

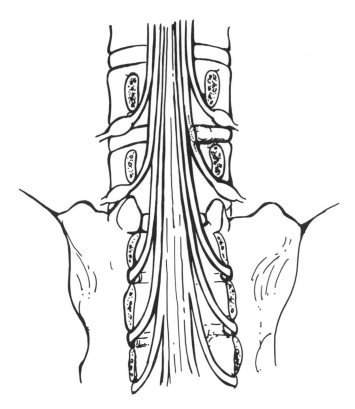

Fig. 11-14. This drawing shows the bulge in relationship to the nerves. Note that the nerve that is descending to make its exit from the spinal column at the level below the bulging disc is the one that is irritated or impinged.

the nerves. Usually, the nerve that is descending to make its exit from the spinal column at the level below the bulging disc is the one that is irritated or impinged.

Acute injuries involving muscle strain and joint sprain usually result from automobile accidents, falls or falling objects. It should be stressed that every worker should always practice the rules of safety and utilize safety equipment. Almost all muscle strains and joint sprains heal in time. It is important that good posture be maintained as healing is taking place. This often involves the use of a soft collar for a neck injury or a lumbosacral corset for a back injury. After healing has taken place, it is important that full strength and flexibility be restored. If this is not done other problems can develop that are more serious. For example, if one is off work for several weeks because of a muscle strain or joint sprain, loss of flexibility and strength will result. One should gradually exercise to restore full strength and normal flexibility. The restoration of strength and flexibility is the important point that should be made. Healing of the injury will eventually take place despite what one does, but exercise to

restore full strength and flexibility must be done or one will not achieve full recovery.

Chronic muscle strains and joint sprains often develop following acute muscle strains and joint sprains because flexibility, strength and good posture were not restored. Neck injuries are a good example. Because of pain, one tends to sit in a slumped, forward head posture during the acute injury stage. As healing takes place, the ligaments and muscles become adapted to the new position. This eventually causes pain because of the strain of the abnormal posture and the loss of flexibility.

Poor posture can also lead to chronic muscle strains and joint sprains. Sway back and weak abdominal muscles contribute to chronic facet joint strain. Neck strain can also develop because of poor posture and faulty work habits. Later, exercises will be discussed which can be shown to the participants to help correct these conditions.

As previously mentioned, joint stiffness and loss of flexibility can cause a back disorder. Because of stiffness, the discs and joints in the back do not receive their normal nutritional supply. This causes weakening of the discs and, over a long period of time, can contribute to a disc disorder and/or degenerative arthritis. Studies show that joint stiffness is directly related to many common spinal disorders.

Other less common back disorders include:

1) Osteoarthritis occurs in everyone to some degree with aging and is usually asymptomatic as long as one maintains normal flexibility and good posture. Severe cases require special attention.

2) Facet joint locking occurs when the joint lining is nipped or pinched between the joint surfaces. It is uncommon and is usually self-limiting with spontaneous recovery. Occasionally it requires manipulation or traction treatments.

3) Joint instability involves overstretched or torn ligaments caused by severe injuries (whiplash). Occasionally it is seen as a result of a birth deformity or a stress fracture.

4) Traumatic fractures are the rare but serious result of traumatic injury. Even though they are uncommon, x-rays should be taken with all traumatic injuries.

5) Stress fractures occur as a result of high levels of repeated stress without sufficient recovery time. They are rare and are usually seen in weekend athletes or heavy laborers. Spondylolisthesis is thought to occur as the result of a stress fracture.

6) Compression fractures occur in older people

(especially women) as the result of inactivity and metabolic changes or through trauma.

7) Tumors are very rare in the spine unless one has a previous history of cancer.

8) Sacroiliac sprain may result from heavy lifting, twisting, a fall or childbirth.

9) Coccyx fracture or sprain may occur as the result of a fall, a direct blow to the tailbone or childbirth.

10) Inflammation can occur in muscles, joints or discs, usually secondary to injury or aggravation. It is present to a certain degree with most of the disorders described earlier.

11) Congenital birth defects such as spina bifida occulta are often of no significance and have nothing to do with the real problem but, because they are seen on x-ray, they are often mistakenly blamed for the problem.

12) Diseases and illnesses elsewhere in the body sometimes cause backache and should always be considered if pain persists beyond a reasonable amount of time.

Treatment — If severe trauma has occurred, ice is often helpful in reducing initial swelling, pain and muscle guarding. It is important to rest the injured area and avoid aggravating it further. If at work, the injury should be reported to a supervisor. Most experts agree that strict bed rest is not helpful in most cases of back injury and that as one begins to improve careful movement and exercise should be started. The nature of the injury should be considered and one should pay attention to back care principles. Flexibility and strength should be restored as healing takes place and a normal balanced posture should be maintained throughout the course of management. Medications are sometimes helpful in reducing the pain and muscle guarding. They actually do very little or nothing to correct the disorder itself, however. Physical therapy modalities are sometimes used to relieve pain and muscle guarding and certain modalities, such as traction, are given to help correct the actual disorder. Rest and relaxation are also important in recovery. Ultimately, in addition to eliminating the cause of the disorder, exercises to restore strength, flexibility and fitness are the answer.

Thus far, we have emphasized what the individual can do to prevent or manage a back injury. What, then, is the role of the medical practitioner in the management of back disorders? Medical evaluation varies depending upon the doctor or therapist that one sees. During medical evaluation, the prac-

titioner is searching for the cause of the disorder and is trying to determine what the actual disorder may be.

It is wise for an individual to use a common sense approach when managing a back disorder. What he does to manage his own back problem is usually more important than what the doctor does. Often, tests such as x-rays, myelograms, CT scans and EMG's are done unnecessarily. These tests seldom show what the real disorder is and they are expensive. Elaborate testing also tends to make one think that the doctor will cure the problem. A back care program should discourage this attitude and should emphasize self-responsibility.

Stop looking for magic answers. How many times have we seen newspapers, magazines and television commercials depicting another "magic answer" for the treatment of a lower back disorder? It seems that as soon as one magic answer is proven to be ineffective another takes its place. Many "back specialists" perpetuate this type of thinking and often it is not the patient's fault that he continues to search for a magic answer. Some medical practitioners seem to encourage this passive attitude as if there actually is a pill, pop, twist, stretch or surgery that will cure the problem.

Prevention — What can be done to prevent a back disorder? With posture, balance is the key. Sitting in a slumped, forward head posture can cause stress. When one is sitting the back should be supported in the normal arched position. The head and shoulders are held in an erect, well balanced position. In this position the weight of the head and shoulders is evenly distributed throughout the structures of the back and neck. It is often helpful to place a rolled towel, small pillow or cushion behind the back to maintain the normal arched position (Fig. 11-15).

When standing, keep work at a proper height so that the neck and lower back are held in an upright balanced position. Work that is too low will cause a forward head strain on the neck and increase disc loading and pressure on the lower back. Work that is too high may cause the opposite problem — a sway back and a strain on the facet joints. This position may be changed by placing one foot on a bar or step stool occasionally (Fig. 11-16). It is wise to move frequently when one is standing or sitting, especially if the position is a stressful one.

One should sleep in a balanced position. This means firm support that is soft enough on the surface to accommodate the normal curvatures of

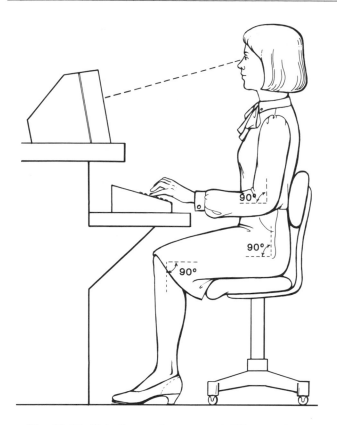

Fig. 11-15. This figure shows good sitting posture.

the body, especially since sleeping positions will change during the night. While sleeping it is best to change positions frequently (Fig. 11-17). A king or queen size bed is often helpful because it allows more freedom to move and change positions. Waterbeds are often recommended for persons with back problems, but it has been this author's experience that they are not beneficial for everyone. When a

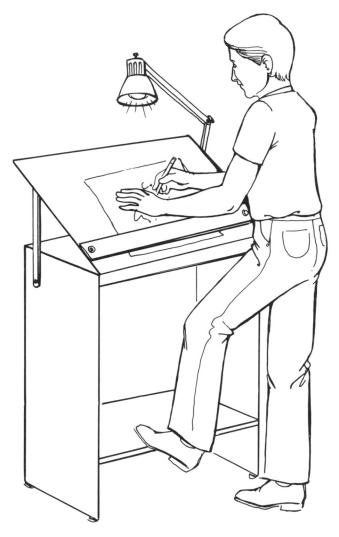

Keep Work At "Balanced" Height

Fig. 11-16. This figure shows good standing posture.

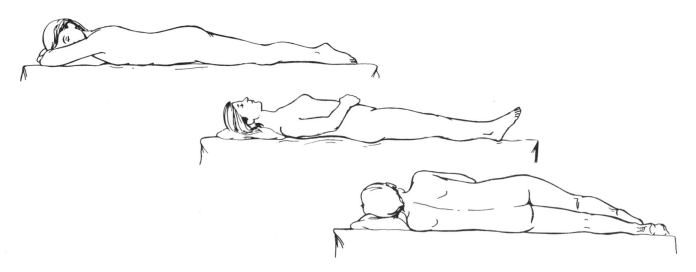

Fig. 11-17. Sleep in a balanced position on a mattress that is firm but not extremely hard. It is best to change positions frequently.

waterbed is used it should be kept relatively full of water to maintain a firm foundation of support. Sleeping on the stomach is not necessarily bad positioning. When getting out of bed one should roll to one side and sit up sideways, using the arms for support.

The most important principle to remember when lifting is to keep the back in an arched position. This arched position tends to put the muscles in a short, strengthened position. It also distributes the weight more evenly between the disc and facet joints and places a more balanced weight on the disc. Professional and olympic weight lifters are taught to squat and bend their legs in order to get as much lift with their legs as possible. They are also taught to keep their heads up and their backs arched to avoid disc injuries in the lower back. Additionally, they wear a belt around their abdomens and are taught to push into the belt to increase intra-abdominal pressure. It is often helpful to place one foot ahead of the other when lifting to get the object being lifted closer to the body. This position is especially important when lifting large, bulky items. This diagonal lifting position also balances the weight within a wide, safe base of support (Fig. 11-18).

Often stress to the lower back is caused by lifting a load that is too heavy. Even when good body mechanics are used there is a limit to the stress that the back can stand. More than one person may be required or a mechanical hoist or lifting device may be needed for heavy objects. Injuries often occur in industry as a result of forward bending and lifting when mechanical lifting devices are readily available but are not being used.

It is always a good idea to slide heavy objects rather than lift them. The same body mechanics principles apply when pushing or pulling, in that a balanced, arched back posture is desirable. Teamwork is important. When two or more people are carrying something, good communication is essential. In addition, it is essential to keep the weight close to the body. A ten pound weight can produce a 100 pound force in the lower back if poor body mechanics are used (Fig. 11-19). Also, when the arms are used as the lever arm, the force will be seven to ten times greater if the weight is held at arm's length.

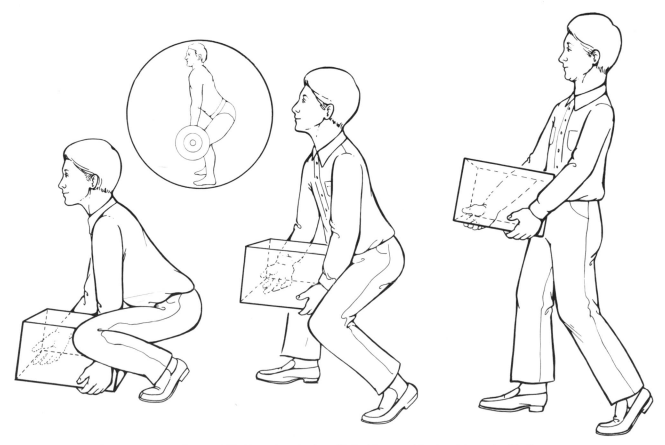

Fig. 11-18. The diagonal lift. Note that the head is held up and the back is arched in the same manner that weight lifters are taught to lift.

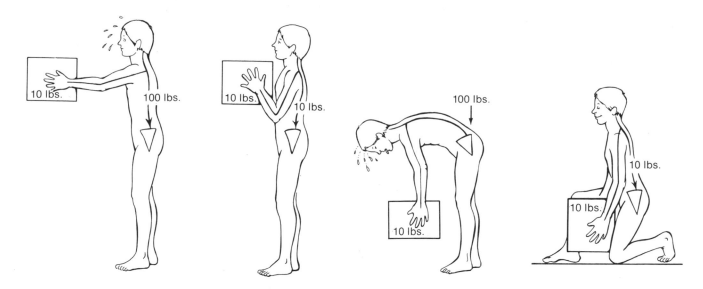

Fig. 11-19. Keep weight close to the body.

Twisting the trunk, especially in a forward bent position, is particularly harmful to both the disc and the facet joints. Pivoting rather than twisting is essential in avoiding a lower back injury. Lifting with a sudden, jerking motion is also potentially harmful and should be avoided.

When carrying heavy objects for long distances it is sometimes a good idea to carry the weight on the shoulder. This permits a worker to keep his back in an arched position. Long objects should be carried with most of the weight to the front so that the worker can observe and control the object properly.

Always allow for proper clearance through doorways and down aisles. If there is insufficient clearance the worker can lose his grip and might be forced into a situation where he could strain his back while trying to secure the load. It is always a good idea to wear protective equipment and clothing.

Interrupt or reverse positions which are stressful as often as possible. This should be one of the key points of any educational program. Many jobs require stressful positions and activities, but if they are interrupted frequently injury will be prevented (Fig. 11-20).

Emotional stress and nutrition also play an important role in prevention of back injuries. People who are emotionally upset or who are under a lot of stress will have a higher incidence of back injury. This is not to say that stress causes back disorders but that stress may magnify an existing back problem. Nutrition plays an important part in our general health and affects the way our body heals when injured.

It is important for the participants to realize that the ultimate responsibility for good health lies with the individual. Low back injuries are no exception.

Exercises — After participating in an educational program for back care, many individuals will want to start an exercise program that will help them maintain a healthy back. At this point, the instructor must stress that there is a difference between hard work and exercise. Many participants in a preventive back care program will feel that because they work hard at their jobs they do not need to exercise. However, people who work at jobs requiring considerable physical labor may still be in poor cardiovascular condition. They may have poor flexibility and may have developed strength only in certain muscle groups, while others may be weak and underdeveloped.

The most important exercise program that one can do to prevent or cure a back disorder is to maintain a regular physical fitness program (Fig. 11-21). There is hardly any type of physical fitness program that is harmful for the back if the exercise is approached in a sensible manner. Exercise should always be started mildly and gradually increased in intensity. Another key to success with a physical fitness program is regularity. Most people who injure themselves with an exercise program do so because they start out with too much too soon or

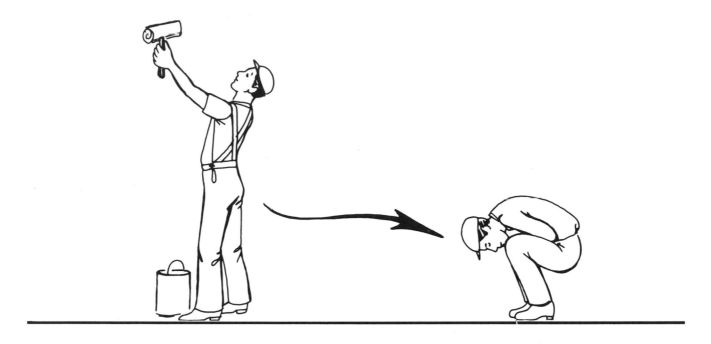

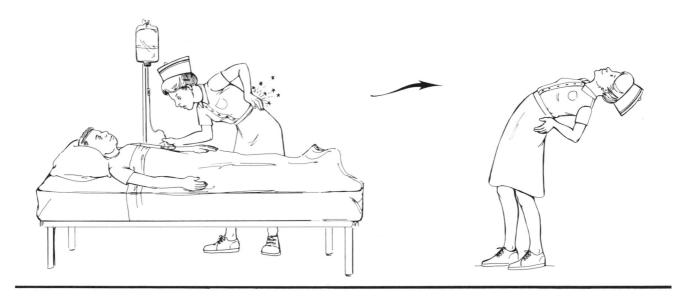

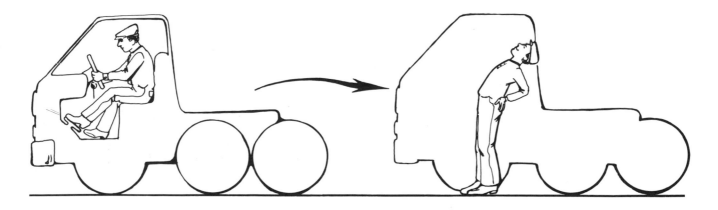

Fig. 11-20. Interrupt or change stressful positions frequently.

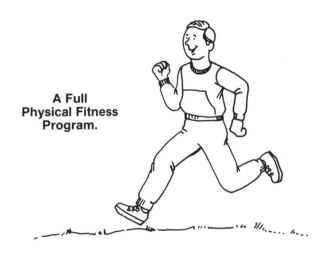

A Full Physical Fitness Program.

Fig. 11-21. The most important exercise anyone can do to prevent or cure a back disorder is to participate regularly in a physical fitness program.

they do not participate on a regular basis. Running, walking, swimming, bicycling and sports activities are all good for the back if approached in a common sense way.

Exercises that increase flexibility and strengthen the trunk and hips are helpful if one is to maintain a healthy back. All of the following exercises are good if one has a healthy back. If a back disorder is already present, however, only a limited number of these exercises should be emphasized while others may cause increased stress to the back.

Tight hamstring muscles prevent the pelvis from rolling forward. As one forward bends, tight hamstrings will cause increased stress on the lower back while forward bending. If one has tight hamstring muscles he will feel a pulling in the back of the thighs with forward bending (Fig. 11-22). An exercise can be done to stretch tight hamstring muscles. While lying supine one should be able to completely extend the leg, keeping the knee straight and forming a 90° angle at the hip. If this cannot be done, tight hamstrings are present and the exercise should be done as shown. Simply hold the leg extended keeping it as straight as possible for five to ten seconds. Repeat the exercises five to ten times, one or two sessions per day.

The slumped, forward head posture is a common cause of neck and upper back pain and headaches. A good exercise to do periodically throughout the day for the forward head posture is the head-back, chin-in exercise as shown in Fig. 11-23.

If one has an excess curve in the lower back (sway back), exercises that stretch the lower back

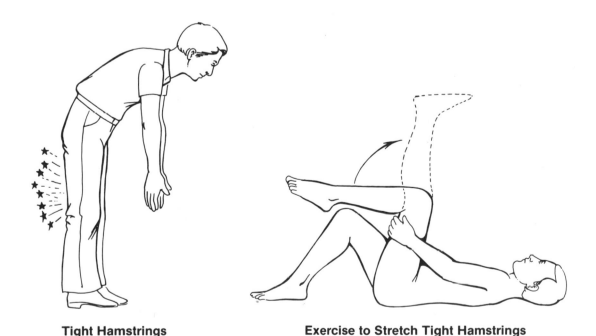

Tight Hamstrings

Exercise to Stretch Tight Hamstrings

Fig. 11-22. Tight hamstring muscles prevent the pelvis from rolling forward as one forward bends. This causes an increased stress on the lower back. An exercise to stretch tight hamstrings is shown on the right.

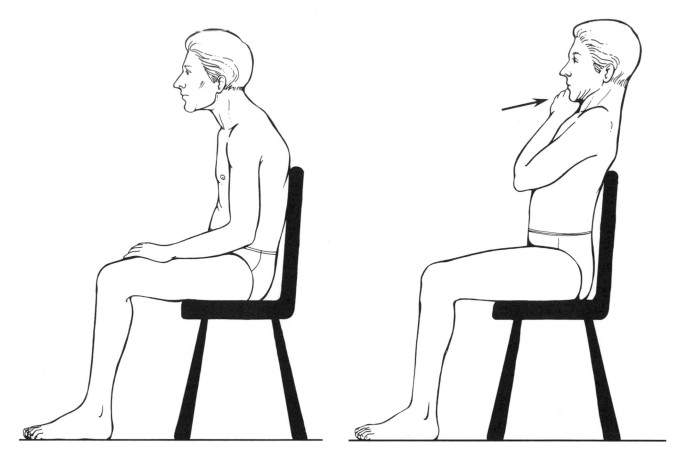

Fig. 11-23. The slumped, forward head posture is shown on the left. A good exercise to do to correct this posture is shown on the right.

muscles and strengthen the abdominal muscles will be beneficial (Fig. 11-24). The exercises that stretch the lower back muscles are the single and double knee-to-chest exercises. Single knee-to-chest exercises are done alternately. They should be held five to ten seconds when the knee is flexed as close to the chest as possible. Double knee-to-chest exercises are done with a five to ten second hold. Five to ten of each of these should be done as often as necessary to keep the back flexible. This exercise may aggravate a disc strain or bulge and should not be done if such a disorder is present.

Partial sit-ups are done to strengthen the abdominal muscles. It is important to have strong abdominal muscles because they help increase intra-abdominal pressure when lifting. This takes some of the weight bearing and stress off of the disc. Partial sit-ups are done correctly with the hips and knees bent. One should raise the arms, head and shoulders off the floor, holding the position for five to ten seconds. One should not raise the trunk far enough

to lift the lower back from the floor. This causes too much pressure on the disc and really does not exercise the abdominal muscles. The feet should not be stabilized because this tends to cause the leg muscles to do the work and lessens the amount of effective abdominal strengthening. It is often helpful to place a small rolled towel under the lower back to support the spine in a normal curved position. In addition to doing the partial sit-ups in a straight position, they may be done in slight diagonal patterns to each side, lifting one shoulder toward the opposite hip. This will strengthen the oblique abdominal muscles. The number of repetitions should be gradually increased as the muscles get stronger, and the exercises should be done at least once a day starting with the arms extended, progressing to arms folded across the chest and, finally, to hands clasped behind the head. This exercise causes increased pressure on the disc and should not be done by a person with an active disc disorder.

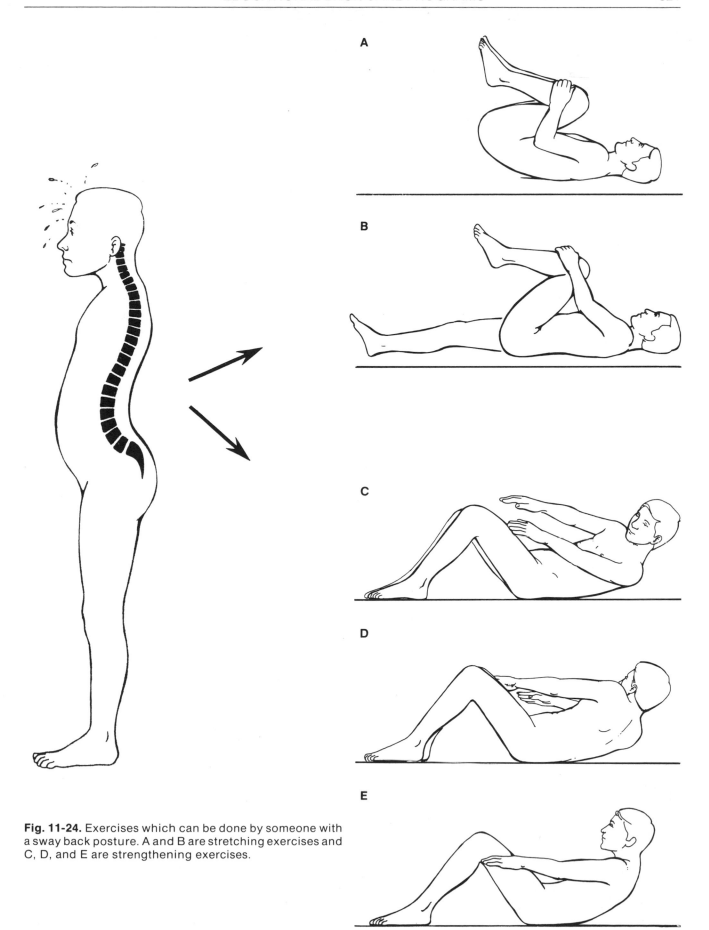

Fig. 11-24. Exercises which can be done by someone with a sway back posture. A and B are stretching exercises and C, D, and E are strengthening exercises.

If one has a flat back or if one is stiff in backward bending because of standing or sitting in a forward bent posture or because of doing a lot of forward bending or lifting, exercises which increase backward bending flexibility and strengthen the back muscles will be beneficial (Fig. 11-25). The press-up exercise is done by pushing up with the arms while the back and abdominal muscles are relaxed. This causes a passive stretch on the lower back. The backward bending stretch can also be done standing. These exercises should each be done five to ten times throughout the day, especially after prolonged sitting or forward bending and lifting. These exercises would not benefit someone with a sway back or someone with excessive flexibility in backward bending.

If one does a lot of sitting or forward bending and lifting, the strengthening exercises shown in Fig. 11-25 will be especially beneficial. These exercises should be started gradually and should be done once or twice a day. The number may be increased to as many as forty to fifty repetitions of each. Small ankle and wrist weights can be added to make these exercises more advanced.

It should be stressed that exercises should be done regularly. One should always start out mildly and increase them as tolerated. A little pain with exercise is usually normal but exercise should not cause pain that lingers afterward.

The following discussion concerns points that should be made with management and supervisory level personnel concerning management of industrial back problems.

Medical literature shows that our present management techniques have failed. Numerous studies show that patients often do just as well with placebo treatment as they do with the various types of treatments that are available and are commonly used today. What are some of the reasons we have failed? Many medical practitioners, although they commonly treat persons with low back problems, openly admit that they have no interest in conservative treatment of back patients. The emphasis of tests and examinations tends to cause the person to think that his problem is more serious than it may actually be. This tends to shift the responsibility for management of the disorder to the attorneys and medical practitioners rather than to the individual.

There is a basic lack of knowledge about conservative management techniques. This is especially true with certain groups of medical practitioners. Improvement is being made, however,

and recent interest and advancements in conservative management techniques have been encouraging. Also, the understanding that medical practitioners cannot "cure" back disorders and the emphasis on patient responsibility and self management have made considerable contributions to better care of back disorders.

Diagnosis and treatment often depend upon the educational background and type of medical practitioner one visits rather than the patient's signs and symptoms. Some practitioners tend to utilize adjustments and manipulations to treat all types of back and neck disorders, while others may almost exclusively utilize drugs, bedrest and/or surgery. Some practitioners may utilize only one type of exercise to treat all types of disorders. Hopefully, these trends are changing. Unfortunately, however, this type of practice is still occurring in some areas.

We are often overly suspicious of the patient with the back problem. This is especially true if the patient does not respond to our favorite type of treatment. Medical practitioners are reluctant to admit that their treatment is wrong and therefore, if the patient does not respond in a timely fashion, it must be the patient's fault and he may be referred for psychological counseling. Initially, when a person experiences a back injury he may be somewhat apprehensive and may be interested in knowing what to do and where to go for help. At this point his attitude is good and all he is concerned about is recovery. He does not have an attorney, he is not angry and he is not trying to "get out of something." At this point we should show sincere interest in him and treat him as if the problem is real. Many persons with back injuries are treated at the very beginning as if they are exaggerating or faking their condition. This causes them to become angry and to work against those who are trying to help them.

It is common for lower back and neck disorders to follow a pattern of intermittent acute flare-ups. Patients are often treated only during the acute episodes. Too much attention is directed toward treatment of pain and muscle spasm and very little is ever done to treat the real cause of the disorder.

What can be done to improve the care of the patient with lower back pain? Obviously, preventing the injury rather than treating it after it occurs is the correct approach. It has already been mentioned that only 3% of American medical care money is spent on prevention. This percentage is far below what it needs to be. Preventative medicine has been shown to work effectively with cardiovascular disease and

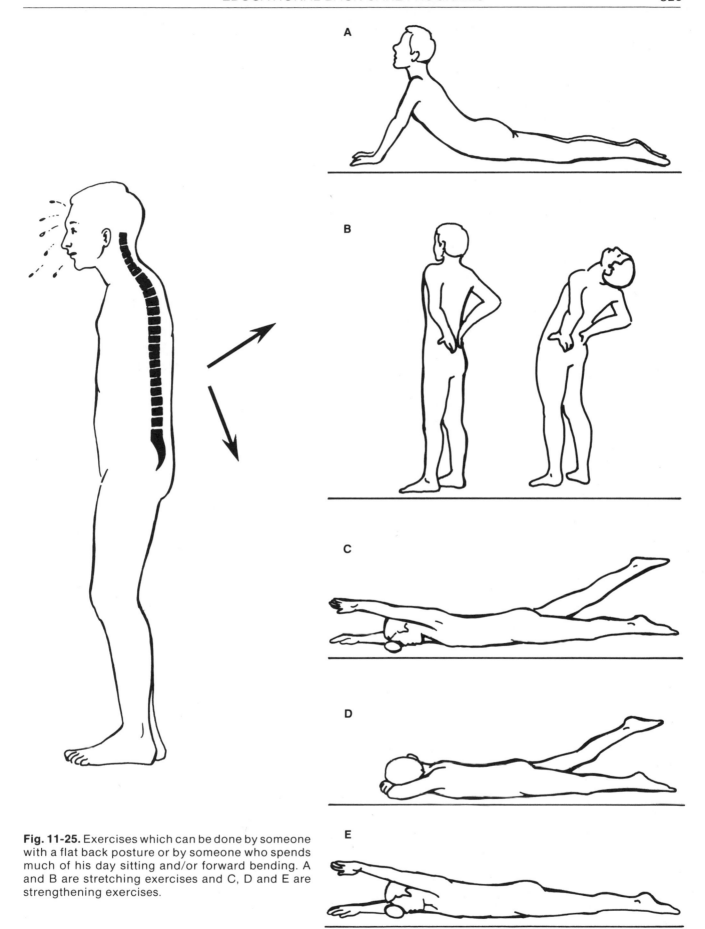

Fig. 11-25. Exercises which can be done by someone with a flat back posture or by someone who spends much of his day sitting and/or forward bending. A and B are stretching exercises and C, D and E are strengthening exercises.

diabetes. The same can be done with back disorders if the effort is made.

We must recognize that there are many types of lower back and neck disorders. It seems as though some medical practitioners diagnose everything without neurological signs as a muscle strain, whereas everything with neurological signs is diagnosed as a disc disorder. Or worse, the patient is told that there is nothing wrong with his back because the x-ray is normal. This kind of medical care causes the patient to feel frustration and anger.

The most common back disorders involve disc strains and acute and chronic muscle strains and joint sprains. The possibility of one of these disorders existing should be explored first and appropriate management should be instituted. Extensive tests and examinations that are looking for rare, infrequently seen disorders are inappropriate, at least in the initial stages of management.

Keep injuries "low profile." Emphasize that expensive tests and examinations only make the patient think he has a serious problem. By keeping the injury low profile, the patient has a realistic outlook toward recovery.

Do something early in the way of positive treatment. The patient, at this point, has a positive attitude toward recovery and returning to work. If something is done initially to encourage this positive attitude everyone will be better off. Avoid sending the patient home for rest without any treatment or instructions. Many times a patient will do things at home that are worse for him than if he were kept at work on light duty. If a patient's condition is such that he cannot work, even on light duty, he should at least have instructions concerning his posture, rest positions and activities that he should or should not be doing.

Keep the patient in the habit of working. If possible, workers should be kept at work and light duties should be provided. It is better for most patients with back disorders to be up and moving around. Light duty situations at work can accommodate this type of environment. One should remember that individuals with disc problems should not be given light duties that involve sitting, riding in an automobile or truck or forward bending, even though the work appears to be light. Keeping the individual at work also removes the reward for a disorder and does help discourage individuals from taking advantage of worker's compensation benefits.

Summary — In conclusion, the important points that a back care program should teach are: 1) Back pain is no joke; 2) Back disorders are seldom caused by a single injury; 3) Almost all back disorders are the result of poor posture, faulty body mechanics, stressful living and working habits, loss of flexibility and a general decline in physical fitness; 4) Disc disorders are the most common and potentially the most serious of all back disorders; 5) One must be in good physical condition to do many jobs; 6) One should keep the back arched when lifting; 7) Medical treatment has failed; 8) The ultimate treatment and prevention program involves eliminating the cause and doing exercises to restore strength, flexibility and physical fitness; 9) One should interrupt or change stressful positions frequently and 10) Balance is the key.

References:

1. Snook, S; Campanelli, R and Hart, J: A Study of Three Preventive Approaches to Low Back Injury. Joul of Occ Med. 20:478-481, 1978.
2. Snook, S; Irvine, C and Bass, S: Maximum Weights and Work Loads Acceptable to Male Industrial Workers: A Study of Lifting, Lowering, Pushing, Pulling, Carrying and Walking Tasks. Am Ind Hyg Assoc, 31:579-586, 1970.
3. Snook, S and Ciriello, V: Maximum Weights and Work Loads Acceptable to Female Workers. Occup Med, 16:527-534, 1974.
4. Cady, L, et al: Strength and Fitness and Subsequent Back Injuries in Firefighters. Joul of Occ Med 21:269-272, April 1979.
5. Kramos, P: New Rules Fight Back Injuries. Health and Safety, 44:42-44, 1975.
6. Biering-Sorenson, F: Physical Measurements as Risk Indicators for Low Back Trouble Over a One-Year Period. Spine 9:106-119, 1984.
7. Tak-Sun, Y, et al: Low Back Pain in Industry. Joul of Occ Med, 26:517-524, 1984.
8. Fisk, J; DiMonte, P and Courington, S: Back Schools. Clinical Orthopaedics, 179:18-23, 1983.
9. Lepore, B; Olson, C and Tomer, G: The Dollars and Sense of Occupational Back Injury Prevention Training. Clinical Management, 4:38-41, 1984.
10. Fitzler, S and Berger, R: Attitudinal Change: The Chelsea Back Program. Occ Health and Safety, 51:24-26, 1982.
11. Fitzler, S; Berger, R: Chelsea Back Program: One Year Later. Occ Health and Safety, 52:52-54, 1983.
12. Isenhagen, S: Personal Communication, Functional Capacities Assessment. Duluth, MN, 1984.
13. Key, G: Personal Communications, Key Functional Assessments. Minneapolis, MN, 1984.
14. Nordby, E: Epidemiology and Diagnosis in Low Back Injury. Occ Health and Safety, 52:52-54, 1983.

INDEX